CDiC Textbook of
PEDIATRIC DIABETES

CDiC Textbook of
PEDIATRIC DIABETES

Editors

Ashok K Das MD FAMS FICP PhD FRCP
Professor and Head
Department of Medicine and Endocrinology
Pondicherry Institute of Medical Sciences
Puducherry, India

Sanjay Kalra MD DM
Consultant
Department of Endocrinology
Bharti Hospital
Karnal, Haryana, India

Foreword

Raghupathy Palany

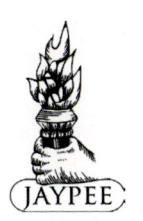

The Health Sciences Publisher

New Delhi | London | Panama

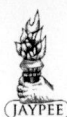

Jaypee Brothers Medical Publishers (P) Ltd

Headquarters

Jaypee Brothers Medical Publishers (P) Ltd
4838/24, Ansari Road, Daryaganj
New Delhi 110 002, India
Phone: +91-11-43574357
Fax: +91-11-43574314
Email: jaypee@jaypeebrothers.com

Overseas Offices

J.P. Medical Ltd
83 Victoria Street, London
SW1H 0HW (UK)
Phone: +44 20 3170 8910
Fax: +44 (0)20 3008 6180
Email: info@jpmedpub.com

Jaypee-Highlights Medical Publishers Inc
City of Knowledge, Bld. 237, Clayton
Panama City, Panama
Phone: +1 507-301-0496
Fax: +1 507-301-0499
Email: cservice@jphmedical.com

Jaypee Brothers Medical Publishers (P) Ltd
17/1-B Babar Road, Block-B, Shaymali
Mohammadpur, Dhaka-1207
Bangladesh
Mobile: +08801912003485
Email: jaypeedhaka@gmail.com

Jaypee Brothers Medical Publishers (P) Ltd
Bhotahity, Kathmandu
Nepal
Phone: +977-9741283608
Email: kathmandu@jaypeebrothers.com

Website: www.jaypeebrothers.com
Website: www.jaypeedigital.com

© 2018, Jaypee Brothers Medical Publishers

The views and opinions expressed in this book are solely those of the original contributor(s)/author(s) and do not necessarily represent those of editor(s) of the book.

All rights reserved. No part of this publication and Interactive DVD-ROM may be reproduced, stored or transmitted in any form or by any means, electronic, mechanical, photocopying, recording or otherwise, without the prior permission in writing of the publishers.

All brand names and product names used in this book are trade names, service marks, trademarks or registered trademarks of their respective owners. The publisher is not associated with any product or vendor mentioned in this book.

Medical knowledge and practice change constantly. This book is designed to provide accurate, authoritative information about the subject matter in question. However, readers are advised to check the most current information available on procedures included and check information from the manufacturer of each product to be administered, to verify the recommended dose, formula, method and duration of administration, adverse effects and contraindications. It is the responsibility of the practitioner to take all appropriate safety precautions. Neither the publisher nor the author(s)/editor(s) assume any liability for any injury and/or damage to persons or property arising from or related to use of material in this book.

This book is sold on the understanding that the publisher is not engaged in providing professional medical services. If such advice or services are required, the services of a competent medical professional should be sought.

Every effort has been made where necessary to contact holders of copyright to obtain permission to reproduce copyright material. If any have been inadvertently overlooked, the publisher will be pleased to make the necessary arrangements at the first opportunity. The **CD/DVD-ROM** (if any) provided in the sealed envelope with this book is complimentary and free of cost. **Not meant for sale.**

Inquiries for bulk sales may be solicited at: jaypee@jaypeebrothers.com

CDiC Textbook of Pediatric Diabetes / Ashok K Das, Sanjay Kalra

First Edition: **2018**

ISBN: 978-93-5270-086-8

Printed at: Paras Offset Pvt. Ltd., New Delhi

CONTRIBUTORS

EDITORS

Ashok K Das MD FAMS FICP PhD FRCP
Professor and Head
Department of Medicine and Endocrinology
Pondicherry Institute of Medical Sciences
Puducherry, India

Sanjay Kalra MD DM
Consultant
Department of Endocrinology
Bharti Hospital
Karnal, Haryana, India

SECTION EDITORS

KM Prasanna Kumar MD DM
Consultant
Bangalore Diabetes Hospital
Centre for Diabetes and
Endocrine Care
Bengaluru, Karnataka, India

Nalini Shah MD DM
Professor and Head
Department of Endocrinology
King Edward Hospital
Mumbai, Maharashtra, India

Nikhil Tandon MD DM PhD
Department of Endocrinology
and Metabolism
All India Institute of Medical
Sciences
New Delhi, India

PV Rao MD PhD FRCP FACE
Director
Kumudini Devi Diabetes
Research Center
Ramdevrao Hospital
Hyderabad, Telangana, India

Raghupathy Palany BSc MD DCH FRCP
Professor
Department of Pediatric
Endocrinology
Indira Gandhi Institute of
Child Health
Bangalore, Karnataka, India

Rakesh Sahay MD DNB DM FICP FACE
Professor and Head
Department of Endocrinology
Osmania Medical College and
Osmania General Hospital
Hyderabad, Telangana, India

Subhankar Chowdhury
DTM&H MD DM MRCP
Professor and Head
Department of Endocrinology
Institute of Post Graduate
Medical Education and Research
Kolkata, West Bengal, India

Vaman Khadilkar MD DNB MRCP DCH
Consultant Pediatric and
Adolescent Endocrinologist
Ira Clinic
Pune, Maharashtra, India

CONTRIBUTING AUTHORS

Aashima Dabas MD
Assistant Professor
Department of Pediatrics
Chacha Nehru Bal Chikitsalaya
New Delhi, India

Abilash Nair MD DM
Assistant Professor
Department of Endocrinology
Government Medical College
Thiruvananthapuram, Kerala, India
All India Institute of Medical Sciences
New Delhi, India

Abraham Paulose MD MRCPCH
Associate Professor
Department of Pediatrics
Malankara Orthodox Syrian Church Medical College
Kochi, Kerala, India

Alok Kanungo MB PhD
Head, Department of Diabetes
Kanungo Institute of Diabetes Specialities
Bhubaneswar, Odisha, India

Anjana Hulse MRCPCH MSc
Consultant, Department of Pediatrics, Apollo Hospitals
Bengaluru, Karnataka, India

Archana S Sarda MD
Director
Sarda Centre for Diabetes and Self Care
Aurangabad, Maharashtra, India

Ashok K Jhingan MD
Chairman
Consultant Physician and Diabetologist
Diabetes Education and Research Foundation
New Delhi, India

Bandgar Tushar MD DM
Additional Professor
Department of Endocrinology
King Edward Hospital
Mumbai, Maharashtra, India

Banshi D Saboo MD PhD
Chief Diabetologist and Director
Dia Care – Diabetes Care and Hormone Clinic
Ahmedabad, Gujarat, India

Bipin K Sethi MD DM
Consultant and Head
Department of Endocrinology
CARE Hospital
Hyderabad, Telangana, India

BV Reshma
Consultant Diabetologist and Endocrinologist
Dr S Srikanta and the Diabetes Collaborative Study Group
Samatvam Endocrinology Diabetes Center, Jnana Sanjeevini Diabetes Hospital and Medical Center, Samatvam: Science and Research for Human Welfare Trust
Bangalore, Karnataka, India

Daruru Ranganath
Former Professor of Pediatrics
Osmania Medical College
Medical Superintendent
Niloufer Hospital
Hyderabad, Telangana, India

Deep Dutta MD DM DNB MNAMS MRCP FACE
Consultant
Department of Endocrinology, Diabetology and Metabolic Disorders
Venkateshwar Hospitals
New Delhi, India

Harsh Y Parekh MD
Senior Resident
Department of Endocrinology
CARE Hospital
Hyderabad, Telangana, India

J Jayannan
Junior Resident, Department of General Medicine, Pondicherry Institute of Medical Sciences
Puducherry, India

Jabbar Khadar MD DM DNB
Professor
Department of Endocrinology
Indian Institute of Diabetes
Trivandrum, Kerala, India

Jayant V Kelwade MD
Senior Resident
Department of Endocrinology
CARE Hospital
Hyderabad, Telangana, India

Kavitha Muniraj
Consultant Diabetologist and Endocrinologist
Dr S Srikanta and the Diabetes Collaborative Study Group
Samatvam Endocrinology Diabetes Center, Jnana Sanjeevini Diabetes Hospital and Medical Center, Samatvam: Science and Research for Human Welfare Trust
Bangalore, Karnataka, India

KM Chandrika PGDD FACE
Diabetologist and Endocrinologist
Dr S Srikanta and the Diabetes Collaborative Study Group
Samatvam Endocrinology Diabetes Center, Jnana Sanjeevini Diabetes Hospital and Medical Center, Samatvam: Science and Research for Human Welfare Trust
Bangalore, Karnataka, India

Contributors

Kranti S Khadilkar MD DM
Consultant
Department of Endocrinology
and Bariatric Medicine
Mazumdar Shaw Medical Centre
Narayana Health City
Bengaluru, Karnataka, India

L Reddy
Dr S Srikanta and the Diabetes
Collaborative Study Group
Samatvam Endocrinology
Diabetes Center
Jnana Sanjeevini Diabetes
Hospital and Medical Center,
Samatvam: Science and Research
for Human Welfare Trust
Bangalore, Karnataka, India

Lila Anurag MD DM
Associate Professor
Department of Endocrinology
King Edward Memorial Hospital
Mumbai, Maharashtra, India

Manash P Baruah MD DM FACE
Director and Consultant
Department of Endocrinology
Excel Center (A Unit of Excelcare Hospitals)
Guwahati, Assam, India

Manoj D Chadha MD DM
Consultant
Department of Endocrinology
PD Hinduja Hospital
Mumbai, Maharashtra, India

Meha Sharma MD DM
Consultant and Head
Department of Rheumatology
Venkateshwar Hospitals
New Delhi, India

Mohd Ashraf Ganie MD DM
Professor
Department of Endocrinology
Institute of Medical Sciences
Srinagar, Jammu & Kashmir, India

Mudita Dhingra MD FIAP
Consultant, Department of
Endocrinology, Rotary Hospital
Ambala, Haryana, India
Radhakishan Hospital
Kurukshetra, Haryana, India

Neera Gupta MD
Head, Medical Education and
Scientific Affairs
Novo Nordisk Education
Foundation
Bangalore, Karnataka, India

Rajesh Khadgawat MD DM DNB MNAMS
Additional Professor
Department of Endocrinology
and Metabolism
All India Institute of Medical Sciences
New Delhi, India

Rajesh R Joshi MD DNB
Professor
Department of Pediatrics
BJ Wadia Hospital for Children
Mumbai, Maharashtra, India

Ranjini Sen MD
Medical Advisor, Novo Nordisk
Education Foundation
Bangalore, Karnataka, India

Rishi Shukla MD DM
Head
Department of Endocrinology
Regency Hospital Ltd.
Centre for Diabetes and
Endocrine Diseases
Kanpur, Uttar Pradesh, India

S Geetha Rao
Dr S Srikanta and the Diabetes
Collaborative Study Group
Samatvam Endocrinology
Diabetes Center
Jnana Sanjeevini Diabetes
Hospital and Medical Center,
Samatvam: Science and Research
for Human Welfare Trust
Bangalore, Karnataka, India

Sangeeta Das MA PhD
Assistant Professor
Department of Psychology
Tagore Arts College
Pondicherry, Tamil Nadu, India

Sathya Prakash MD Dip CBT
Consultant, Department of
Psychiatry, Institute of Brain and
Spine/Sitaram Bhartia Institute
of Science and Research
New Delhi, India

Shivane Vyankatesh
Consultant
Department of Diabetology and
Endocrinology, King Edward
Hospital, Shushrusha Citizens'
Co-operative Hospital
Mumbai, Maharashtra, India

Shuchy Chugh
Diabetes Education Specialist
Novo Nordisk Education
Foundation
Bangalore, Karnataka, India

SK Hammadur Rahaman MD
Senior Resident, Department of
Endocrinology and Metabolism
All India Institute of Medical Sciences
New Delhi, India

Sneha M Kothari MD DNB
Consultant, Department of
Endocrinology, Global Hospitals
Mumbai, Maharashtra, India

SS Srikanta MD PhD FEDM FACE
Medical Director and Senior
Consultant, Department of
Endocrinology, Jnana Sanjeevini
Diabetes and Medical Centre
Bengaluru, Karnataka, India

Sujoy Ghosh DM FRCP FACE FICP
Associate Professor
Department of Endocrinology
Institute of Post Graduate
Medical Education and Research
Kolkata, West Bengal, India

Sunil M Jain MD DM
Chief Endocrinologist and
Managing Director
TOTALL Diabetes Hormone
Institute
Indore, Madhya Pradesh, India

Sweety Agrawal MD DM
Senior Resident, Department of
Endocrinology and Metabolism
All India Institute of Medical
Sciences
New Delhi, India

Usha Rangaraj
Dr S Srikanta and the Diabetes
Collaborative Study Group
Samatvam Endocrinology
Diabetes Center

Jnana Sanjeevini Diabetes
Hospital and Medical Center,
Samatvam: Science and Research
for Human Welfare Trust
Bangalore, Karnataka, India

V Sri Nagesh MD DM
Consultant
Department of Endocrinology,
CARE Hospital
Hyderabad, Telangana, India

Vasanthi Nath
Dr S Srikanta and the Diabetes
Collaborative Study Group
Samatvam Endocrinology
Diabetes Center, Jnana Sanjeevini
Diabetes Hospital and Medical
Center, Samatvam: Science and
Research for Human Welfare Trust
Bangalore, Karnataka, India

Vijay Viswanathan MD PhD
FICP FRCP (London) FRCP (Glasgow)
Head and Chief Diabetologist
MV Hospital for Diabetes
Chennai, Tamil Nadu, India

Yashdeep Gupta MD DM
Assistant Professor
Department of Endocrinology
and Metabolism
All India Institute of Medical
Sciences
New Delhi, India

Yatan PS Balhara MD DNB
MNAMS MSc
Associate Professor
Department of Psychiatry
National Drug Dependence
Treatment Centre
WHO Collaborating Centre on
Substance Abuse
All India Institute of Medical
Sciences
New Delhi, India

FOREWORD

India has a huge burden of approximately 69.2 million people with diabetes. Of all people with diabetes, approximately 95% are estimated to have type 2 diabetes mellitus. This has led to overlooking of children with type 1 diabetes mellitus (T1DM) with terrible consequences. In an attempt to address the critical gap in the management of children with T1DM in India, Novo Nordisk A/S, through the Novo Nordisk Education Foundation, in collaboration with the International Society for Paediatric and Adolescent Diabetes has launched Changing Diabetes in Children (CDiC) program.

The CDiC program was unveiled in India, in September 2011, by our former President Dr APJ Abdul Kalam. The vision of the program is "to initiate and strive for giving access to comprehensive diabetes care for the economically under-privileged children with type 1 diabetes in India."

The program focuses on six needed elements which includes "infrastructure and equipment, insulin and supplies, capacity building and raising awareness, patient education, advocacy and sharing learnings, and the outcomes."

There are 21 CDiC centers operational across India, and these centers are taking care of 4,063 children with T1DM from economically underprivileged families providing them with opportunity to manage their diabetes better through access to care and support.

Type 1 diabetes mellitus is one of the most common endocrine and metabolic conditions in childhood. Incidence is rapidly increasing, especially among the youngest children. As reported by International Diabetes Federation in 2015, in India there are approximately 70,200 children with T1DM in age group 0–14 years. Insulin treatment is lifesaving and lifelong need for these children. Management also requires learning self-discipline, adherence to a balanced diet, exercise, and treatment.

Through "CDiC Textbook of Pediatric Diabetes," we intend to support and strengthen management of children with diabetes by sharing practical aspects of diabetes care including recent advances. I am confident that this initiative will engrave a new milestone in diagnosis and management of childhood diabetes.

Raghupathy Palany BSc MD DCH FRCP
Chairperson, Changing Diabetes in Children, India
Professor, Department of Pediatric Endocrinology
Indira Gandhi Institute of Child Health
Bangalore, Karnataka, India

PREFACE

A Legacy Begins

*"Start children off on the way they should go, and
even when they are old they will not turn from it"*

–Proverbs 22:6

All children deserve a good start in life, and children with diabetes are no exception. Children living with diabetes need good care, to help them grow as productive members of society. For this, they need diabetes care providers who are aware of their special needs, and are empowered to deliver the required support.

In today's adult dominated type 2 diabetes mellitus and metabolic syndrome epidemic, however, we often find children with diabetes fighting for their rightful place under the sun (Prasanna et al). Changing Diabetes in Children (CDiC) has lent support to these children, providing clinical care, education, counseling, and advocacy. This book on Pediatric Diabetology adds to this collective effort.

Eminent and experienced authors from across India have contributed their best, writing chapters which explain the diagnosis, evaluation, and management of childhood diabetes. Clinical and laboratory evaluation is covered, as is nonpharmacological and pharmacological management of its acute/chronic complications.

The Diabetes Control and Complications Trial (DCCT) proved that complications of type 1 diabetes mellitus can be prevented. Our textbook, we hope, will do the same for thousands of children it reaches through their care providers. The Epidemiology of Diabetes Interventions and Complications Study at 30 years (EDIC) showed that the benefits of DCCT were durable. Both DCCT and EDIC provided evidence to support the wisdom shared in the Book of Proverbs, quoted above.

This book, we hope, will provide benefits as robust as those of DCCT, and as long-lasting as those of EDIC. Humbly, we pray that this begins a new legacy: a legacy of empowerment, a legacy of health, a legacy of happiness, for children with diabetes, and for their care providers. We thank the Almighty for having given us the opportunity to be of service.

Ashok K Das

Sanjay Kalra

ACKNOWLEDGMENTS

This book is a collaborative effort of many individuals. In our philanthropic journey of Changing Diabetes in Children (CDiC), we have always focused to improve the clinical care of underprivileged children with diabetes. Our efforts have been directed to give them a better tomorrow. Through this book, our endeavor is to present our experiences in this journey and share the advances in the field of managing diabetes in children. We are indebted to all the contributing authors who have toiled incessantly without which the fruition of this task was impossible.

We wish to thank Melvin Oscar D'souza, Managing Trustee, Novo Nordisk Education Foundation and CDiC team for their constant support. We want to extend our sincere thanks to Dr MV Srishyla, Dr Neera Gupta, Dr Ranjini Sen, and Dr Shuchy Chugh for their scientific support, and Vinay Ransiwal and Dinakaran P for their technical and administrative support. We also wish to place on record our heartfelt thanks to Ulrik Uldall Nielsen, Senior Program Manager, Novo Nordisk A/S, Denmark, on his special support for this effort.

We also want to thank Jaypee Brothers Medical Publishers (P) Ltd. for publishing this book and special thanks to Dr Neeraj Choudhary and Neha Bakshi for their persistent efforts and support.

We are grateful to the "Changing Diabetes in Children Program" for this wonderful initiative and helping us in making innovative changes in improving patient care specially children with diabetes.

CONTENTS

Section 1: Introduction

Section Editor: KM Prasanna Kumar

1. Childhood Diabetes — 3
   Ashok K Jhingan

2. Epidemiology of Childhood Diabetes — 8
   Subhankar Chowdhury, Sujoy Ghosh

3. Monogenic Diabetes: Perspectives and Clinical Implications from Pediatric to Adult Endocrinology — 21
   BV Reshma, Kavitha Muniraj, KM Chandrika, S Geetha Rao, L Reddy, Usha Rangaraj, Vasanthi Nath, Neera Gupta, Ranjini Sen, Mudita Dhingra, Sanjay Kalra, Ashok K Das, SS Srikanta; The Diabetes Collaborative Study Group

4. Growth and Development in Children with Type 1 Diabetes Mellitus — 31
   Raghupathy Palany, Abraham Paulose

Section 2: Clinical and Laboratory Approach

Section Editor: Raghupathy Palany

5. Clinical Examination of Type 1 Diabetes Mellitus — 41
   Rishi Shukla

6. Initial and Annual Laboratory Investigations — 48
   Bipin K Sethi, V Sri Nagesh, Jayant V Kelwade, Harsh Y Parekh

7. Glycemic Monitoring in Children — 53
   Meha Sharma, Deep Dutta, Sanjay Kalra

8. Childhood Diabetes: Common Pitfalls in Diagnosis and Management — 59
   Sweety Agrawal, Nikhil Tandon

Section 3: Nonpharmacological Management

Section Editor: PV Rao

9. Medical Nutrition Therapy in Children with Type 1 Diabetes Mellitus — 67
   Anjana Hulse, KM Prasanna Kumar

10.	**Exercise in Children and Adolescents with Type 1 Diabetes Mellitus** *Rajesh R Joshi*	76
11.	**Diabetes Education** *Archana S Sarda*	82
12.	**Biopsychosocial Dimensions in Diabetes: A Brief Outline** *Sangeeta Das*	94

Section 4: Pharmacological Management

Section Editor: Subhankar Chowdhury

13.	**Insulin Therapy** *Ashok K Das*	105
14.	**Noninsulin Therapy** *Sanjay Kalra, Manash P Baruah*	123
15.	**Continuous Glucose Monitoring System and Insulin Pump** *Sunil M Jain*	131
16.	**Pancreas and Islet Cell Transplant in Children** *Sujoy Ghosh*	148

Section 5: Acute Complications

Section Editor: Nalini Shah

17.	**Diabetic Ketoacidosis in Children** *Alok Kanungo*	159
18.	**Management of Diabetes in Hospitalized Children** *PV Rao, Daruru Ranganath*	172
19.	**Surgery in a Child with Diabetes** *Sneha M Kothari, Manoj D Chadha*	177
20.	**Hypoglycemia** *Kranti S Khadilkar, Shivane Vyankatesh,* *Lila Anurag, Bandgar Tushar, Nalini Shah*	191

Section 6: Chronic Complications

Section Editor: Vaman Khadilkar

21.	**Lipid Disorders in Type 1 Diabetes Mellitus** *Bipin K Sethi, V Sri Nagesh*	201
22.	**Hypertension** *Sanjay Kalra, Mudita Dhingra, Rakesh Sahay*	207

23.	Microvascular Complications *Vijay Viswanathan*	215
24.	Future Metabolic Risk among Subjects with Type 1 Diabetes Mellitus *SK Hammadur Rahaman, Mohd Ashraf Ganie*	222

Section 7: Special Situations

Section Editor: Nikhil Tandon

25.	Sick Day Management *Banshi D Saboo*	231
26.	Managing Diabetes in Neonates and Toddlers *Aashima Dabas, Rajesh Khadgawat*	238
27.	Psychiatric Management *Yatan PS Balhara, Sathya Prakash*	249

Section 8: Miscellaneous

Section Editor: Rakesh Sahay

28.	Diabetes Education Material *Archana S Sarda, Shuchy Chugh*	263
29.	Genetics of Type 1 Diabetes Mellitus *Mudita Dhingra, J Jayannan, Ashok K Das, Sanjay Kalra*	280
30.	Type 2 Diabetes Mellitus in Children *Jabbar Khadar, Abilash Nair*	288
31.	Type 1 Diabetes Mellitus: A Perspective from Guidelines *Sanjay Kalra, Yashdeep Gupta*	299
	Appendix	*309*
	Index	*313*

PLATE 1

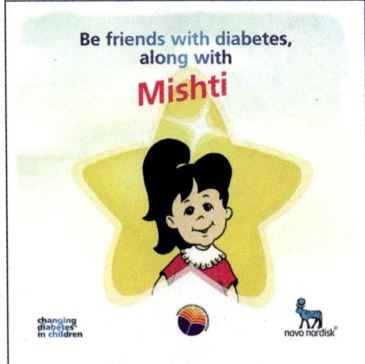
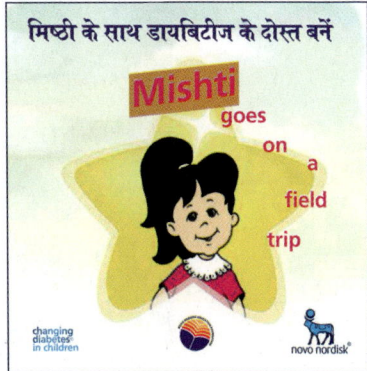
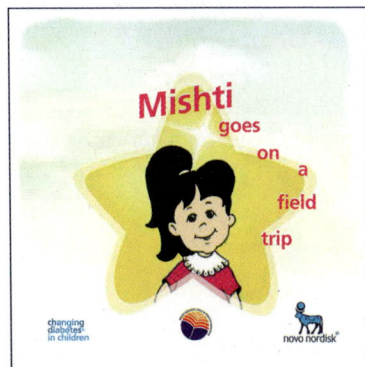
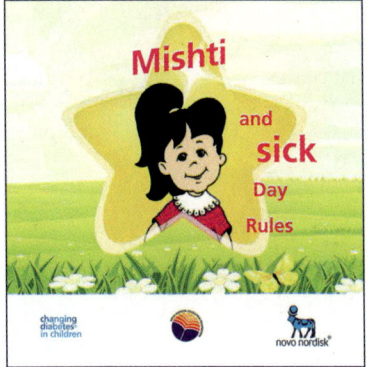

Fig. 1: Mishti story book *(Chapter 28)*

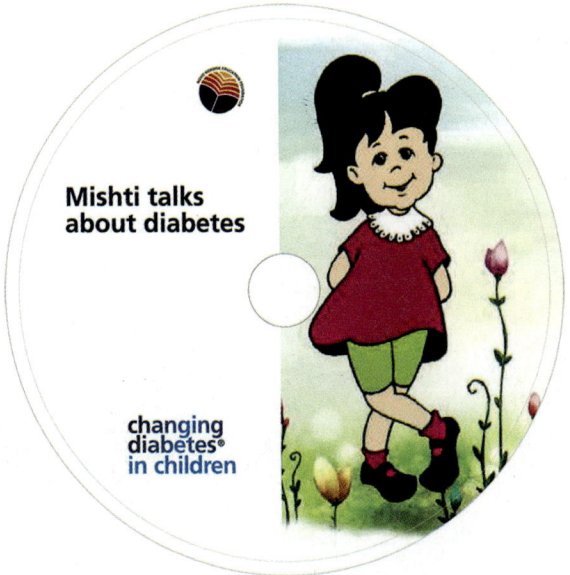

Fig. 2: Cover of Mishti video *(Chapter 28)*

PLATE 2

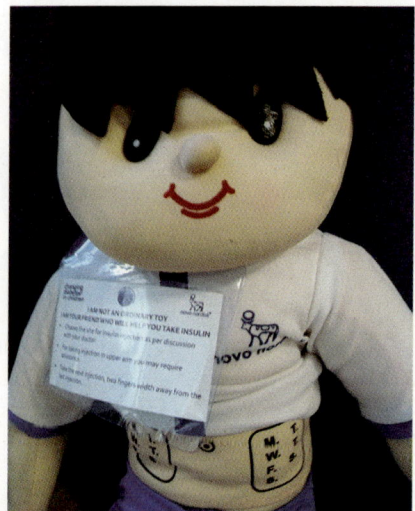

Fig. 3: NOTTI doll presenting sites of injection *(Chapter 28)*

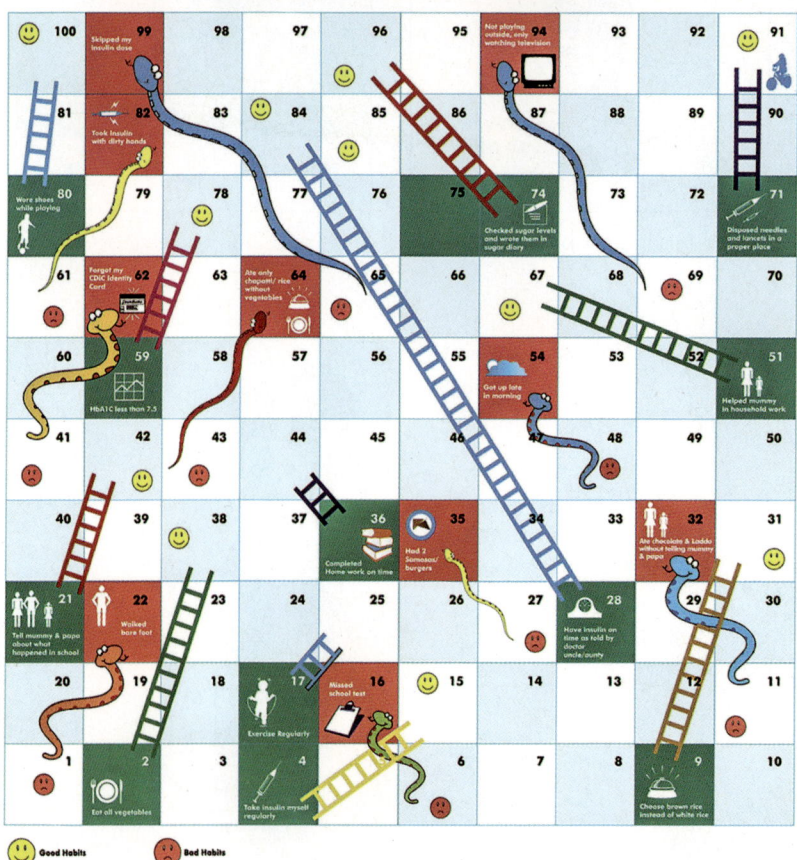

Fig. 4: Snake and ladder game *(Chapter 28)*

PLATE 3

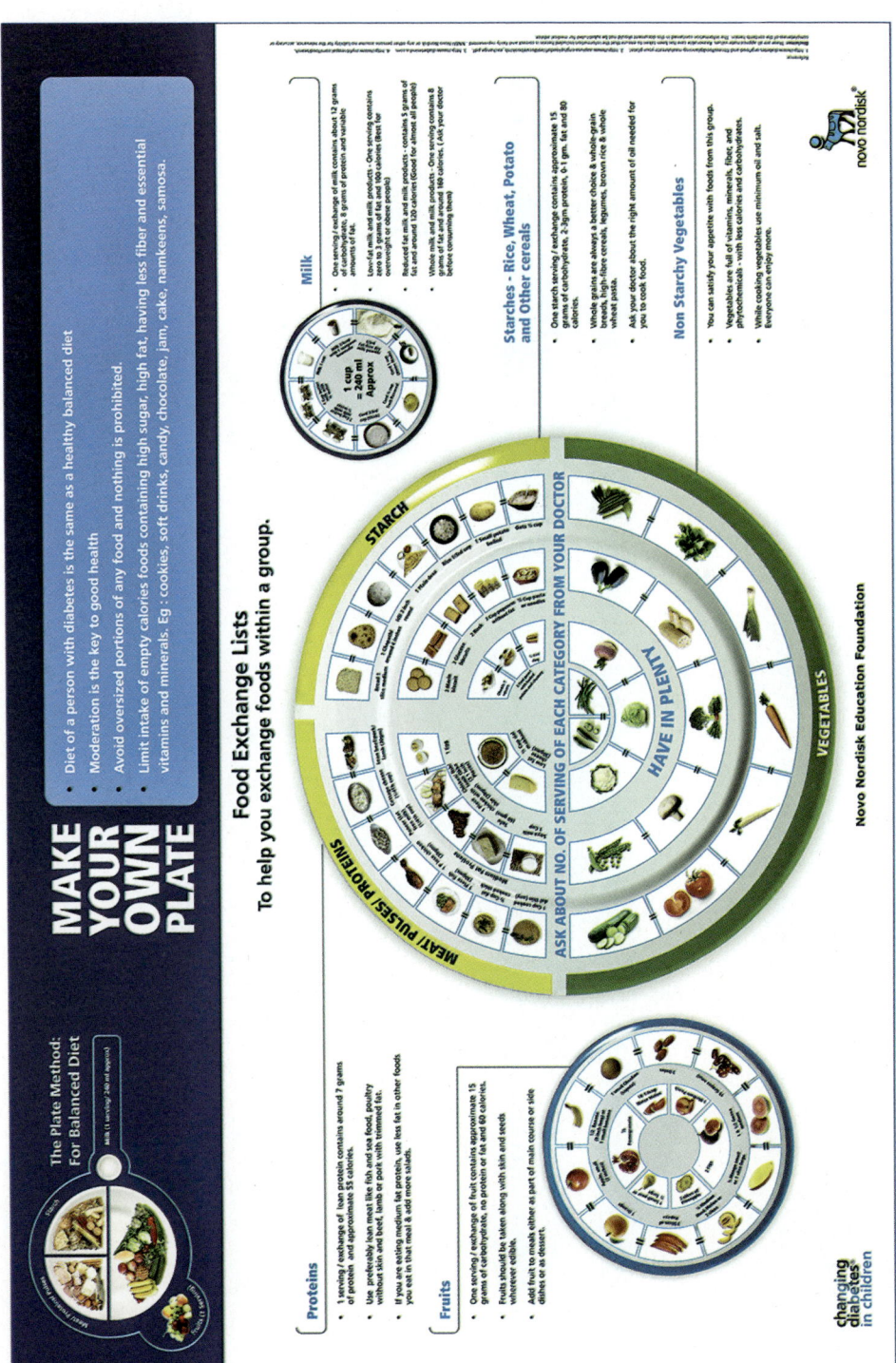

Fig. 5: Make your own plate poster *(Chapter 28)*

PLATE 4

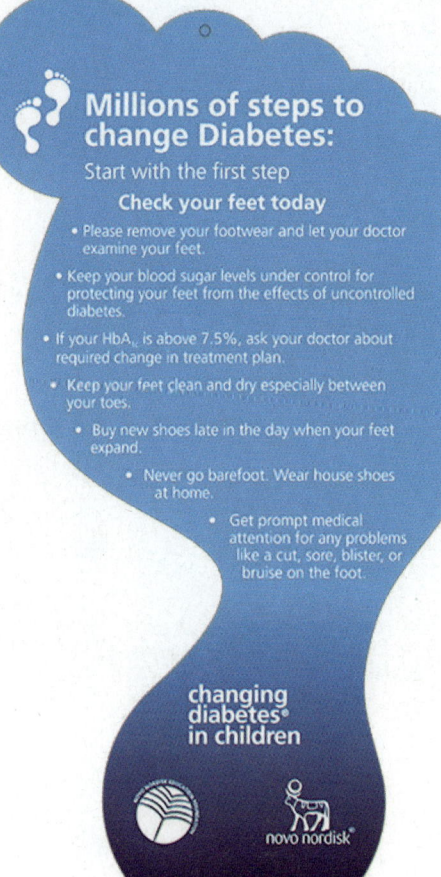

Fig. 6: Foot door knob hanger *(Chapter 28)*

PLATE 5

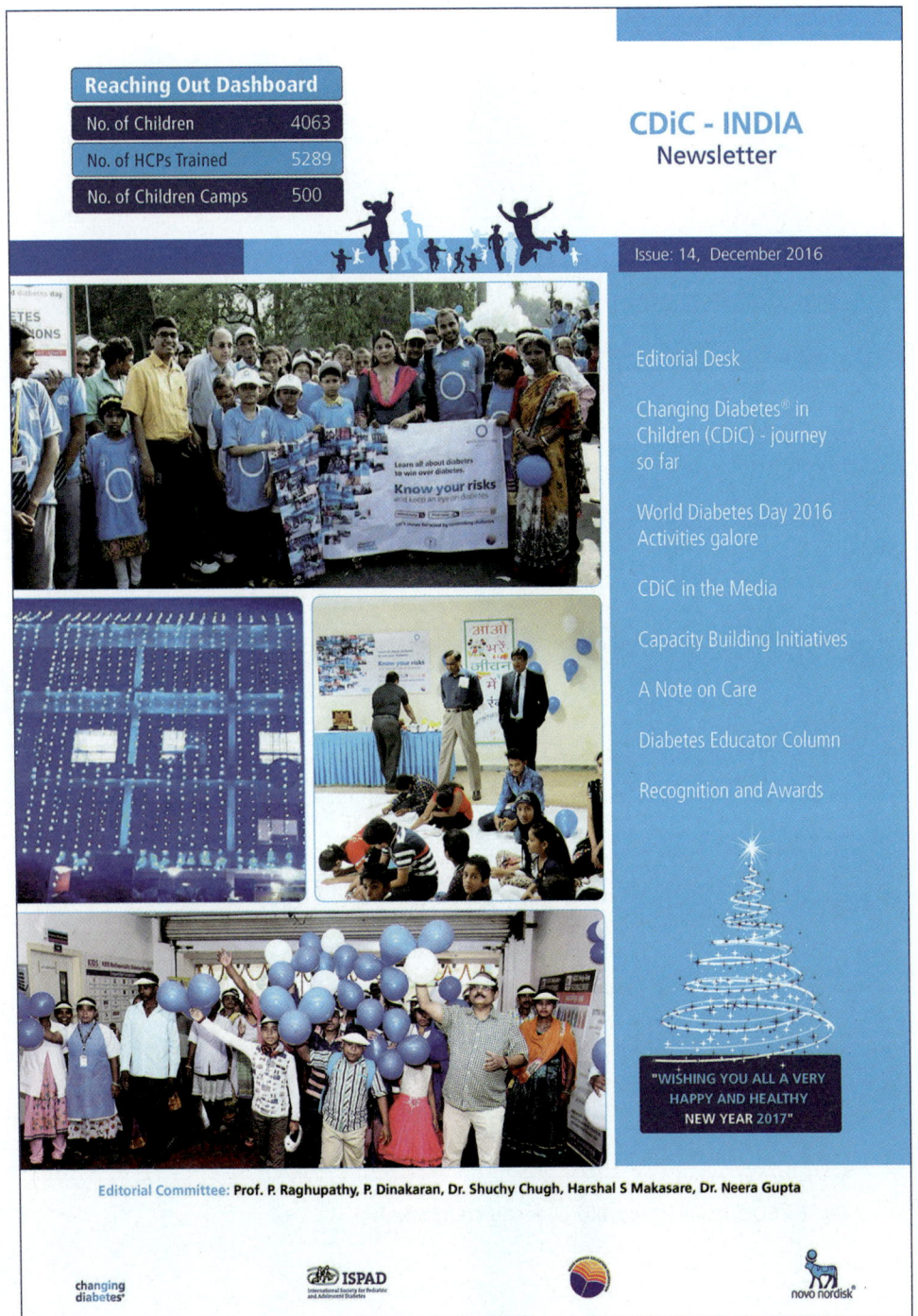

Fig. 7: CDiC newsletter; Table of contents *(Chapter 28)*

PLATE 6

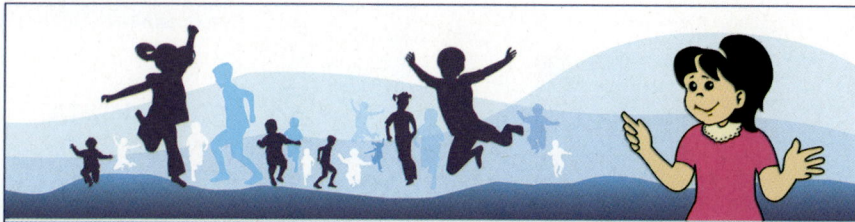

Mishti - Guardian
(a CDiC initiative to empower parents and families of children with type 1 diabetes)

Issue - IV Dec 2016

Editorial Team
Dr P. Raghupathy
P Dinakaran
Dr Shuchy Chugh
Dr Neera Gupta

Advisory Team
Dr A K Das
Dr AK Jinghan
Dr Alok Kanungo
Dr Archana Sarda
Dr Banshi Saboo
Dr Bipin K Sethi
Dr KM Prasanna Kumar
Dr Manoj Chadha
Dr Nalini Shah
Dr Nikhil Tandon
Dr P K Jabbar
Dr P. V. Rao
Dr Rajesh Joshi
Dr Rishi Shukla
Dr Sanjay Kalra
Dr Sanjay Reddy
Dr SS Srikanta
Dr Subhankar Chowdhury
Dr Sunil M Jain
Dr Surendra Kumar
Dr Vaman Khadilkar
Dr Vijay Viswanathan

Diabetes Educators and parents form a crucial component of the diabetes care team. With their support and special attention, we could bring huge change in the lives of many children with type 1 diabetes. In this 4th issue of the Mishti Guardian newsletter, the medium of connecting parents and other care givers of children with type 1 diabetes, we have compiled interesting articles, stories and facts. This is to support in their endevour for offering a good quality of life for these children. It is truly rewarding to see these children with type 1 diabetes, smile & enjoy good quality of life.

Diabetes is a disorder, which affects the child and his/her parents all the time. It is a fact that Type 1 diabetes is a demanding condition to have. It changes the entire life of the child and family members, because it means, not only multiple daily injections for a lifetime but also changes in your lifestyle. This includes food and daily activities, continuous vigil and care along with constant contact with hospitals. There is no holiday for diabetes management. It is definitely a challenging task, but once managed with discipline it gives good results. Given proper treatment and education, these children can grow up to be productive adults. You all will agree that, diabetes self – management education and awareness is the most effective mean to empower children with type 1 diabetes to manage diabetes on the long run.

In this issue, continuing our journey of strengthening the knowledge and education, we have an interesting article on "Management of diabetes in playground" by Prof. P Raghupathy, which gives insights how a child can manage diabetes while enjoying and playing. Along with that we have an article by Dr Sanjay Kalra which explains how right growth is an important indicator of good metabolic control and the role of right nutrition for it. We get a close view of life of a child with type 1 diabetes by a story from the IID CDiC center by Dr P K Jabbar. In the end, we have an article emphasizing on "Prevention is always better than cure" as how to "prevent acute complications for children with type 1 diabetes" by Dr A K Das. In the last page, we have BMI chart to know how healthy we are as an individual and about our requirement to follow a healthy lifestyle.

We look forward to your valuable feedback and suggestions. This is your magazine, so please do send in your feedback and contributions.

With best wishes,

Editorial Team

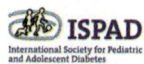 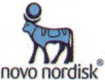

Fig. 8: CDiC newsletter; Editorial section *(Chapter 28)*

PLATE 7

Knowing about Carbs

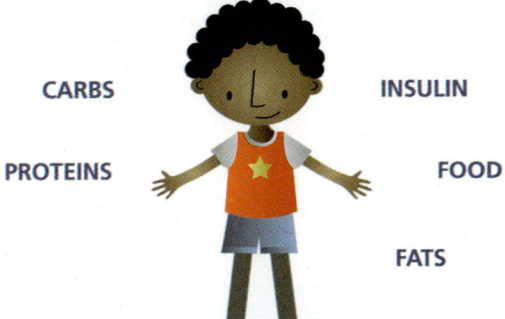

CARBS INSULIN
PROTEINS FOOD
FATS

All children need energy
to grow | play | study | do all other activities

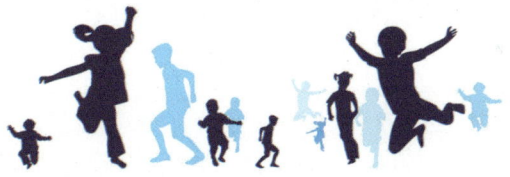

Our body is a wonderful machine,
which gets energy from the food we eat

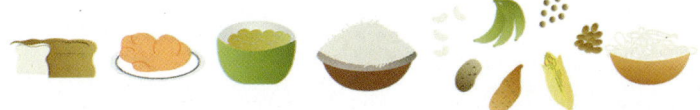

Carbohydrates present in food
are the main source of energy, others being proteins and fats. Children with type 1 diabetes need to take insulin according to the carbohydrate intake.

 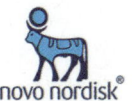

Continued

Continued

Knowing about Carbs

Carbohydrates and their relationship with insulin

Carbohydrates are main source of energy in food that fuels children's metabolism, supports growth and maintains overall health. Carbohydrates are present in varying amounts in most foods. These includes fruits, vegetables, grains, beans, legumes, milk, milk products and foods with sugar such as candy, soda and other sweets. If there is enough insulin present in the body naturally or provided by injections, it will utilize the carbohydrates. However, if body is producing less or no insulin, then blood sugar is bound to rise.

Types of carbohydrates[1]

- Sugars (also known as simple or fast acting carbohydrates)
- Starches (also known as complex carbohydrates or slow acting carbohydrates)
- Fiber

Good Carbs - Complex carbohydrates which are full of fiber and get absorbed slowly into our systems, resulting in fewer spikes in blood sugar levels are good carbohydrates. E,g whole wheat bread, cereals and veggies like corn, potatoes and carrots.

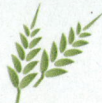
Whole Grain Breads

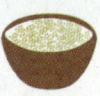
Brown Rice

Vegetables

Fresh Fruits

Bad Carbs - Refined and processed carbohydrates that strip away beneficial fiber or food containing large amount of sugars are bad carbohydrates. Eg

Candy, Sweets & Desserts

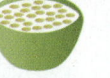
Sugared Cereals

Sweetened Drinks

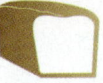
Refined Breads

However all carbs can raise blood sugar levels if there is no insulin or less insulin in the body. It is always good to take good carbs. Allthough children can have every food in moderate quantity if it is balanced by right dose of insulin. It's a little easier for people to control their diabetes if they eat about the same amount of carbs at about the same times each day.

No wonder knowing what kind and how much carbohydrate to eat can be confusing!

Let us learn

1. Ask your Dietician or physician about the carbohydrate content (CHO) of common food items you eat. Here is an example ➝

Menu[2]	Quantity	CHO Content
Cooked Rice	1/3 Cup	15
Chapati 1 medium 6 Inch	1 medium	15
Vegetable (Non Starchy)	1 Cup	5
Poha	½ Cup	15
Curds	½ Cup	6
Milk	1 Cup	12
Apple	1 small	15

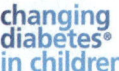

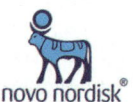

Fig. 9: Leaflet; knowing about carbohydrates *(Chapter 28)*

PLATE 8

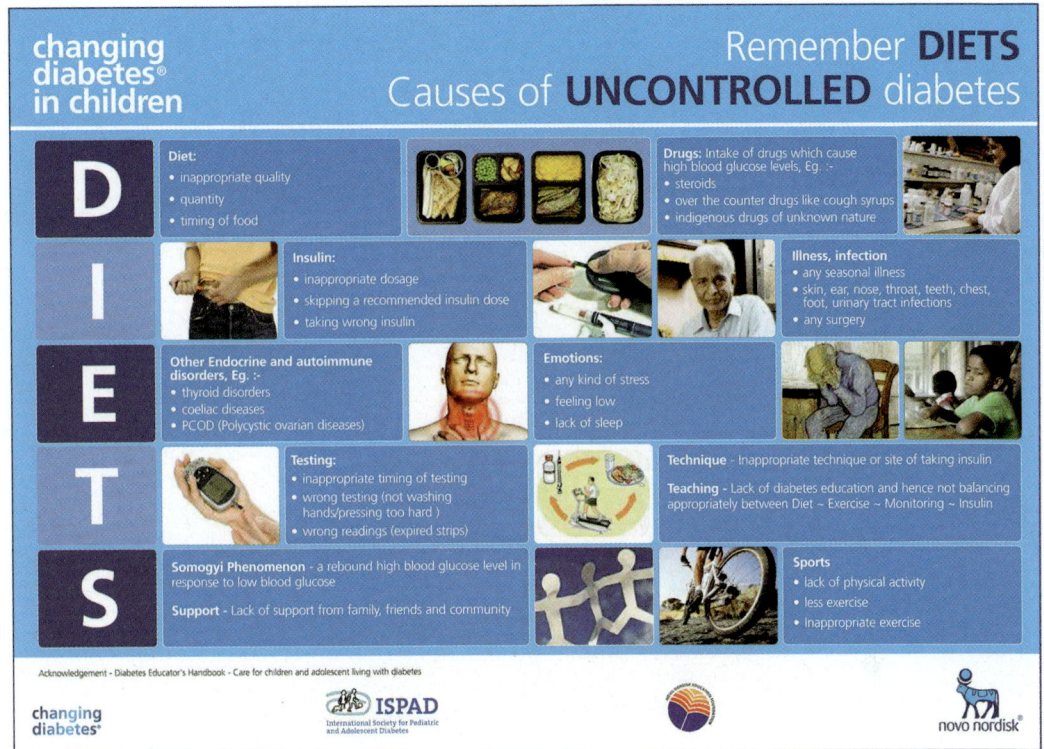

Fig. 10: DIETS leaflet *(Chapter 28)*

PLATE 9

Control Diabetes before it controls you

Average blood glucose (mg/dL)	HbA_{1c}
126	6
140	6.5
154	7
169	7.5
183	8
197	8.5
212	9
226	9.5
240	10
255	10.5
269	11
283	11.5
298	12
312	12.5
326	13
341	13.5
355	14
369	14.5
384	15
398	15.5
412	16
427	16.5
441	17
456	17.5
470	18
484	18.5
499	19

6 - 7% — Diabetes (Good Control)

7- 8.5% — Diabetes (Moderate Control, Monitor Carefully, Visit Doctor)

>8.5% — Diabetes Danger zone, Visit your doctor immediately

HbA_{1c} calculations using the formula: 28.7 X A1C – 46.7 = eAG taken from http://professional.diabetes.org/glucosecalculator.aspx, * 2011 ADA guidelines.
*https://www.aace.com/files/dccwhitepaper.pdf **DCCT[1]/ UKPDS[2]/Kumamoto[3]

changing diabetes® in children

NOVO NORDISK EDUCATION FOUNDATION

novo nordisk®

Fig. 11: Glycosylated hemoglobin calculator *(Chapter 28)*

PLATE 10

Stay fit with healthy weight

Body Mass Index (BMI) is a reliable calculator to evaluate and know whether a person is having healthy weight/ underweight / overweight / or obese. It is a ratio calculated from weight and height.

Metric BMI Formula

BMI^1 = (Weight in kilograms / (height in meters x height in meters)

If you are overweight (with a BMI over 25) and physically inactive, you may develop:
- Type 2 diabetes.
- Cardiovascular (heart and blood circulation) disease.
- Gallbladder disease.
- High blood pressure (hypertension)
- Osteoarthritis.
- Certain types of cancer, such as colon and breast cancer

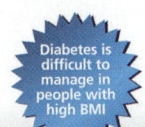
Diabetes is difficult to manage in people with high BMI

HEIGHT		\multicolumn{16}{c}{BODY WEIGHT (kg)}														
ft. in	cm	50	54	58	62	66	70	74	78	82	86	90	94	98	102	106	110
4.7	140	25.5	27.6	29.6	31.6	33.7	35.7	37.8	39.8	41.8	43.9	45.9	48.0	50.0	52.0	54.1	56.1
4.9	144	24.1	26.0	28.0	29.9	31.8	33.8	35.7	37.6	39.5	41.5	43.4	45.3	47.3	49.2	51.1	53.0
4.10	148	22.8	24.7	26.5	28.3	30.1	32.0	33.8	35.6	37.4	39.3	41.1	42.9	44.7	46.6	48.4	50.2
4.12	152	21.6	23.4	25.1	26.8	28.6	30.3	32.0	33.8	35.5	37.2	39.0	407	42.4	44.1	45.9	47.6
5.1	156	20.5	22.2	23.8	25.5	27.1	28.8	30.4	32.1	33.7	35.3	37.0	38.6	40.3	41.9	43.6	45.2
5.3	160	19.5	21.1	22.7	24.2	25.8	27.3	28.9	30.5	32.0	33.6	35.2	36.7	38.3	39.8	41.4	43.0
5.5	164	18.6	20.1	21.6	23.1	24.5	26.0	27.5	29.0	30.5	32.0	33.5	24.9	36.4	37.9	39.4	40.9
5.6	168	17.7	19.1	20.5	22.0	23.4	24.8	26.2	27.6	29.1	30.5	31.9	33.3	24.7	36.1	37.6	39.0
5.8	172	16.9	18.3	19.6	21.0	22.3	23.7	25.0	26.4	27.7	29.1	30.4	31.8	33.1	34.5	35.8	37.2
5.9	176	16.1	17.4	18.7	20.0	21.3	22.6	23.9	25.2	26.5	27.8	29.1	30.3	31.6	32.9	34.2	35.5
5.11	180	15.4	16.7	17.9	19.1	20.4	21.6	22.8	24.1	25.3	26.5	27.8	29.0	30.2	31.5	32.7	34.0
6.0	184	14.8	15.9	17.1	18.3	19.5	20.7	21.9	23.0	24.2	25.4	26.6	27.8	28.9	30.1	31.3	32.5
6.2	188	14.1	15.3	16.4	17.5	18.7	19.8	20.9	22.1	23.2	24.3	25.5	26.6	27.7	28.9	30.0	31.1
6.4	192	13.6	14.6	15.7	16.8	17.9	19.0	20.1	21.2	22.2	23.3	24.4	25.5	26.6	27.7	28.8	29.8
6.5	196	13.0	14.1	15.1	16.1	17.2	18.2	19.3	20.3	21.3	22.4	23.4	24.5	25.5	26.6	27.6	28.6
6.7	200	12.5	13.5	14.5	15.5	16.5	17.5	18.5	19.5	20.5	21.5	22.5	23.5	24.5	25.5	26.5	27.5
6.8	204	12.0	13.0	13.9	14.9	15.9	16.8	17.8	18.7	19.7	20.7	21.6	22.6	23.5	24.5	25.5	26.4
6.10	208	11.6	12.5	13.4	14.3	15.3	16.2	17.1	18.0	19.0	19.9	20.8	21.7	22.7	23.6	24.5	25.4
6.11	212	11.1	12.0	12.9	13.8	14.7	15.6	16.5	17.4	18.2	19.1	20.0	20.9	21.8	22.7	23.6	24.5
7.1	216	10.7	11.6	12.4	13.3	14.1	15.0	15.9	16.7	17.6	18.4	19.3	20.1	21.0	21.9	22.7	23.6
7.3	220	10.3	11.2	12.0	12.8	13.6	14.5	15.3	16.1	16.9	17.8	18.6	19.4	20.2	21.1	21.9	22.7

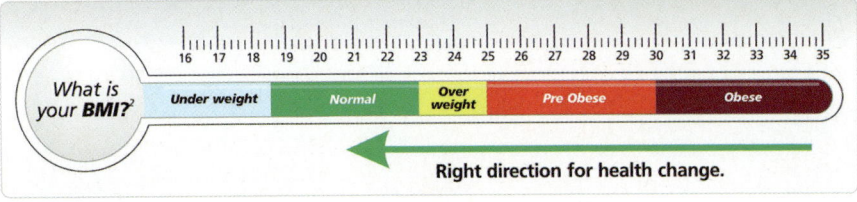

What is your **BMI?**[2] — Under weight | Normal | Over weight | Pre Obese | Obese

Right direction for health change.

1. http://apps.who.int/bmi/index.jsp?introPage=intro_3.html, accessed on 13 April 2016. 2. http://japi.org/february_2009/R-1.pdf, accessed on 14 April 2016

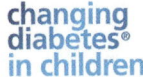
changing diabetes® in children

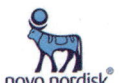
novo nordisk

Fig. 12: Body mass index chart *(Chapter 28)*

SECTION 1

Introduction

Editor

KM Prasanna Kumar

CHAPTER 1

Childhood Diabetes

Ashok K Jhingan

INTRODUCTION

Incidence of diabetes is on steep rise throughout the world and so as diabetes in children. Approximately, 90% of the children with diabetes have type 1 diabetes. Early diagnosis and differentiating the type of diabetes can have therapeutic implications. In this chapter, we will see the etiological and clinical classification of diabetes in children.

DEFINITION

The term diabetes mellitus describes a complex metabolic disorder characterized by chronic hyperglycemia resulting from defects in insulin secretion, insulin action, or both. Inadequate insulin secretion and/or diminished tissue responses to insulin in the complex pathways of hormone action result in deficient insulin action on target tissues, which leads to abnormalities of carbohydrate, fat, and protein metabolism. Impaired insulin secretion and/or action may coexist in the same patient.[1,2]

CLASSIFICATION

The type of diabetes assigned to a young person at diagnosis is typically based on their characteristics at presentation, however, increasingly the ability to make a clinical diagnosis has been hampered by factors including the increasing prevalence of overweight in young people with type 1 diabetes,[3,4] and the presence of diabetic ketoacidosis in some young people at diagnosis of type 2 diabetes.[5,6]

In addition, the presentation of a familial form of mild diabetes during adolescence should raise the suspicion of monogenic diabetes, which accounts for 1–4% of pediatric diabetes cases.[7-10]

SECTION 1: Introduction

The etiological classification of diabetes is shown in box 1, which is based on the American Diabetes Association classification.[2]

BOX 1: Etiological classification of diabetes[2]
Type 1
Beta-cell destruction, usually leading to absolute insulin deficiency
• Immune mediated
• Idiopathic
Type 2
It may range from predominantly insulin resistance with relative insulin deficiency to a predominantly secretory defect with or without insulin resistance
Other specific types   • Genetic defects of β-cell function <ul><li>Chromosome 12, *HNF1A* (MODY3)</li><li>Chromosome 7, *GCK* (MODY2)</li><li>Chromosome 20, *HNF4B* (MODY1)</li><li>Other rare forms of MODY including:<ul><li>Chromosome 13, *IPF-1* (MODY4);</li><li>Chromosome 17, *HNF1B* (MODY5);</li><li>Chromosome 2, *NEUROD1* (MODY6);</li><li>Chromosome 2, *KLF11* (MODY7);</li><li>Chromosome 9, *CEL* (MODY8);</li><li>Chromosome 7, *PAX4* (MODY9)</li><li>Others</li></ul></li><li>Transient neonatal diabetes mellitus (most commonly *PLAGL1/HYMAI* imprinting defect on 6q24)</li><li>Permanent neonatal diabetes mellitus (most commonly *KCNJ11* gene encoding Kir6.2 subunit of β-cell KATP channel)<ul><li>Mitochondrial DNA mutation</li><li>Others</li></ul></li></ul> • Genetic defects in insulin action <ul><li>Type A insulin resistance</li><li>Leprechaunism</li><li>Rabson-Mendenhall syndrome</li><li>Lipoatrophic diabetes</li><li>Others</li></ul> • Diseases of the exocrine pancreas <ul><li>Pancreatitis</li><li>Trauma/pancreatectomy</li><li>Neoplasia</li><li>Cystic fibrosis</li><li>Hemochromatosis</li><li>Fibrocalculous pancreatopathy</li><li>Others</li></ul> • Endocrinopathies <ul><li>Acromegaly</li><li>Cushing's syndrome</li><li>Glucagonoma</li><li>Pheochromocytoma</li><li>Hyperthyroidism</li><li>Somatostatinoma</li><li>Aldosteronoma</li><li>Others</li><li>Porphyria</li><li>Prader-Willi syndrome</li><li>Others</li></ul>

Continued

Continued

- Drug- or chemical-induced
  - Vacor
  - Pentamidine
  - Nicotinic acid
  - Glucocorticoids
  - Thyroid hormone
  - Diazoxide
  - β-adrenergic agonists
  - Thiazides
  - Dilantin
  - α-interferon
  - Others
- Infections
  - Congenital rubella
  - Cytomegalovirus
  - Enterovirus
  - Others
- Uncommon forms of immune-mediated diabetes
  - "Stiff-man" syndrome
  - Anti-insulin receptor antibodies
  - Autoimmune polyendocrine syndrome types I and type II
  - Immunodysregulation polyendocrinopathy enteropathy X-linked syndrome
  - Others
- Other genetic syndromes sometimes associated with diabetes
  - Down syndrome
  - Klinefelter syndrome
  - Turner syndrome
  - Wolfram syndrome
  - Friedreich's ataxia
  - Huntington's chorea
  - Laurence-Moon-Biedl syndrome
  - Myotonic dystrophy

Gestational diabetes mellitus

CEL, carboxyl ester lipase; HNF, hepatocyte nuclear factor; IPF, insulin promoter factor; KLF11, Kruppel-like factor 11; MODY, maturity-onset diabetes of the young; PAX4.

The differentiation between type 1, type 2, monogenic, and other forms of diabetes has important implications for both therapeutic decisions and educational approaches. Differentiating the type of diabetes is very important as it has therapeutic implications. There are specific tests that can help in confirming the type of diabetes:
- Detection of autoantibodies: The presence of glutamic acid decarboxylase, IA2, IAA, and/or ZnT8 for type 1 diabetes. These autoantibodies are present in 85–90% cases with fasting hyperglycemia
- Elevated fasting C-peptide: To distinguish young people with non-autoimmune, insulin resistant type 2 diabetes from type 1 diabetes.

Measuring C-peptide levels is not recommended in early stage or acute phase as there can be an overlap in insulin or C-peptide between type 1 and type 2 in first year after diagnosis. In insulin treated patients measuring C-peptide when the glucose is sufficiently high (>8 mmol/L) to stimulate C peptide will detect if endogenous insulin secretion is still present. This is not common beyond the remission phase (2–3 years) in children with T1D.

SECTION 1: Introduction

TABLE 1: Clinical characteristics of type 1 diabetes, type 2 diabetes, and monogenic diabetes in children and adolescents[11-13]

Characteristic	Type 1	Type 2	Monogenic
Genetics	Polygenic	Polygenic	Monogenic
Age of onset	6 months to young adulthood	Usually pubertal (or later)	Often postpubertal
Clinical presentation	Most often acute, rapid	Variable; from slow, mild (often insidious) to severe	Variable (may be incidental in *GCK*)
Associations			
• Autoimmunity	Yes	No	No
• Ketosis	Common	Uncommon	Common in neonatal diabetes mellitus and rare in other forms
• Obesity	Population frequency	Increased frequency	Population frequency
• Acanthosis nigricans	No	Yes	No
Frequency (% of all diabetes in young people)	Usually >90%	<10%	1–4%
Parent with diabetes	2–4%	80%	90%

In cases where autoantibodies are not detected, one should look for the following:
- Family history of diabetes if anybody in the family has autosomal dominant diabetes
- Diagnosis of diabetes in first 6 months of life
- Nonprogressing mild fasting plasma glucose (100–150 mg/dL), in young, non-obese, and asymptomatic
- Associated conditions such as deafness, optic atrophy, or syndromic features
- A history of exposure to drugs, toxic to β-cells.

Immediate molecular genetic testing should be done in all patients diagnosed with diabetes in the first 6 months of life to define if it is neonatal diabetes mellitus, as type 1 diabetes is extremely rare in this subgroup. Beyond the age of 6 months, genetic testing should be limited to those patients who are negative for autoantibodies.

Characteristic features of youth onset type 1 diabetes in comparison with type 2 diabetes and monogenic diabetes are shown in table 1.

CONCLUSION

Genetic testing plays an important role in defining the type of childhood diabetes. Even in resource limited settings, full efforts should be made for performing all necessary tests in order to reach at correct diagnosis.

CHAPTER 1: Childhood Diabetes

REFERENCES

1. World Health Organization. Definition and Diagnosis of Diabetes Mellitus and Intermediate Hyperglycaemia: Report of a WHO/IDF Consultation. Geneva, Switzerland: World Health Organization; 2006.
2. American Diabetes Association. Diagnosis and classification of diabetes mellitus. Diabetes Care. 2014;37:S81-90.
3. Islam ST, Abraham A, Donaghue KC, Chan AK, Lloyd M, Srinivasan S, et al. Plateau of adiposity in Australian children diagnosed with type 1 diabetes: a 20-year study. Diabet Med. 2014;31:686-90.
4. Kapellen TM, Gausche R, Dost A, Wiegand S, Flechtner-Mors M, Keller E, et al. Children and adolescents with type 1 diabetes in Germany are more overweight than healthy controls: results comparing DPV database and CrescNet database. J Pediatr Endocrinol Metab. 2014;27:209-14.
5. Rewers A, Klingensmith G, Davis C, Petitti DB, Pihoker C, Rodriguez B, et al. Presence of diabetic ketoacidosis at diagnosis of diabetes mellitus in youth: the Search for Diabetes in Youth Study. Pediatrics. 2008;121:e1258-66.
6. Dabelea D, Rewers A, Stafford JM, Standiford DA, Lawrence JM, Saydah S, et al. Trends in the prevalence of ketoacidosis at diabetes diagnosis: the SEARCH for diabetes in youth study. Pediatrics. 2014;133:e938-45.
7. Fendler W, Borowiec M, Baranowska-Jazwiecka A, Szadkowska A, Skala-Zamorowska E Deja G, et al. Prevalence of monogenic diabetes amongst Polish children after a nationwide genetic screening campaign. Diabetologia. 2012;55:2631-5.
8. Irgens HU, Molnes J, Johansson BB, Ringdal M, Skrivarhaug T, Undlien DE, et al. Prevalence of monogenic diabetes in the population-based Norwegian Childhood Diabetes Registry. Diabetologia. 2013;56:1512-9.
9. Pihoker C, Gilliam LK, Ellard S, Dabelea D, Davis C, Dolan LM, et al. Prevalence, characteristics and clinical diagnosis of maturity onset diabetes of the young due to mutations in HNF1A, HNF4A, and glucokinase: results from the SEARCH for Diabetes in Youth. J Clin Endocrinol Metab. 2013;98:4055-62.
10. Galler A, Stange T, Muller G, Näke A, Vogel C, Kapellen T, et al. Incidence of childhood diabetes in children aged less than 15 years and its clinical and metabolic characteristics at the time of diagnosis: data from the Childhood Diabetes Registry of Saxony, Germany. Horm Res Paediatr. 2010;74:285-91.
11. Zeitler P, Fu J, Tandon N, Nadeau K, Urakami T, Barrett T, et al. Type 2 diabetes in the child and adolescent. Pediatr Diabetes. 2014;15 (Suppl 20):26-46.
12. Rubio-Cabezas O, Hattersley AT, Njølstad PR, Mlynarski W, Ellard S, White N, et al. ISPAD Clinical Practice Consensus Guidelines 2014. The diagnosis and management of monogenic diabetes in children and adolescents. Pediatr Diabetes. 2014;15 (Suppl 20):47-64.
13. Craig ME, Jefferies C, Dabelea D, Balde N, Seth A, Donaghue KC, et al. ISPAD Clinical Practice Consensus Guidelines 2014. Definition, epidemiology, and classification of diabetes in children and adolescents. Pediatr Diabetes. 2014;15 (Suppl 20):4-17.

CHAPTER 2

Epidemiology of Childhood Diabetes

Subhankar Chowdhury, Sujoy Ghosh

INTRODUCTION

Diabetes is a chronic disorder characterized by hyperglycemia, which may result from absolute insulin deficiency or inadequate insulin action and/or both.[1] Worldwide, there are 415 million people with diabetes. Diabetes management involves a close collaboration between those who are affected and their healthcare providers in order to prevent a range of costly and dangerous complications, which if left untreated may result in death. In the year 2013, 5.1 million deaths were associated with diabetes. Diabetes is not only a health concern, but also a big financial threat. About 548 billion US dollars were spent for treatment of diabetes related health conditions (12% of global health expenditure). The population most commonly affected by diabetes (worldwide) is generally aged between 40 and 59 years, and majority (three quarters) of them live in low- and middle-income countries. Among the different types of diabetes, a rapid increase in incidence of type 2 diabetes mellitus (T2DM) has occurred over the last few years and is anticipated to increase the number of people suffering with diabetes to 642 million by 2040. The presence of diabetes is increasing in children as well. This is occurring in parallel to the childhood obesity epidemic. In this chapter, the epidemiology of childhood diabetes with emphasis on incidence and prevalence, risk factors, and clinical course of diabetes has been discussed.

DIABETES MELLITUS IN CHILDREN

The diagnosis of diabetes in children has become increasingly complex with the emergence of increased rates of childhood-onset T2DM, monogenic and medication-induced diabetes.[2] Differentiating between different types of childhood diabetes is challenging, and requires a basic understanding of pathophysiology of various types of diabetes and associated risk factors. Overlapping clinical features and conflicting findings on laboratory investigations

CHAPTER 2: Epidemiology of Childhood Diabetes

sometimes complicate the picture. The clinician must pay careful attention to family history, laboratory evidence of endogenous insulin production or pancreatic autoimmunity, and the natural progression of the disease, in order to make an accurate diagnosis and choose the most appropriate and effective treatment regimen.[3] Diabetes in children can be classified into the following general categories:

- Type 1 diabetes mellitus: It is characterized by destruction of pancreatic β-cells, culminating in absolute insulin deficiency. The destruction of pancreatic β-cells is mostly autoimmune-mediated, though idiopathic type 1 diabetes mellitus (T1DM) is now a not uncommonly encountered clinical entity[4-6]
- Type 2 diabetes mellitus: It is characterized by relative lack of insulin action; eventually many progress to develop absolute insulin deficiency as well. Type 1 diabetes mellitus is still the most common type of diabetes in children; however, there is progressive increase in prevalence of T2DM in this age group.

Because of the commonness of genetic background of T2DM in our country, some children have so-called 'double diabetes', i.e., T1DM along with a significant component of insulin resistance.

Other types of diabetes: These include maturity onset diabetes in young (MODY), which are monogenic forms of diabetes affecting β-cell function and many being generally responsive to oral secretagogues. The diagnosis is challenging because of overlapping clinical features and lack of genetic testing facilities (except for few specialized centers).

A rare, but interesting, group of disorders is identified as neonatal diabetes mellitus.

One can still see fibrocalculous pancreatopathy with secondary diabetes in different pockets of India.

Besides these, there are diabetes secondary to endocrinopathies, e.g., Cushing's syndrome, maternally inherited diabetes with deafness, and various rare genetic syndromes.

EPIDEMIOLOGY OF TYPE 1 DIABETES MELLITUS IN CHILDREN

Incidence and Prevalence of Type 1 Diabetes Mellitus

Worldwide prevalence of T1DM is 5-10% among all individuals with diabetes. There is, however, a wide geographic variation in the reported incidence and prevalence of T1DM. These are seen in some of the large studies such as EURODIAB, World Health Organization (WHO) Multinational Project for Childhood Diabetes (known as the DiaMond Project) and the SEARCH for Diabetes in Youth (SEARCH) study.[7,8]

The EURODIAB ACE study group during the period 1989-94 identified 16,362 cases of T1DM in 44 centers throughout Europe and Israel. It reported annual increase in the incidence rate of 3.4% [95% confidence interval (CI) 2.5-4.4%) in T1DM patients. Few central European countries reported higher incidence. Highest rate of increase was in the youngest age group: age 0-4 years (6.3%, 95% CI 1.5-8.5%), 5-9 years (3.1%, 95% CI 1.5-4.8%), and 10-14 years (2.4%, 95% CI 1.0-3.8%), with earlier onset implying a longer burden of disease and greater need for care in younger.

SECTION 1: Introduction

The DiaMond project was initiated by the WHO in 1990 with the objective to investigate and monitor the patterns in incidence of childhood T1DM worldwide. A total of 19,164 T1DM children less than or equal to 14 years of age from 100 centers in 50 countries from 1990 to 1994 were included in the project. It was noticed that there is more than 350-fold difference in the incidence of T1DM amongst different populations worldwide, with age-adjusted incidences ranging from a low of 0.1/100,000 per year in China and Venezuela to a high of 36.5/100,000 in Finland and 36.8/100,000 in Sardinia. The lowest incidence (<1/100,000 per year) was reported in the populations from China and South America and the highest incidence (>20/100,000 per year) was reported in Sardinia, Finland, Sweden, Norway, Portugal, United Kingdom, Canada, and New Zealand. Incidence rates reported from the United States (US) populations were 10–20/100,000 per year. Whereas, approximately half of the European populations reported incidence between 5–10/100,000 per year, rates were higher in the remainder. Incidence was correlated with age, highest in the 10–14 year old. Male-to-female ratio was reported at 3 centers; none reported higher incidence for female patients. The authors considered genetic or environmental/behavioral factors to be the reason for variation in incidence within ethnic groups.[9]

The SEARCH for Diabetes in Youth study was conducted by Liese AD et al. in 2001 to estimate the prevalence and type of diabetes mellitus in youth less than 20 years of age in the US. A total of 6,379 US youth with diabetes were identified for the study. Crude prevalence was estimated to be 1.82 cases per 1,000 youth. Patients within age group of 0–9 years had lower prevalence (0.79 cases per 1,000 youth) than for those 10–19 years of age (2.80 cases per 1,000 youth). Non-Hispanic white youth had the highest prevalence (1.06 cases per 1,000 youth) in the younger group. The study also reported that among younger children T1DM accounted for more than or equal to 80%. Incidence rates depicted in SEARCH study were higher than previous US reports from Allegheny County, Philadelphia but lower than for African American children.[10]

The International Diabetes Federation 2015 atlas states that T1DM prevalence in children has increased to half a million (542,000) and that the prevalence of T1DM is increasing by 3% every year. United States tops the number of cases of T1DM with 84,100 followed by India with 70,200.

Risk Factors for Development of Type 1 Diabetes Mellitus in Children

Age

Worldwide T1DM accounts for more than or equal to 85% of all diabetes cases in children less than 20 years of age.[11] While peak incidence is noted between the ages of 10–14 years (peripuberty), it may have its onset at all ages, even as late as the 9th decade of life.[12,13] Incidence rates decline after puberty and appear to stabilize in young adulthood (15–29 years). Approximately, 10% of diabetes cases in adults are found to have antibodies associated with T1DM. However, β-cell destruction is often slower in these cases as compared to T1DM in children, which often delay the requirement of insulin therapy. These individuals diagnosed with autoimmune diabetes when they are adults have been referred to as having latent autoimmune diabetes of adults (LADA).[14,15]

Gender

In young population with T1DM, on an average girls and boys are equally affected.[16] Incidence rate seems to be different according to the region. Among populations of European origin with higher incidence rates, male affliction is more, whereas those with lower incidence rate tend to have female predilection.[17,18] However, studies have reported that after puberty (especially in adulthood), males are more commonly affected.[19]

Race/Ethnicity

The SEARCH for Diabetes in Youth Study presented data in which race and ethnic specific issues in diabetes were evaluated. The incidence of T1DM in Hispanic youth in the SEARCH study was 15.0/100,000 and 16.2/100,000 for females and males, respectively of age group 0–14 years. The incidence of T1DM was lower among Asian and Pacific Islander youth, 6.4 and 7.4/100,000 person years in 0–9 and 10–19 years old, respectively.

Genotype

Amongst the wide range of genes implicated in pathogenesis of T1DM, the most important are the human leukocyte antigen (HLA) complex on chromosome 6, in particular, the HLA class II. They are considered to be the principal susceptibility markers for T1DM.[20] About 90–95% of young children with T1DM carry either or both susceptibility haplotypes.

However, only 5% or fewer children with HLA-conferred genetic susceptibility actually develop clinical disease.[21] An association between T1DM and other autoimmune diseases, such as autoimmune thyroid disease, Addison's disease, celiac disease, and autoimmune gastritis is well-established. The clustering of these autoimmune diseases is related to genes within the major histocompatibility complex.[22,23]

Other Risk Factors

Environmental factors appear to trigger the immune-mediated process in genetically susceptible individuals. However, these environmental triggers which initiate pancreatic β-cell destruction remain largely unknown. Few studies even highlight the role of nongenetic factors including seasonal influences. Nutritional factors, like vitamin D and early introduction of cow's milk in diet, have also been implicated.

Seasonal Variation

Several studies have suggested a peak in the reported cases in autumn and winter and smaller number of cases in spring and summer, consistently in both the hemispheres. This association with seasonal variation seems particularly strong in those children diagnosed with T1DM between ages 10 and 14 years. Changes in vitamin D status or affliction with viruses during these seasons have been postulated as possible underlying factors. However, others have refuted such theories on the basis of long/variable preclinical latent disease period prior to disease manifestation.

SECTION 1: Introduction

Familial Clustering and Twin Studies

About 4-6% of siblings of T1DM probands have been reported to develop T1DM, compared to 0.2-1% background population. Offsprings of affected fathers have 1.5-3 times greater risk of T1DM compared to affected mothers. It is estimated that by age of 20 years, 5-8% of offspring of men with T1DM and 2-5% of offspring of women with T1DM would develop T1DM.

There is high concordance of incidence of T1DM in twins, with monozygotic twins being more commonly afflicted as compared to dizygotic twins. In one study, the cumulative risk of T1DM in monozygotic twins was almost 25-32% (compared to 3.2-10% in dizygotic twins). Data highlights the fact that genetic susceptibility is important, but not exclusive for development of T1DM.

Environmental Risk Factors

Several putative environmental factors have been implicated in the pathogenesis of T1DM.

Viral infections: Several studies have implicated various viral infections (rubella virus, *Enterovirus*) in the pathogenesis of T1DM. The so called hygiene hypothesis, which proposes that decline in microbial exposure in populations leads to altered immunity may also account for increased susceptibility to T1DM.

Toxins: Evidence of possible environmental toxins in pathogenesis of T1DM is less robust. However, the rodenticide Vacor and other toxins, like bafilomycin, and increased exposure to nitrates and nitrites which may be converted to N-nitroso compounds have been suggested as possible culprits.

Nutritional Factors

Molecular mimicry has been suggested as a possible mechanism by which exposure to cow's milk (bovine serum albumin) may trigger an immune reaction resulting in T1DM. Some studies have also suggested evidence for the role of age at introduction of cereals or gluten with occurrence of T1DM.

Vitamin D is known for its immunomodulatory effects. Lower level of vitamin D is shown to be associated with greater risk of T1DM. Additionally, a case control study found an association between intakes of cod liver oil and lower risk of T1DM.

Type 1 Diabetes Mellitus: Status in India

The South-East Asia Region has a high prevalence of T1DM in children. About 77,900 children were found to be affected. The International Diabetes Federation (IDF) 2015 data suggest that the prevalence of T1DM is increasing by 3% annually and that there are 70,200 patients suffering from T1DM in India. Menon PSN et al., in year 1990, presented an overview on "childhood onset diabetes mellitus in India".[24] According to this, the prevalence of T1DM in children aged below 15 years ranged from 0.8 to 3.61%. Several studies were conducted thereafter looking at the same issue (Table 1).[25]

Incidence rate of 10.5/100,000 per year, was predicted from a study conducted in South India for about 4 years. Similarly, a study from Karla et al., from Karnal district in 2008, showed a prevalence of 18.3/100,000 in the 0-14 years age group.[26]

CHAPTER 2: Epidemiology of Childhood Diabetes

TABLE 1: Incidence and prevalence/percentage of type 1 diabetes mellitus reported in India

Author name	Place	Year or period of study	Number of T1DM in children reported and given as % where applicable	Total sample studied	Age at diagnosis
Incidence of T1DM					
Bai et al. Ramachandran et al. Kalra et al.	Chennai Karnal	1991 1991–1994 2008	10.5/100,000 person-years 3.82/100,00 24.22/100,000	10513 IDDM registry Endocrine center registry	School children <15 years 0–6 years 5–15 years
Prevalence/percentage of T1DM (clinic based)					
Verma IC	New Delhi	1980–84	44 (80.0)	55	5–12 years
Venkataraman et al.	Chennai	1979–89	126 (7.88%)	160	<20 years
Mohan et al.		1990	165 (63.9)	258	<20 years
Ramachandran et al.		1991	0.26/100 (30 children)	116, 486	<15 years
Ramachandran et al.		2000	617	–	<20 years
Kumar et al.		1991–2001	8 (0.01%)	70,000	≤1 year
Mohan et al.		2007	286 (65.9%)	434	<16 years
Ganesh et al.		2003–2007	4 (0.05)	83	≤1 years
Poovazhagi et al.		1999–2010	350 (81%)	432	<12 years
Amutha et al.		1992–2009	940 (68.5)	1,372	≤19 years
Poovazhagi et al.		1999–2012	40 (7.9)	506	≤1 year
Kota et al.	Hyderbad	1997–2011	260	–	10.5 ± 7.2 years
Sahay et al.		1999–2002	28 (59.6)	47	<20 years
Abraham et al.	Central Kerala	1985–1989	39 (67%)	58	<20 years
Bhadada SK et al.	Chandigarh	2002–2008	189	–	10.8 ± 7.3
Unnikrishnan et al.	Multicentric study	2006–2008	535 (89%)	603	<20 years
Bhatia et al.	Lucknow	2004	130 (81%)	160	<18 years
Balasubramanian et al.		10 year period	55 children	–	<20 years
Singh et al.		1992–1997	83 (57.2)	145	13.8 ± 7.3
Samal et al.	Cuttack	1983–1988	54 (60%)	90	<15 years
Mazumder et al.	Kolkata	2004–2006	41 (70.7)	58	<18 years
Kumar P et al.	Karnataka	1995–2008	134 (43%)	311	9–14 years
Zargar et al.	Srinagar	1990–1999	84 (90.3)	93	<20 years

T1DM, type 1 diabetes mellitus; IDDM, insulin dependent diabetes mellitus.

SECTION 1: Introduction

EPIDEMIOLOGY OF TYPE 2 DIABETES MELLITUS IN CHILDREN

Incidence and Prevalence

Type 2 diabetes mellitus is influenced by behavioral, nutritional, and environmental factors. It has emerged as the leading cause of mortality and morbidity. There is also an increase in the incidence of T2DM in children and adolescents. Among all the newly diagnosed cases in adolescents, one-third of them are T2DM. Pinhas-Hamiel et al. was amongst the few who reported the rising trend of T2DM in young patients with diabetes. In their study, they observed that during the period of two years 1992–1994, there was a fourfold increase in the proportion of young diabetes patients having T2DM. However, when they analyzed data from 1982–1994, they observed a 10-fold increase. The SEARCH study group (a United States multicenter observational study conducting population based ascertainment of cases of diabetes mellitus in individuals <20 years) found that the incidence of T2DM was highest among American Indian individuals aged 15–19 years, followed by Asian-Pacific Islanders and Black individuals of the same age group. Fagot-Campagna et al., noted the prevalence of T2DM in North American Indian children aged 15–19 year. They reported the prevalence of 50.9 per 1,000 for Pima Indians, 4.5 for all US American Indians, and 2.3 for Canadian Creed, and Ojibway Indians in Manitoba. Between 8 and 45% of recently diagnosed cases of diabetes among children and adolescents in the United States is T2DM. Those developing T2DM were more likely to be obese, physically inactive, have a family history of T2DM, and signs of insulin resistance.

Insulin and C peptide levels are often raised and antibodies are absent, which may help differentiate T1DM from T2DM, but insulin secretion may well be blunted at diagnosis of T2DM. Glycosylated hemoglobin levels may range from 10 to 13%, and a sizeable proportion of patients have hypertension, hypertriglyceridemia, albuminuria, sleep apnea, and depression, and these factors may worsen over time. However, treatment protocols vary considerably, and several of the drugs used for glycemic, blood pressure, and lipid control are not approved for use in children.

Increasing incidence is also reported in studies from Japanese, Asian-American, British, Chinese, Libyan, Bangladeshi, Australian, and Maori populations.

Type 2 Diabetes Mellitus in Children: Status in India

Studies have reported an increasing trend of T2DM in India. Most of these are from Southern India. Amutha et al., studied the clinical profile of diabetes in the young between 1992 and 2009. It was observed that there was an overall increase in percentage of young diabetes from 0.55% in 1992 to 2.5% in 2009. Of the registered 2,630 patients, 1,135 (43.2%) had T1DM, 1,262 (48.0%) had T2DM, and 233 had other types.

The Diabetes Epidemiology Study Group in India (DESI) conducted National Urban Diabetes Survey (NUDS) in 2001 and Mohan et al. conducted the Chennai Urban Rural Epidemiology Study (CURES) in 2004; these are among the two most comprehensive studies for diabetes in India. Both, NUDS and CURES show that there has been a shift towards diagnosis of T2DM in childhood, even within the 4-year time gap between these studies.[27]

Ramachandran et al. reported 18 children (5 boys and 13 girls) with T2DM diagnosed below the age of 15 years at their clinic. About 9 were obese and 12 had high waist hip ratio, indicating visceral obesity. Of note is the fact that 9 patients were asymptomatic and picked up on screening which was performed due to strong family history of diabetes mellitus and/or because of obesity. They had good glycemic control on treatment with metformin or sulfonylurea or a combination of both. In a study by Bhatia et al., T2DM accounted for 12% of cases (total 160 cases) of diabetes mellitus in children below 18 years of age. At Dr Mohan's Diabetes Specialities Centre, a tertiary diabetes center in Chennai, the proportion of childhood-onset T2DM (age <16 years) showed an increasing trend from 1999 to 2006. However, this could reflect referral bias as cases of youth-onset diabetes tend to get referred earlier to tertiary care centers. According to their analysis in 2006, of 434 children with diabetes who had an age at onset less than 16 years, 116 (26.7%) had youth-onset T2DM.

Causes of Increasing Type 2 Diabetes Mellitus in Children in India

Changes in Lifestyle (Urbanization)

With improving standards of living, and availability of food in plenty, the traditional micronutrient rich foods are being replaced by unhealthy energy dense, highly processed, micronutrient-poor foods. Increase in sedentary habits is also a significant contributor.

Obesity and Type 2 Diabetes Mellitus in Youth

An important factor for obesity in India is the intense competition for admissions to schools and colleges with flourishing tuition classes, right from nursery levels. Children are forced to use their playtime for additional studies. Games or physical training sessions are restricted or nonexistent in many schools. Some schools do not have any playgrounds. Also, due to unsafe roads (traffic, crime) children are discouraged from walking or cycling to school. Poor availability of parks, swimming pools, gymnasiums, and play areas limits physical activity further. Obesity, especially of visceral fat further increases the risk. For a similar total body fat content, Indians have higher truncal fat (subscapular, suprailiac, abdominal skin folds) than Caucasians. The Y-Y paradox or the concept of 'thin fat' Indians states that at body mass index similar to Western counterparts, Indians tend to have higher body fat content, which might account for higher risk of metabolic disease in Indians.

Genetic/Constitutional Predisposition

Modern environment may have unmasked previously silent obesogenic genes or the 'thrifty genotypes' (i.e., programming of previously malnourished populations to accumulate fat more intensely in an attempt to store for future starvation). In addition, familial pattern of eating, exercise, and behaviour also contributes to increased incidence in families.

High and Low Birth Weights as Risk Factors for Diabetes

Both low and high birth weight have been implicated in the association with the future risk of T2DM. Additionally, history of gestational diabetes mellitus (GDM) increases future risk of diabetes in offspring.

SECTION 1: Introduction

Other Factors

Various other factors may contribute to increased childhood T2DM including formula feeding and intake of calorie dense diet, and the high glycemic index of our predominantly carbohydrate diet have also been implicated.

MATURITY ONSET DIABETES OF THE YOUNG

Maturity onset diabetes of the young is an inherited, monogenic, autosomal dominant, non-insulin dependent, early-onset diabetes mellitus. It is diagnosed usually before the age of 25 years. These patients are generally nonobese and present with mild asymptomatic hyperglycemia. The existence of a mild form of familial diabetes was recognized as early as 1928, however, only after 1964 the term MODY came into use.

Genetic Basis of Maturity Onset Diabetes of the Young

Regarding the genetic basis of MODY, the era of major discoveries started in 1991 when Graeme Bell et al. described the apparent association of MODY with a deoxyribonucleic acid polymorphism in the adenosine deaminase gene located on chromosome 20. It took another 5 years to identify the first gene associated with MODY, namely the transcription factor known as hepatocyte nuclear factor-4α (HNF-4α gene). This form of MODY was named MODY1 in order to distinguish it from other MODY cases not carrying mutations in this gene. Till date 12 different forms have been identified, table 2 denotes these 12 forms and genetic abnormalities associated with each.

TABLE 2: Genetic characteristics of different Maturity onset diabetes of the young types

Disease	Gene	Frequency	Locus	Protein
MODY 1	HNF-4α (TCF-14)	~4–5%	20q 12-q13.1	Hepatocyte nuclear factor 4α (transcription factor 14)
MODY 2	GCK	~20–60%	7p15-p13	Glucokinase (hexokinase-4)
MODY 3	HNF-1α (TCF1)	~30–60%	12q24.2	Hepatocyte nuclear factor 4α (transcription factor I)
MODY 4	IPF-1 (PDX1)	<1%	13q12.1	Insulin promoter factor 1, pancreatic and duodenal homeobox 1
MODY 5	HNF-1β (TCF-2)	~2–5%	17q12	Hepatocyte nuclear factor 1β (transcription factor 2)
MODY 6	NEUROD-1	<1%	2q32	Neurogenic differentiation 1
MODY 7	KLF11	<1%	2p25	Kruppel-like factor 1
MODY 8	CEL	<1%	9q37	Carboxylester hydroxylase/lipase
MODY 9	PAX4	<1%	7q32	Paired box gene 4
MODY 10	INS	<1%	11p15.5	Insulin
MODY 11	BLK	<1%	8p23-p22	Tyrosine kinase, B-lymphocyte specific
MODY 12	ABCC8	<1%	11p15.1	ATP-binding cassette, subfamily C, member 8

MODY, maturity onset diabetes of the young.

Prevalence of Maturity Onset Diabetes of the Young

Worldwide estimate suggests that MODY accounts for 1-2% of all cases of diabetes. It is underdiagnosed and many a times incorrectly classified as T1DM or T2DM. Maturity onset diabetes of the young-2 is thought to account for 10-60% of total cases, whereas MODY-3 accounts for approximately 20% cases. Thus, screening asymptomatic youth with a strong family history of diabetes or women with mild diabetes diagnosed during pregnancy is recommended if facilities are available.

EPIDEMIOLOGY OF MONOGENIC FORMS OF DIABETES

Monogenic forms of β-cell diabetes account for approximately 1-2% of all cases of diabetes. Its true prevalence is underestimated due to underdiagnoses. Most of the times, diagnosis is difficult, as clinical features overlap with other common forms of diabetes.[28] Diagnosis should be considered in children with

- Family history of diabetes (especially, evidence of vertical transmission over 3 generations) without typical features of T2DM
- Mild fasting hyperglycemia (100-150 mg/dL especially if young and nonobese)
- Negative autoantibodies without signs of obesity or insulin resistance
- Other associated features specific for a particular variety of monogenic diabetes
- Single gene defects produce monogenic β-cell diabetes.[29]

NEONATAL DIABETES MELLITUS

Neonatal diabetes mellitus (NDM) is a rare (1:300,000-400,000 newborns) form of diabetes diagnosed in the first 6 months of life. It is characterized by hyperglycemia along with low levels of insulin.

Types of Neonatal Diabetes Mellitus

Neonatal diabetes mellitus based on clinical aspects can be categorized as: transient NDM (TNDM) and permanent NDM (PNDM). Both differ in the duration of insulin dependence early in the disease. Transient neonatal diabetes mellitus develops due to improper insulin production but resolves spontaneously. About 50-60% of cases of NDM are found to have TNDM. Although molecular mechanism remains unknown, intrauterine growth retardation is usually present with absence of anti-islet antibodies and HLA class II haplotypes. Very few patients show presence of exocrine pancreatic insufficiency. Patient usually recovers within 1 year, but recurrences are consistent with non-autoimmune T1DM. Permanent neonatal diabetes mellitus is less common compared to TNDM. It is difficult to differentiate between the two types at diagnosis.[30] Mutations in adenosine triphosphate-sensitive potassium channel genes (KCNJ11, ABCC8) and the insulin gene (INS) are the most common causes of PNDM.

SECTION 1: Introduction

Incidence and Prevalence of Neonatal Diabetes Mellitus

Kanakatti Shankar et al. estimated the prevalence of PNDM among SEARCH study participants, which was carried out from 2001 to 2008. From the 15,829 SEARCH participants with diabetes, 39 were diagnosed before 6 months of age. Total 35 had PNDM (0.22% of all diabetes cases in SEARCH), 3 had TNDM, and 1 was unknown. Almost 66.7% had a clinical diagnosis of T1DM. The prevalence rate of PNDM in youth less than 20 years was estimated at 1 in 252,000.[31]

From Southern India, Varadarajan et al. studied etiology, clinical presentation, and outcome of NDM. He included 40 infants with infantile onset diabetes. Of this, 8% were with onset of DM at less than 12 weeks of age, 67.5% presented with diabetic ketoacidosis (DKA) and 30% had a provisional diagnosis of DM or DKA at first physician contact. Low C-peptide levels were observed in 85%. Wolcott Rallison syndrome was the commonest type encountered. Some of the common problems were missed diagnosis and recurrent admissions for metabolic instability. Mortality at 12.5-year follow-up was 32.5%. Fever (60%) and polyuria (50%) were the two most common clinical features noticed in these patients.[32]

TRENDS IN INDIA

The Indian Council for Medical Research (ICMR) established the Young Diabetes Registry (YDR) with the primary objective to understand the disease pattern and disease burden. The ICRM YDR registry, being hospital based, has its own limitations and may not reflect the actual population burden.

All cases reported after 1st January 2000 were included if they had a diagnosis of diabetes at age less than or equal to 25 years. At the end of phase 1 (i.e., upto 31st july 2011), the registry enrolled 5,546 patients of which T1DM was the most prevalent type, accounting for 63.9% of all patients followed by youth onset T2DM which accounts for 25.3%. Other forms of diabetes such as GDM (3.9%), MODY (3.1%), chronic pancreatitis (1.3%), and LADA (1%) were also reported. Of the eight collaborating centers, there was variation in the subtypes of diabetes, with Chennai and Dibrugarh reporting T2DM being the subtype in up to 40% of the patients, whereas other centers reported higher prevalence of T1DM (accounting for 71.5 to 94.4%).

The mean age of diagnosis of T1DM was 12.9 ± 6.5 years while that for T2DM was 21.6 ± 3.7 years. About 49.5% were males and 50.5% were females. About 23.3% of patients belonged to low socioeconomic strata. Family history of diabetes was common (paternal 22.6%, maternal 18.7%, grandparents 27.9%, siblings 3.9%).

Common modes of presentation for T1DM were weight loss, osmotic symptoms, and/or ketosis, whereas one-third of T2DM detection was incidental. The T2DM patients were more likely to be obese and had features of insulin resistance including acanthosis, polycystic ovarian syndrome.

About 15.4% of patients (including 26.4% of T2DM and 11.1% of T1DM patients) had at least one chronic complication of diabetes at registration. Retinopathy was the most common complication (3.1% in T1DM and 10.4% in T2DM). Nephropathy was the next common complication in T1DM and neuropathy was the next common complication in T2DM.

Individuals with diabetes for longer than 20 years, the prevalence of coronary artery disease were 9.8% in T2DM as compared to 4.8% in T1DM.

Type 2 diabetes mellitus was commonly associated with other comorbidities, such as dyslipidemia (11.3%), hypertension (7.4%), and hypothyroidism (2.1%). Significant number of patients even with a diagnosis of T2DM (32.6%) were on insulin therapy.

CONCLUSION

The incidence and prevalence of diabetes in childhood is on the rise worldwide and India is no different. This could be due to many factors but primarily because in the rise in obesity and also because of greater awareness of the disease amongst physicians and lay public. Previously T1DM was perhaps the most important cause of diabetes in young. Of late there has been a greater prevalence of T2DM. This change in trend is particularly remarkable in the urban areas. However when evaluating a child with diabetes in addition to T1DM and T2DM we have to consider other less common causes including MODY, FCPD and other rarer disorders.

REFERENCES

1. International Diabetes Federation. IDF Diabetes Atlas. 7th ed. Brussels: International Diabetes Federation; 2015. [online] Available from: http://www.idf.org/diabetesatlas. Accessed July 2016.
2. Prasad AN. Type 2 diabetes mellitus in young need for early screening. Indian Pediatr. 2011;48(9):683-8.
3. Amed S, Hamilton J. The emerging landscape of childhood diabetes: unraveling the diagnosis. Diabetes Management. 2012;2(6):521-35.
4. American Diabetes Association. Standards of Medical Care in Diabetes-2015. Diabetes Care. 2015;38(Suppl 1):S1-2.
5. American Diabetes Association. Diagnosis and classification of diabetes mellitus. Diabetes Care. 2009;32 Suppl 1:S62-7.
6. Liese AD, D'Agostino RB Jr, Hamman RF, Kilgo PD, Lawrence JM, Liu LL, et al. The burden of diabetes mellitus among US youth: prevalence estimates from the SEARCH for Diabetes in Youth Study. Pediatrics. 2006;118(4):1510-8.
7. DIAMOND Project Group. Incidence and trends of childhood Type 1 diabetes worldwide 1990–1999. Diabet Med. 2006;23:857-66.
8. Levy-Marchal C, Patterson CC, Green A; EURODIAB ACE Study Group. Europe and Diabetes. Geographical variation of presentation at diagnosis of type I diabetes in children: the EURODIAB study. European and Diabetes. Diabetologia. 2001;44 (Suppl 3):B75-80.
9. Variation and trends in incidence of childhood diabetes in Europe. EURODIAB ACE Study Group. Lancet. 2000;355:873-6.
10. Dabelea D, Bell RA, D'Agostino RB Jr, Imperatore G, Johansen JM, Linder B, et al. Incidence of diabetes in youth in the United States. JAMA. 2007;297(24):2716-24.
11. Thunander M, Petersson C, Jonzon K, Fornander J, Ossiansson B, Torn C, et al. Incidence of type 1 and type 2 diabetes in adults and children in Kronoberg, Sweden. Diabetes Res Clin Pract. 2008;82:247-55
12. Karvonen M, Viik-Kajander M, Moltchanova E, Libman I, LaPorte R, Tuomilehto J. Incidence of childhood type 1 diabetes worldwide. Diabetes Mondiale (DiaMond) Project Group. Diab Care. 2000;23:1516-26.
13. Haller MJ, Atkinson MA, Schatz D. Type 1 diabetes mellitus: etiology, presentation, and management. Pediatr Clin North Am. 2005;52:1553-78.
14. Leslie RD, Williams R, Pozzilli P. Clinical review: Type 1 diabetes and latent autoimmune diabetes in adults: one end of the rainbow. J Clin Endocrinol Metab. 2006;91:1654-9.
15. Naik RG, Palmer JP. Latent autoimmune diabetes in adults (LADA) Rev Endocr Metab Disord. 2003;4:233-41.
16. Soltesz G, Patterson CC, Dahlquist G. Worldwide childhood type 1 diabetes incidence--what can we learn from epidemiology? Pediatr Diabetes. 2007;8(Suppl 6):6-14.

SECTION 1: Introduction

17. Green A, Gale EAM, Patterson CC. Incidence of childhood-onset insulin-dependent diabetes mellitus: the EURODIAB ACE Study. Lancet. 1992;339:905-9.
18. Karvonen M, Pitkaniemi M, Pitkaniemi J, Kohtamaki K, Tajima N, Tuomilehto J. Sex difference in the incidence of insulin-dependent diabetes mellitus: an analysis of the recent epidemiological data. World Health Organization DIAMOND Project Group. Diabetes Metab Rev. 1997;13:275-91.
19. Kyvik KO, Nystrom L, Gorus F, Songini M, Oestman J, Castell C, et al. The epidemiology of Type 1 diabetes mellitus is not the same in young adults as in children. Diabetologia. 2004;47:377-84.
20. Mehers KL, Gillespie KM. The genetic basis for type 1 diabetes. Br Med Bull. 2008;88:115-29.
21. Concannon P, Erlich HA, Julier C, Morahan G, Nerup J, Pociot F, et al. Type 1 diabetes: evidence for susceptibility loci from four genome-wide linkage scans in 1,435 multiplex families. Diabetes. 2005;54:2995-3001.
22. Tsirogianni A, Pipi E, Soufleros K. Specificity of islet cell autoantibodies and coexistence with other organ specific autoantibodies in type 1 diabetes mellitus. Auto immun Rev. 2009;8:687-91.
23. Barker JM. Type 1 diabetes associated autoimmunity: Natural History, Genetic Associations and Screening. J Clin Endocrinol Metab. 2006;91(4):1210-7.
24. Menon PSN, Virmani A, Shah P, Raju R, Sethi AK, Sethia S, et al. Childhood onset diabetes mellitus in India: an overview. Int J Diab Dev Countries. 1990;10:11-6.
25. Amutha A, Thai K, Viswanathan M. Childhood and Adolescent Onset Type 1 Diabetes in India. MGM J Med Sci. 2013;1(1):46-53.
26. Kalra S, Kalra B, Sharma A. Prevalence of type 1 diabetes mellitus in Karnal district, Haryana state, India. Diabetol Metab Syndr. 2010;2:14.
27. Ramachandran A, Snehalatha C, Krishnaswamy CV. Incidence of IDDM in children in urban population in Southern India. Madras IDDM Registry Group Madras, South India. Diabetes Res Clin Pract. 1996;34:79-82.
28. Murphy R, Ellard S, Hattersley AT. Clinical implications of a molecular genetic classification of monogenic beta-cell diabetes. Nat Clin Pract Endocrinol Metab. 2008;4(4):200-13.
29. Vaxillaire M, Bonnefond A, Froguel P. The lessons of early-onset monogenic diabetes for the understanding of diabetes pathogenesis. Best Pract Res Clin Endocrinol Metab. 2012;26(2):171-87.
30. Polak M, Cave H. Neonatal diabetes mellitus: a disease linked to multiple mechanisms. Orphanet J Rare Dis. 2007;2:12.
31. Kanakatti Shankar R, Pihoker C, Dolan LM, Standiford D, Badaru A, Dabelea D, et al. Permanent neonatal diabetes mellitus: prevalence and genetic diagnosis in the SEARCH for Diabetes in Youth Study. Pediatr Diabetes. 2013;14(3):174-80.
32. Varadarajan P, Sangaralingam T, Senniappan S, Jahnavi S, Radha V, Mohan V. Clinical profile and outcome of infantile onset diabetes mellitus in southern India. Indian Pediatr. 2013;50(8):759-63.

CHAPTER 3

Monogenic Diabetes: Perspectives and Clinical Implications from Pediatric to Adult Endocrinology

BV Reshma, Kavitha Muniraj, KM Chandrika, S Geetha Rao, L Reddy, Usha Rangaraj, Vasanthi Nath, Neera Gupta, Ranjini Sen, Mudita Dhingra, Sanjay Kalra, Ashok K Das, SS Srikanta; The Diabetes Collaborative Study Group

INTRODUCTION

Diabetes in childhood and adolescence currently comprises a wide range of different types of diabetes: (i) type 1 diabetes mellitus (T1DM), (ii) type 2 diabetes mellitus (T2DM), (iii) other specific types, (iv) gestational diabetes mellitus (GDM). The "other specific types" include the following:[1]

- Monogenic defects of β-cell function
- Mitochondrial diabetes
- Genetic defects in insulin action
- Drug- or chemical-induced
- Infections
- Diseases of the exocrine pancreas
- Endocrinopathies
- Uncommon forms of immune-mediated diabetes
- Other genetic syndromes sometimes associated with diabetes.

The most common forms of diabetes—T1DM and T2DM—are polygenic, meaning the risk of developing these forms of diabetes is related to multiple genes. Polygenic forms of diabetes often run in families. Environmental factors, like increase in body weight due to unhealthy eating habits, physical inactivity, and other wrong lifestyle practices, play an important role for the development of T2DM.

MONOGENIC DIABETES—DEFINITION

Monogenic diabetes results from one or more defects in a single gene. The disease may be inherited within families as a dominant, recessive, or non-Mendelian trait or may present as a spontaneous case due to a *de novo* mutation. Well over 40 different genetic subtypes of monogenic diabetes have been identified to date, each having a typical phenotype and a specific pattern of inheritance.[2,3]

SECTION 1: Introduction

Monogenic forms of diabetes account for about 1–5% of all cases of diabetes in young people. It is very important to differentiate monogenic from polygenic forms of diabetes, as the treatment approaches may be different. Also, counseling can be rendered to the families on the consequences and nature of the disorder, the probability of transmitting it, and the options available in treatment. Genetic testing needs to be carried out to avoid misdiagnosing "monogenic" to "polygenic" form.

MONOGENIC DIABETES—GENE MUTATIONS (TABLE 1)

- Beta-cell dysfunction monogenic diabetes (most common):
  - Genes that regulate β-cell function/development (transcription factors)

TABLE 1: Monogenic diabetes: Classification and characteristics

Classification	Characteristics
Beta-cell dysfunction monogenic diabetes	
Group A: Neonatal diabetes diagnosed within 6–12 months of life	
Transient neonatal diabetes mellitus	Transient neonatal diabetes from imprinting anomalies on 6q24
Permanent neonatal diabetes mellitus	Neonatal diabetes due to mutations in the *KATP* channel genes
	Neonatal diabetes due to mutations in *INS* gene
	Wolcott-Rallison syndrome
	Neonatal diabetes due to *GCK* mutations
	Immunodysregulation polyendocrinopathy enteropathy X-linked (IPEX) syndrome
	Other causes of neonatal diabetes
Group B: Familial mild hyperglycemia or diabetes—autosomal dominant (MODY)	
	Mild fasting hyperglycemia due to glucokinase gene mutations (GCK-MODY, MODY2)
	Familial diabetes due to HNF1A-MODY (MODY3) and HNF4A-MODY (MODY1)
Group C: Genetic syndromes—diabetes with extrapancreatic features	
	Diabetes insipidus, diabetes mellitus, optic atrophy, and deafness syndrome (Wolfram syndrome)
	Renal cysts and diabetes syndrome (HNF1B-MODY or MODY5)
	Mitochondrial diabetes
	Diabetes secondary to monogenic diseases of the exocrine pancreas
Insulin resistance monogenic diabetes	
	Primary insulin signaling defects due to mutations in the insulin receptor gene
	Monogenic lipodystrophies
	Ciliopathy-related insulin resistance and diabetes

MODY, maturity-onset diabetes of the young; KATP, adenosine triphosphate-sensitive potassium.

- Insulin resistance monogenic diabetes (rare):
  - Genes that regulate insulin action.

MONOGENIC DIABETES—DIAGNOSIS

The majority of patients with genetically proven monogenic diabetes are initially incorrectly diagnosed as T1DM or T2DM. The correct diagnosis is crucial: To predict the clinical course of the patient; to explain other associated clinical features; to guide the most appropriate treatment; and for clinical implications for other family members—often correcting the diagnosis and treatment. Thus, correct clinical and genetic diagnosis facilitates optimum diagnosis, genetic counseling, and therapy.

BETA-CELL DYSFUNCTION MONOGENIC DIABETES

It can be classified as:
- Group A: Neonatal diabetes (NDM)
  - Diagnosed within 6–12 months of life
- Group B: Familial mild hyperglycemia or diabetes
  - Autosomal dominant
- Group C: Genetic syndromes—diabetes
  - With extrapancreatic features.

Group A: Neonatal Diabetes—Diagnosed within 6–12 Months of Life

- Neonatal diabetes is insulin requiring diabetes which is usually diagnosed in the first 6–12 months of life
- Transient neonatal diabetes mellitus (TNDM)
  - That resolved at a median of 12 weeks and then did not require any treatment, although as many as 50% of cases would ultimately relapse
- Permanent neonatal diabetes mellitus (PNDM)
  - Required continual treatment from diagnosis.

Neonates who are diagnosed as having NDM usually have low birth weight compared to neonates of same gestational age. Insulin apart from its effects on glucose metabolism also contributes to growth promotion during fetal development, and hence, decrease in insulin during this period can be one of the causes of low weight compared to neonates of same gestational age. Two types of NDM exist: PNDM and TNDM. In PNDM category, these neonates will require lifelong treatment to control their blood glucose levels. In neonates whose diabetes remits within few weeks or months are classified as TNDM. Diabetes may relapse later in life in TNDM. Clinical features including type of presentation, associated features will guide during planning for genetic testing The details of the monogenic subtypes of neonatal and infancy onset diabetes are given in appendix table A1.

Transient Neonatal Diabetes Mellitus[4,5]

Characteristics of transient neonatal diabetes mellitus have been mentioned in table 2.

SECTION 1: Introduction

TABLE 2: Characteristics of transient neonatal diabetes mellitus

Gene/inheritance	Age (weeks)/diagnosis	Other features	Pancreas appearance
ZAC/HYAMI (imprinting defect on 6q24), 70%	0.5/(0–4)	Macroglossia (23%)	Normal
Kir6.2 (KCNJ11), 25%	6/(0–260)	Developmental delay (20%) Epilepsy (6%) Diabetic ketoacidosis (30%)	Normal
SUR1 (ABCC8)	6/(0–17)	Developmental delay	Normal
HNF-1β dominant (60%), spontaneous	–	Renal developmental disorders	Atrophy

Permanent Neonatal Diabetes Mellitus[6-11]

Sulfonylurea receptor mutations

Sulfonylurea receptor mutations are given in table 3.
Phenotypes of sulfonylurea mutations:
- Transient neonatal diabetes mellitus
- Permanent neonatal diabetes mellitus
    - Developmental delay and neonatal diabetes [intermediate DEND (iDEND)]
    - Developmental delay, epilepsy, and neonatal diabetes (DEND).

Neonatal Diabetes Due To Mutations in the Adenosine Triphosphate-Sensitive Potassium Channel Genes

Sulfonylurea medications can be started (transfer from insulin as per an inpatient protocol), and are effective (improvement in glycemic control, without increasing hypoglycemia) in up to 90% of patients who have mutation in adenosine triphosphate-sensitive potassium (KATP) channel genes. Sulfonylurea (e.g., glibenclamide) dose requirement is usually high in this group, requiring about 0.5 mg/kg/day to even 2.3 mg/kg/day in few subjects; however, the dose requirement usually decreases over a period of time and these patients can maintain their target blood glucose range. Type 2 diabetes mellitus patients do not require such high doses of sulfonylurea. Also, per information from few brains imaging studies, it is observed that sulfonylurea may cross the blood brain barrier and improve neurological symptoms to some extent. Discoloration of teeth and diarrhea, though transient, are the side effects noted with this group of drugs.

TABLE 3: Sulfonylurea receptor mutations

Gene/inheritance	Age (weeks)/diagnosis	Other features	Pancreas appearance
Kir6.2 (KCNJ11) (50%)	6/(0–260)	Developmental delay (20%) Epilepsy (6%) Diabetic ketoacidosis (30%)	Normal
SUR1 (ABCC8)	6/(0–17)	Developmental delay	Normal

Other Mutations

Other mutations are given in table 4.

Neonatal Diabetes Due to Mutations in INS Gene[12,13]

Commonest cause of PNDM is KATP channel mutations. Next in line is mutation in the coding region of the *INS* gene (heterozygous). Beta-cell death occurs due to trapping and accumulation of misfolded proinsulin molecules in the endoplasmic reticulum (endoplasmic reticulum stress and β-cell apoptosis). Genetic *INS* mutations testing should be considered in other antibody negative "T1DM" infants/children, as sometimes *INS* gene mutation may cause diabetes onset after 6 months of age.

Wolcott-Rallison Syndrome[14]

Mutations—biallelic, in the gene encoding EIF2AK3 (eukaryotic translation initiation factor α-2-kinase 3) causes Wolcott-Rallison syndrome. This syndrome is a rare type of recessively inherited disease. This syndrome is characterized by early onset diabetes, spondyloepiphyseal dysplasia leading to growth retardation, and recurrent hepatic and/or renal dysfunction. In most of the cases, the onset of diabetes is seen in the first few months of life, however, it might present after 3–4 years of age also. Diagnosis of Wolcott-Rallison syndrome should be considered in children with PNDM and born of consanguineous marriage, and from a highly inbred population.

TABLE 4: Other mutations

Gene/inheritance	Age (weeks)/diagnosis	Other features	Pancreas appearance
INS	9/(0–26)	None	Normal
EIF2AK3 Wolcott-Rallison syndrome/recessive	13 (6–65)	Epiphyseal dysplasia (90%), osteopenia (50%), acute liver failure (75%), developmental delay (80%), hypothyroidism (25%); insulin requiring	Atrophy of pancreas (?), exocrine dysfunction (25%)
FOXP3	6 (0–30)	Only boys affected	?
GCK (glucokinase)/recessive (homozygous/compound heterozygous)	–	Parents have fasting hyperglycemia as heterozygotes	Normal
IPF1/recessive	–	Parents may have early-onset diabetes as heterozygotes	Absent
PTF1A/recessive	–	Severe neurological dysfunction and cerebellar hypoplasia	Atrophy
IPEX syndrome/X linked (monogenic autoimmune diabetes)	–	Chronic diarrhea with villous atrophy (95%); pancreatic and thyroid autoantibodies (75%), thyroiditis (20%), eczema (50%); anemia (30%), often die young (first year)	–

IPEX, immunodysregulation polyendocrinopathy enteropathy X-linked syndrome

SECTION 1: Introduction

Neonatal Diabetes Due to GCK Mutations[15]

The *GCK* mutations can also cause PNDM (2–3% of cases). This should be considered in children born to parents with mild fasting hyperglycemia. Parents do not display any symptoms of hyperglycemia, and hence, fasting blood glucose should be checked in parents of children having NDM, irrespective of consanguinity or family history of diabetes. Treatment with sulfonylurea has not produced any clear results in these children.

Immunodysregulation Polyendocrinopathy Enteropathy X-linked Syndrome[16]

Immunodysregulation polyendocrinopathy enteropathy X-linked (IPEX) syndrome is the only established form of "autoimmune" (β-cell autoimmunity and pancreatic islet autoantibodies) PNDM and occurs due to mutations in the *FOXP3* gene. This is X-linked and characterized by immune dysregulation, polyendocrinology, and enteropathy. The IPEX syndrome should be considered in young male infants presenting with diabetes, immune deficiency, severe infections, and diarrhea. Treatments include insulin for diabetes, and steroids and sirolimus for enteropthy. Allogeneic bone marrow transplant with reduced intensity conditioning can be considered. Gene therapy approaches are in the experimental stage.

Other Causes of Neonatal Diabetes

The clinical features in other causes of neonatal and infancy-onset diabetes have been described.[2,3] Fecal elastase and fecal fats are the best tests, functional, to assess the exocrine pancreas (pancreas imaging not reliable). Pancreatic supplements can be used if pancreatic hypoplasia/aplasia is detected. All causes of NDM, apart from KATP channel mutations, need insulin therapy.

Group B: Familial Mild Hyperglycemia or Diabetes— Autosomal Dominant (Maturity-onset Diabetes of the Young)[17]

Each genetic subtype of maturity-onset diabetes of the young (MODY) has its own pattern of hyperglycemia, age of onset, associated symptoms, hereditary or consanguinity component, and response to treatment, etc. Though MODY has a strong family history, first time genetic mutations (sporadic *de novo*) are also observed.

Common subtypes of MODY and additional clinical features are outlined in table 5. The clinical and molecular characteristics of "Maturity Onset Diabetes of Young" subtypes are given in appendix table A2.

Group C: Genetic Syndromes— Diabetes with Extrapancreatic Features[2,3]

A monogenic disorder should be considered in any child with diabetes associated with multisystem extrapancreatic features. These syndromes may either cause NDM or present in later life (Tables 5 and 6).

CHAPTER 3: Monogenic Diabetes: Perspectives and Clinical Implications...

TABLE 5: Common subtypes of maturity-onset diabetes of the young and additional clinical features

Gene/inheritance	Age (years)/diagnosis	Glucose at diagnosis (mmol/L)	Other features
HNF1α (MODY3)	14/(4–18)	17/(11–26)	• Large increment in an OGTT (2-h–0 h usually >5 mmol/L) • Low renal threshold • Progressive hyperglycemia with age • Sensitive to sulfonylureas
HNF4α (MODY1)	17/(5–18)	15/(9–20)	• Similar to HNF-1α, but renal threshold normal • Macrosomia very common and 20% have prolonged neonatal hypoglycemia • Sensitive to sulfonylureas
GCK (MODY2)	10/(0–18)	11/(5.5–16)	• Usually incidental finding at diagnosis • Fasting glucose in range 5.5–8 mmol/L • Small increment in an OGTT (2h–0 h usually <3.5 mmol/L) • Little deterioration in glycemia with age

MODY, maturity-onset diabetes of the young; OGTT, oral glucose tolerance test.
- HNF1α /HNF4α-MODY: Sulfonylureas as first-line drug; insulin
- GCK-MODY, -MODY2: Most frequent form in pediatric patients; fasting hyperglycemia or mild diabetes; low birth weight. Diet only; insulin during pregnancy
- GCK-PNDM: GCK (glucokinase) recessive (homozygous/compound heterozygous), insulin + sulfonylureas; parents have fasting hyperglycemia as heterozygotes.

TABLE 6: Genetic syndromes—diabetes with extrapancreatic features

Gene/inheritance	Age (years)/diagnosis	Treatment	Other features
WFS1; recessive (Wolfram syndrome)	<16	Insulin (nonautoimmune β-cell death)	DIDMOAD: Optic atrophy, diabetes insipidus, sensory neural deafness, dilated renal tracts, truncal ataxia, other neurological signs; death 30 years median age
HNF1β (MODY5)	–	Insulin requiring	Renal development disorders, renal cysts, renal dysplasia, uterine and genital anomalies, hyperuricemia, gout, abnormal liver function test. Pancreas atrophy, subclinical exocrine deficiency Not sensitive to sulfonylureas; insulin requiring
mtDNA: 3242 (A to G) tRNA$^{Leu(UUR)}$; mitochondrial diabetes: Maternal transmission	> Pediatric range	Insulin	Sensory neural deafness, short stature Mitochondrial myopathy, encephalopathy, lactic acidosis, and stroke (MELAS) syndrome
SLC19A2; recessive (Roger syndrome)	–	Insulin Thiamine ±	Thiamine responsive megaloblastic anemia, sensorineural deafness

MODY, maturity onset diabetes of the young; DIDMOAD, Diabetes Insipidus, Diabetes Mellitus, Optic Atrophy and Deafness.

SECTION 1: Introduction

TABLE 7: Monogenic diabetes—insulin resistance syndromes: Additional clinical features

Gene/inheritance	Age (years)/diagnosis	Other features
Insulin receptor; leprechaunism (recessive)	Congenital	Abnormal facies, large genitalia; small for gestational age and growth retardation; rarely survive infancy
Insulin receptor; Rabson-Mendenhall (recessive)	Congenital	Extreme growth retardation, abnormal dentition
Insulin receptor; type A (recessive)	Adolescence	Insulin resistance in absence of obesity
Total: Seipin and *AGPAT2* (recessive) Partial: Lamin *AC* and *PPARG* (dominant); lipodystrophy	Congenital or adolescence	Loss of subcutaneous fat—partial or total

INSULIN RESISTANCE MONOGENIC DIABETES

Monogenic Diabetes—Insulin Resistance Syndromes[18]

These syndromes are summarized in table 7.
- Acanthosis nigricans
- Androgen excess
  - Hypertrichosis, polycystic ovarian syndrome
- Hyperinsulinemia—massive
  - In the absence of obesity
  - Hypertriglyceridemia
- Treatment (severe insulin resistance): very difficult
  - Metformin, thiazolidinediones ±: U 500 insulin—pumps
  - Recombinant leptin (total lipodystrophy).

In addition, insulin resistance syndrome subtypes, gene inheritance, leptin/adiponectin levels and associated clinical features are summarized in appendix table A3.

POPULATION PREVALENCE OF MONOGENIC DIABETES[19,20]

A challenging study has tried to evaluate dynamic changes in the prevalence of different types of diabetes in pediatric populations in Poland, with a specific focus on monogenic diabetes. The prevalence of monogenic diabetes in the pediatric population with a low prevalence of obesity remained stable and was nearly fivefold higher than that of T2DM and cystic fibrosis related diabetes (CFRD), justifying a need for increased access to genetic diagnostic procedures in diabetic children.
- Population of Polish children 0–18 years (December 2011)[19]
  - Prevalence of T1DM: 138/100,000
  - Prevalence of T2DM: 1.01/100,000
  - Prevalence of CFRD: 0.95/100,000
  - Prevalence of all monogenic diabetes: 4.6/100,000
  - Prevalence of PNDM: 1/300 000 = 0.3/100,000
  - Monogenic diabetes: 3.1–4.2% [5%] children with diabetes; 83% *GCK*-MODY

- Population of United Kingdom Polish children 0–20 years: A large systematic study confirmed a prevalence of 2.5% of patients with monogenic diabetes who were less than 20 years of age in six United Kingdom clinics. This figure suggests that approximately 50% of the estimated 875 United Kingdom pediatric patients with monogenic diabetes have still not received a genetic diagnosis. This biomarker screening pathway is a practical approach that can be used to identify pediatric patients who are most appropriate for genetic testing.

MONOGENIC DIABETES: WHAT IT TEACHES US ON THE COMMON FORMS OF TYPE 1 AND TYPE 2 DIABETES MELLITUS?[21-23]

To date, more than 30 genes have been linked to monogenic diabetes. Candidate gene and genome-wide association studies have identified more than 50 susceptibility loci for common T1DM and approximately 100 susceptibility loci T2DM. About 1–5% of all cases of diabetes result from single gene mutations and are called monogenic diabetes. Pathophysiological basis of the role of monogenic diabetes genes that have also been found to be associated with common T1DM and/or T2DM are being elucidated.

GLUCOKINASE MONOGENIC DIABETES AND GESTATIONAL DIABETES MELLITUS[24]

Glucokinase monogenic diabetes (*GCK*-MODY) should be differentiated from "standard" GDM because management differs. In particular, intensive glycemic control, may adversely affect the fetus of a pregnant woman with *GCK*-MODY. In contrast to GDM, which is associated with a greatly increased risk for subsequent diabetes, women with *GCK*-MODY, and their affected offspring, have a low prevalence of diabetes complications and do not require treatment outside of pregnancy.

CONCLUSION

Monogenic forms of diabetes should be expected with the frequency of about 5% of all children/patients with diabetes. Diabetes with unusual course of the disease or other coexisting disorders in children or young adults may suggest monogenic diabetes. Some forms of monogenic diabetes may require specific method of treatment.

Many clinical subgroups and specific entities of monogenic diabetes are now known, due to identification of the gene causing the disease through advanced molecular genetic testing. This method of testing is nowadays used to confirm the specific disease type. However, since these tests are costly, in resource limited settings, they should be ordered only if these will be value addition to the strong suspicion of the clinician, based on the overall clinical presentation and profile. Genetically determined wide clinical heterogeneity and spectrum of "monogenic diabetes" are becoming increasingly apparent, extending across all ages of diabetes onset—from neonate and infancy, to childhood, adolescence and youth, and even adults. Accumulating new science in this field can lead to future practical implementation of "diabetes pharmacogenomics" and "personalized medicine".[2,3]

SECTION 1: Introduction

REFERENCES

1. Global IDF/ISPAD Guideline for Diabetes in Childhood and Adolescence 2011. [online] Available from: http://www.idf.org/sites/default/files/Diabetes-in-Childhood-and-Adolescence-Guidelines.pdf;http://web.ispad.org/sites/default/files/idf-ispad_diabetes_in_childhood_and_adolescence_guidelines_2011.pdf.
2. ISPAD Clinical Practice Consensus Guidelines 2009 Compendium. The diagnosis and management of monogenic diabetes in children and adolescents. Pediatr Diabetes. 2009;10(Suppl. 12):33-42.
3. ISPAD Clinical Practice Consensus Guidelines 2014 Compendium. The diagnosis and management of monogenic diabetes in children and adolescents. Pediatr Diabetes. 2014:15(Suppl. 20): 47-64.
4. Temple IK, Gardner RJ, Mackay DJ, Barber JC, Robinson DO, Shield JP. Transient neonatal diabetes: widening the understanding of the etiopathogenesis of diabetes. Diabetes. 2000;49:1359-66.
5. Rubio-Cabezas O, Ellard S. Diabetes mellitus in neonates and infants: genetic heterogeneity, clinical approach to diagnosis, and therapeutic options. Horm Res Paediatr. 2013;80:137-46.
6. Ashcroft FM. ATP-sensitive potassium channelopathies: focus on insulin secretion. J Clin Invest. 2005;115:2047-58.
7. Babenko AP, Polak M, Cavé H, Busiah K, Czernichow P, Scharfmann R, et al. Activating mutations in the ABCC8 gene in neonatal diabetes mellitus. N Engl J Med. 2006;355:456-66.
8. Hattersley AT, Ashcroft FM. Activating mutations in Kir6.2 and neonatal diabetes: new clinical syndromes, new scientific insights, and new therapy. Diabetes. 2005;54:2503-13.
9. Greeley SA, Tucker SE, Naylor RN, Bell GI, Philipson LH. Neonatal diabetes mellitus: a model for personalized medicine. Trends Endocrinol Metab. 2010;21:464-72.
10. Klupa T, Skupien J, Mirkiewicz-Sieradzka B, Gach A, Noczynska A, Zubkiewicz-Kucharska A, et al. Efficacy and safety of sulfonylurea use in permanent neonatal diabetes due to KCNJ11 gene mutations: 34-month median follow-up. Diabetes Technol Ther. 2010;387-91.
11. Gurgel LC, Crispim F, Noffs MH, Belzunces E, Rahal MA, Moises RS. Sulfonylurea treatment in permanent neonatal diabetes due to G53D mutation in the KCNJ11 gene: improvement in glycemic control and neurological function. Diabetes Care. 2007;30: e108.
12. Colombo C, Porzio O, Liu M, Massa O, Vasta M, Salardi S, et al. Seven mutations in the human insulin gene linked to permanent neonatal/infancy-onset diabetes mellitus. J Clin Invest. 2008;118:2148-56.
13. Molven A, Ringdal M, Nordbo AM, Raeder H, Stoy I, Lipkind GM, et al. Mutations in the insulin gene can cause MODY and autoantibody-negative type 1 diabetes. Diabetes. 2008;57:1131-5.
14. Rubio-Cabezas O, Patch AM, Minton JA, Flanagan SE, Edghill EL, Hussain K, et al. Wolcott-Rallison syndrome is the most common genetic cause of permanent neonatal diabetes in consanguineous families. J Clin Endocrinol Metab. 2009;94:4162-70.
15. Njolstad PR, Sagen JV, Bjorkhaug L, Odili S, Sheha-deh N, Bakry D, et al. Permanent neonatal diabetes caused by glucokinase deficiency: inborn error of the glucose-insulin signaling pathway. Diabetes. 2003;52:2854-60.
16. Verbsky JW, Chatila TA. Immune dysregulation, polyendocrinopathy, enteropathy, X-linked (IPEX) and IPEX-related disorders: an evolving web of heritable autoimmune diseases. Curr Opin Pediatr. 2013;25:708-14.
17. Shields BM, Hicks S, Shepherd MH, Colclough K, Hattersley AT, Ellard S. Maturity-onset diabetes of the young (MODY): how many cases are we missing? Diabetologia. 2010;53:2504-8.
18. Parker VE, Semple RK. Genetics in endocrinology: genetic forms of severe insulin resistance: what endocrinologists should know. Eur J Endocrinol. 2013:R71-80.
19. Fendler W, Borowiec M, Baranowska-Jazwiecka A, Szadkowska A, Skala-Zamorowska E, Deja G, et al. Prevalence of monogenic diabetes amongst Polish children after a nationwide genetic screening campaign. Diabetologia. 2012;55(10):2631-5.
20. Shepherd M, Shields B, Hammersley S, Hudson M, McDonald TJ, Colclough K, et al.; The UNITED Team. Systematic population screening, using biomarkers and genetic testing, identifies 2.5% of the U.K. pediatric diabetes population with monogenic diabetes. Diabetes Care. 2016;dc160645.
21. Vaxillaire M1, Froguel P. Monogenic diabetes in the young, pharmacogenetics and relevance to multifactorial forms of type 2 diabetes. Endocr Rev. 2008;29(3):254-64.
22. Yang Y, Chan L. Monogenic Diabetes: What It Teaches Us on the Common Forms of Type 1 and Type 2 Diabetes. Endocr Rev. 2016;37(3):190-222.
23. Tallapragada DSP, Bhaskar S, Chandak GR. New insights from monogenic diabetes for "common" type 2 diabetes. Front Genet. 2015;6:251.
24. Rudland VL, Hinchcliffe M, Pinner J, Cole S, Mercorella B, Molyneaux L, et al. Identifying glucokinase monogenic diabetes in a multiethnic gestational diabetes mellitus cohort: New pregnancy screening criteria and utility of HbA1c. Diabetes Care. 2016;39(1):50-2.

CHAPTER 4

Growth and Development in Children with Type 1 Diabetes Mellitus

Raghupathy Palany, Abraham Paulose

INTRODUCTION

Growth disorders among children with type 1 diabetes mellitus (T1DM) were fairly common in the pre-insulin era. Even in the early years after insulin became available, Mauriac syndrome with the characteristic features of stunted growth, hepatomegaly, obesity, pallor, and delayed skeletal maturation was commonly encountered.[1,2] This was an extreme example of a growth disorder which resulted from chronic poor control of diabetes over a long period. With appropriate treatment, hepatomegaly would regress promptly and growth will gradually improve, while in some others, once begun, poor growth may continue despite optimal therapy. The delay in the onset of puberty and reduced final height were also reported in the past.[3,4] However, with improved diabetes care and many advances over the years, the outcome for growth in children with T1DM has been largely favorable. A majority of children have achieved normal final adult heights but yet, deviations from normal growth continue to be reported, especially during pubertal years.[5,6] Rare cases of Mauriac syndrome also appear occasionally in the literature.[7]

WEIGHT AND LENGTH AT BIRTH

A number of studies examining the influence of birth weight in developing diabetes have yielded interesting results. In a large population based cohort study, a linear increased incidence of T1DM was found with increasing birth weights.[8] There was no significant association between gestational age and T1DM. In a systematic review and meta-analysis, Harder et al. observed a decreased risk of T1DM with low birth weight (<2,500 g) and increased risk with heavier birth weight, viz., a 7% increase in risk with each 1,000 g increase in birth weight.[9] In the Finnish population registry, it was observed that boys with T1DM were longer and heavier at birth than controls; girls were longer at birth.[10] Low birth weight and short birth length were found to be protective from development of T1DM in another study covering several European centers.[11]

SECTION 1: Introduction

GROWTH IN INFANCY

Increased weight gain by itself or when combined with increased weight and height gain during childhood is known to adversely affect the risk of developing T1DM.[12] Height gain in infancy is not consistently known to increase the risk of T1DM. The lower rate of weight gain in breastfed babies has been considered a protective factor.

GROWTH IN CHILDHOOD

While reviewing several Western studies, weight gain during childhood was found to have no causative role for the increased risk of developing T1DM[13] but others found a positive influence for such risk.[14, 15] Rapid height gain in the prediabetic phase was noted only in boys who were later diagnosed with T1DM.[16] Similar observations were made in the Finnish[17] and Dutch[13] studies. Children with T1DM and their siblings are often seen to be taller than other children in the population. Nevertheless, in a twin study, decreased height velocity was recorded in the twins who later developed diabetes.[18]

Acceleration of growth noted at the initial diagnosis of T1DM has been hypothesized to be caused by hyperinsulinemia in the prediabetic period.

HEIGHT AT DIAGNOSIS

At initial diagnosis, children with T1DM have been reported in several studies to be taller than controls[3, 19] but there are also conflicting reports.[4, 20] The relevance of social class was examined and the data obtained were equivocal for development of T1DM or otherwise. Most of the data are from the developed nations. A study from Southern India reported normal heights in children at the time of diagnosis.[21] Generally, children developing T1DM after the age of 10 years appear to have a normal height at diagnosis.

GROWTH AND PUBERTY AFTER DIAGNOSIS

There are many studies reporting the reduction in height standard deviation score (SDS) in the initial years following diagnosis.[22, 23] Normal prepubertal growth was observed in a Belgian study.[24] The loss of growth potential commonly occurs in the prepubertal years after diagnosis and is highest in those who were the tallest to begin with, although no explanation is available for this phenomenon. Furthermore, patients with onset of T1DM under the age of 5 years showed the greatest loss of height during puberty[25] and an association between poor relative growth and younger age at onset was reported. It is postulated that height loss was noticed more often in children treated in the past with less intensive regimes and loss of height SDS is lower with more intensive insulin schedules.[26]

Delayed puberty is not a common feature nowadays as in the past but this still continues to be reported. No delay in pubertal onset was also found in several studies,[26, 27] e.g., age at menarche was not different in those treated with the recent more intensive treatment as compared to the group less intensively treated in the past.[26]

In the older reports, lesser pubertal growth spurt than normal controls, as also a delay in the onset of peak height velocity were noted but recent data are in favor of normal growth spurt in puberty.

FINAL HEIGHT

There is a general consensus that the overall final height outcome of children with T1DM has shown considerable improvement over the last 30 years, showing no deviation from the midparental height prediction.[22] However, Ahmed et al.[27] noted that girls do not fare well because they were tall at diagnosis, had poor pubertal growth, and their final height was significantly reduced in relation to their midparental height. Such discrepancy in optimal growth may occur even with conventional therapy.[24]

WEIGHT GAIN

Generally, body weights of children and adolescents tend to be normal for age. When compared with controls, increased weight gain in the first few years after diagnosis has been known to occur.[25] Weight gain relative to height during the pubertal years was seen in another study, wherein the girls had acquired increase in fat mass,[27] but the boys had reduction in their total body fat. Intensive insulin therapy may be a causative factor in increased weight gain. Excessive weight gain is often observed in girls during late adolescence[28] and can be associated with menstrual disorders[29] and not with eating disorders.[28]

GLYCOSYLATED HEMOGLOBIN AND GROWTH

A longitudinal study over a 5-year period has clearly demonstrated that higher glycosylated hemoglobin (HbA1c) values are associated with lower height velocity[30] while another longitudinal study has shown a negative relationship with peak height velocity SDS and HbA1c.[25]

ASSOCIATED GROWTH DISORDERS

While poor glycemic control is responsible for poor or slow growth in T1DM, other associated disorders which can significantly affect growth will need to be identified. Autoimmune thyroiditis with hypothyroidism is the most frequent associated disorder seen more often in girls and those with T1DM for long duration. Hence, routine screening for thyroid disease in children has been recommended. Celiac disease known to slow growth has also been reported in children with T1DM from Northern India.[31] Therefore, T1DM children with poor growth will need to be investigated with endomysial or anti-gliadin antibodies. Treatment with thyroxine or gluten-free diet will greatly improve growth in these two disorders and therefore, needs to be diagnosed promptly.

Vitamin D deficiency is widely prevalent in the general population with its effects on bone health and growth. In children with T1DM, microalbuminuria and diabetic nephropathy are reported in vitamin D deficiency states.[32] Regular vitamin D supplementation along with dietary calcium and protein intake is essential for improving growth and reducing the risk of complications. Bone metabolism may be related to varying insulin-like growth factor-1 (IGF-1) bioavailability or persisting hypercalciuria, a frequent feature in T1DM.[33]

Other common causes affecting growth in children with T1DM and delayed puberty are directly related to poor glycemic control due to poor compliance as a result of low socioeconomic status, lack of family support, and emotional disorders. Appropriate insulin dosing, multidose insulin therapy, combined with optimal food intake at the right intervals, and regular physical exercises are known to yield the best results for minimizing growth and pubertal disorders in T1DM. Hypoparathyroidism, adrenal insufficiency, growth hormone or gonadotropin deficiency, and other concurrent chronic illnesses may also cause poor growth.

GROWTH HORMONE AND INSULIN-LIKE GROWTH FACTOR-1 AXIS

Growth hormone secretion is higher and IGF-1 level is lower in children with T1DM,[34,35] with the latter noted especially during puberty. Although IGF-1 levels are lower in both boys and girls, girls are more prone to develop reduced pubertal growth spurt. In other studies, such sex differences were not demonstrable; nor was any relationship between peak height velocity SDS and IGF-1 SDS observed.[27] In this study, low levels of IGF-1 were found during puberty and were thought to be causing the poor pubertal growth.

Total daily insulin dose seems to have an important role in the regulation of growth hormone/IGF-1 axis, as evidenced in newly diagnosed patients by low growth hormone binding protein. Growth hormone binding protein levels and the subsequent rise after 3 months of insulin therapy.[36] Insulin is responsible for increasing hepatic IGF-1 production through its action on growth hormone receptor or post-growth hormone receptor events.

DEVELOPMENT

Infants and Toddlers

Irregular and erratic meal schedules, failure to understand the need for regular blood sugar tests and insulin injections, and family conflicts tend to make diabetes control very difficult. Temper tantrums may result due to difficult behavior. Gentle caring approach with patience and love will be beneficial.

School Age Children

Maintenance of optimal diabetes control is very important in this age group as in any others but normal psychosocial development of the children will greatly help in achieving good control. Parents also need appropriate education in handling these children. Without adequate control, these children are susceptible to develop stunted growth, hepatomegaly, and delayed pubertal onset. Between the ages of 6 and 11 years, the child must master diabetes care regimen, modify the diet while completing common developmental tasks. Diabetes mellitus can affect learning, memory, mental speed, and eye-hand coordination.[37] Children with diabetes scored less compared to controls on all scores (Wechsler's coding, digit span test, and Raven's colored progressive matrices).

Lower scores were attributed to both metabolic control and psychosocial factors.[37] Neuropsychological deficits were observed few years after diagnosis. Children with T1DM had reduced speed of information processing, decrements in conceptual reasoning, weakness in attention executive functioning, defective memory, and acquisition of new knowledge. It was shown that cognitive function was poorer, reaction time longer, memory scale poorer, although intelligence quotient was comparable with control children.[38] Central nervous system vascular or metabolic dysfunction, emotional influence of the chronic illness, or a central neuropathy (analogous to peripheral neuropathy) may all contribute. Major predictors in these changes include onset of diabetes prior to 4 years, recurrent hypoglycemia and hyperglycemia.

Children tend to miss school more often, and obtain lower scores.[39] Therefore, one must consider educational skills in diabetic children when planning diabetic treatment regimens. Children with normal psychosocial development adequately cope with diabetes. Better glycemic control and quality of life are seen in children when parents, school personnel, and friends receive some training in diabetes management and guide these children effectively in preventing and treating diabetes complications.

Adolescents

Depression is very common in children and adolescents with T1DM, with some of them developing somatic complaints, anxiety, antisocial behavior, aggression, etc. Eating disorders are also common, especially with misuse of insulin for controlling hyperglycemia.

Individual psychotherapy through counseling during clinic visits helps the children with stress to overcome their psychological problems. Cognitive behavior treatment is also useful in depressive states to tide over their preconceived notions and ideas to furnish them with accurate and adaptive thoughts which will in turn help in optimal control of diabetes.

RECOMMENDATIONS

Normal growth is one of the major goals in the treatment of children with T1DM. A multidisciplinary team of specialists trained in pediatric diabetes management and sensitive to the challenges of children and adolescents with T1DM should provide care for this population. It is essential that diabetes self-management education and support, medical nutrition therapy, and psychosocial support be provided at diagnosis and regularly thereafter by individuals experienced with the educational, nutritional, behavioral, and emotional needs of the growing child and family. The balance between adult supervision and self-care should be defined at the first interaction and re-evaluated at each clinic visit. This relationship will evolve as the child reaches physical, psychological, and emotional maturity.

Frequent regular follow-up visits every 2-3 months are important for achieving the targets planned with therapy. Clinic visits may have to be more frequent during the first few months following diagnosis. Every clinic visit is an opportunity for continuing and reinforcing diabetes education along with growth and pubertal assessment. Some of the important aspects are summarized below:

- Monitor height and weight carefully and plot on a growth chart, for growth velocity monitoring, at every visit. Any deviation from the norm should be identified early and appropriate remedial measures should be undertaken
- Pubertal assessment is an integral part of examination
- Blood pressure should be measured at each routine visit using an appropriate size cuff with the patient seated and relaxed
- Reinforce the need for a better glycemic control at each visit
- Measuring thyroid-stimulating hormone and anti-thyroid peroxidase antibodies soon after diagnosis of T1DM is reasonable. If normal, consider rechecking every 1-2 years or sooner if patient develops symptoms of thyroid dysfunction, thyromegaly, an abnormal growth rate, or unusual glycemic variations
- Consider screening for celiac disease by measuring tissue transglutaminase in children with a positive family history of celiac disease, growth failure, failure to gain weight, weight loss, diarrhea, flatulence, abdominal pain, or signs of malabsorption or in children with frequent unexplained hypoglycemia or deterioration in glycemic control
- Annual screening for microalbuminuria, with a random spot urine sample for albumin-to-creatinine ratio should be considered once the child has had diabetes for 5 years
- Advice relevant to changing needs, e.g., adequate protein, iron, calcium, and vitamin D intake
- Assess psychosocial distress and family stresses that could impact adherence with diabetes management and provide appropriate referrals to trained mental health professionals. Consider screening for depression and disordered eating behaviors using available screening tools.

CONCLUSION

Optimal glycemic control eventually yields normal physical growth and pubertal growth spurt but yet lack of pubertal growth spurt and lessened final height are still observed, which may be directly related to poor metabolic control. This is, however, difficult to quantify. Intensive insulin therapy has been observed to improve HbA1c values but has not categorically been shown to improve or avoid pubertal growth abnormalities. The feasibility of portal mode of administration of insulin in ameliorating growth disorders in T1DM is being currently examined. Intensive insulin therapy by itself may cause increased weight gain and may not be an answer to prevent growth abnormalities in T1DM. The role of newer analogs of insulin will also need to be studied further in this regard.

CHAPTER 4: Growth and Development in Children with Type 1 Diabetes Mellitus

REFERENCES

1. Justin EP, Root HF, White P. The growth, development and prognosis of diabetic children. JAMA. 1925;85:420-2.
2. Wagner R, White P, Bogan I. Diabetic dwarfism. Arch Dis Child. 1942;63:667-727.
3. Jivani SK, Rayner PH. Does control influence the growth of diabetic children? Arch Dis Child. 1973;48:109-15.
4. Petersen H, Korsgaard B, Deckert T, Nielsen E. Growth, body weight and insulin requirements in diabetic children. Acta Paediatr Scand. 1978;67:453-7.
5. Herber SM, Dunsmore IR. Does control affect growth in diabetes mellitus? Acta Paediatr Scand. 1988;77:303-5.
6. Dunger DB. Insulin and insulin-like growth factors in diabetes mellitus. Arch Dis Child. 1995;72:469-71.
7. Franzese A, Iorio R, Buono P, Mascolo M, Mozzillo E, Valerio G. Mauriac syndrome still exists. Diabetes Res Clin Pract. 2001; 54: 219-21.
8. Stene LC, Magnus P, Lie RT, Søvik O, Joner G. Birth weight and childhood onset type 1 diabetes: population based cohort study. BMJ. 2001;322:889-92.
9. Harder T, Roepke K, Diller N. Birth weight, early weight gain, and subsequent risk of type 1 diabetes: Systematic review and meta-analysis. Am J Epidemiol. 2009;169:1428-36.
10. Podar, T, Onkamo P, Forsen T, Karvonen M, Tuomilehto-Wolf E, Tuomilehto J. Neonatal anthropometric measurements and risk of childhood-onset type 1 diabetes. DiMe Study Group. Diabetes Care. 1999;22:2092-4.
11. Dahlquist GG, Patterson C, Soltesz G. Perinatal risk factors for childhood type 1 diabetes in Europe. The EURODIAB Substudy 2 Study Group. Diabetes Care. 1999;22:1698-702.
12. Virtanen SM, Knip M. Nutritional risk predictors of betal cell autoimmunity and type 1 diabetes at a young age. Am J Clin Nutr. 2003;78:1053-67.
13. Bruining GJ. Association between infant growth before onset of juvenile type-1 diabetes and autoantibodies to IA-2. Netherlands Kolibrie study group of childhood diabetes. Lancet. 2000;356:655-6.
14. Group TESS. Rapid early growth is associated with increased risk of childhood type 1 diabetes in various European populations. Diabetes Care. 2002;25:1755-9.
15. Johansson C, Samuelsson U, Ludvigsson J. A high weight gain early in life is associated with an increased risk of type 1 (insulin-dependent) diabetes mellitus. Diabetologia. 1994;37:91-4.
16. Blom L, Persson LA, Dahlquist G. A high linear growth is associated with an increased risk of childhood diabetes mellitus. Diabetologia. 1992;35:528-33.
17. Hypponen E, Virtanen SM, Kenward MG, Knip M, Akerblom HK. Obesity, increased linear growth, and risk of type 1 diabetes in children. Diabetes Care. 2000;23:1755-60.
18. Leslie RD, Lo S, Millward BA, Honour J, Pyke DA. Decreased growth velocity before IDDM onset. Diabetes. 1991;40:211-6.
19. Drayer NM. Height of diabetic children at onset of symptoms. Arch Dis Child. 1974;49:616-20.
20. Evans N, Robinson VP, Lister J. Growth and bone age of juvenile diabetics. Arch Dis Child. 1872;47:589-93.
21. Ramachandran A, Snehalatha C, Joseph TA, Vijay V, Viswanathan M. Height at onset of insulin-dependent diabetes in children in southern India. Diabetes Res Clin Pract. 1994;23:55-7.
22. Brown M, Ahmed MI, Clayton KL, Dunger DB. Growth during childhood and final height in type 1 diabetes. Diabet Med. 1994;11:182-7.
23. Holl RW, Grabert M, Heinze E, Sorgo W, Debatin KM. Age at onset and long-term metabolic control affect height in type-1 diabetes mellitus. Eur J Pediatr. 1998;157:972-7.
24. Du Caju MV, Rooman RP, op de Beeck I. Longitudinal data on growth and final height in diabetic children. Pediatr Res. 1995;38:607-11.
25. Thon A, Heinze E, Fellen KD, Holl RW, Schmidt H, Koletzko S, et al. Development of height and weight in children with diabetes mellitus: report in two prospective multicentre studies, one cross-sectional, one longitudinal. Eur J Pediatr. 1992;151:258-62.
26. Donaghue KC, Kordonouri O, Chan A, Silink M. Secular trends in growth in diabetes: are we winning? Arch Dis Child. 2001;88:151-4.
27. Ahmed ML, Connors MH, Drayer NM, Jones JS, Dunger DB. Pubertal growth in IDDM is determined by HbA1c levels, sex and bone age. Diabetes Care. 1998;21:831-5.

28. Peveler RC, Fairburn CG, Boller IG, Dunger D. Eating disorders in adolescents with IDDM. A controlled study. Diabetes Care. 1992;15:1356-60.
29. Adcock CJ, Perry LA, Lindsel DR, Taylor AM, Holly JM, Jones J, et al. Menstrual irregularities are more common in adolescents with type 1 diabetes: association with poor glycaemic control and weight gain. Diabetic Med. 1994;11:465-70.
30. Gunczler P, Lanes R, Essa S, Paoli M. Effects of glycemic control on the growth velocity and several metabolic parameters of conventionally treated children with insulin dependent diabetes mellitus. J Pediatr Endocrinol Metab. 1996;9:569-75.
31. Bhadada SK, Kochhar R, Bhansali A, Dutta U, Kumar PR, Poornachandra KS, et al. Prevalence and clinical profile of celiac disease in type 1 diabetes mellitus in north India. J Gastroenterol Hepatol. 2011;26:376-81.
32. Verrotti A, Basciani F, Carle F, Morgese G, Chiarelli F. Calcium metabolism in adolescents and young adults with type 1 diabetes mellitus without and with persistent microalbuminuria. J Endocrinol Invest. 1999;22:198-202.
33. Malone JI, Lowitt S, Duncan JA, Shah SC, Vargas A, Root AW. Hypercalciuria, hyperphosphaturia, and growth retardation in children with diabetes mellitus. Pediatrics. 1986;78:298-304.
34. Edge JA, Dunger DB, Matthews DR, Gilbert JP, Smith CP. Increased overnight growth hormone concentrations in diabetic compared with normal adolescents. J Clin Endoccrinol Metab. 1990;71:1356-62.
35. Amiel SA, Sherwin RS, Hintz RL, Gertner JM, Press CM, Tamborlane WV. Effect of diabetes and its control on insulin-like growth factors in the young subject with type 1 diabetes. Diabetes 1984;33:1175-9.
36. Arslanian SA, Menon RK, Gierl AP, Heil BV, Foley TP Jr. Insulin therapy increases low plasma growth hormone binding protein in children with new-onset type 1 diabetes. Diabetic Med. 1993;10:833-8.
37. Naguib JM, Kulinskaya E, Lomax CL, Garralda ME. Neurocognitive performance in children with type 1 diabetes—A Meta analysis. Journal Pediat Psychol. 2009;34:271-82.
38. Northam E, Anderson P, Werther G, Warne GL, Adler RG, Andrewes D. Neuropsychological complications of IDDM in children 2 years after disease onset. Diabetes Care. 1998;21:379-84.
39. McCarthy AM, Kindgren S, Menegeling M, Tsalikian E, Engvall J. Factors associated with academic achievement in children with type 1 diabetes. Diabetes Care. 2003;26:112-7.

SECTION 2

Clinical and Laboratory Approach

Editor
Raghupathy Palany

CHAPTER 5

Clinical Examination of Type 1 Diabetes Mellitus

Rishi Shukla

INTRODUCTION

Type 1 diabetes mellitus (T1DM) is present in about 5–10% of patients with diabetes mellitus.[1] Type 1 diabetes mellitus can be diagnosed at any age, however, it is most common chronic disease in childhood.[2] The most common age of diagnosis is between 5 and 7 years and or near puberty.[3] People with T1DM usually are asymptomatic as symptoms develop after many years of chronic prolonged hyperglycemia. The classic symptoms include polyuria, polydipsia, polyphagia, and unexplained weight loss. If patients present with diabetic ketoacidosis, they may have Kussmaul respiration, dehydration, hypotension, or sometimes disturbed mental status. In cases, if the disease of prolonged duration, there can be presence of lethargy, blurred vision, numbness, and tingling in both hands and feet usually bilateral, symmetric, and ascending. Clinical examination plays a pivotal role not only in diagnosing the patients with T1DM, but also throughout their lives in monitoring and managing their condition aiming at better treatment outcomes.

Clinical examination or approach to T1DM patient begins with detailed history taking followed by complete physical examination supported by laboratory investigations.

HISTORY

Proper history of patient for classic symptoms should be taken like a several week history of polyuria, polydipsia, polyphagia, and weight loss, with hyperglycemia, glycosuria, ketonemia, and ketonuria may be present. Sudden onset of symptoms in young lean patient with ketoacidosis has also been considered as diagnostic of T1DM. It is an immune mediated form of diabetes. The preclinical disease shows presence of two or more antibodies while an overt clinical disease usually has presence of multiple antibodies.[2] A focused diabetes history in an established disease should also include questions on diabetes control about hypo- or hyperglycemia (near normal glucose levels), microvascular complications (dilated eye examination, urine protein tests), macrovascular complications (hypertension, lipid levels, claudication, stroke, or transient ischemic attack), and about foot infections or ulcers.

PHYSICAL EXAMINATION

All patients should be examined thoroughly for general examination. It should include height, weight, body mass index, weight gain or loss, monitoring growth of child, nutritional status, and signs of dehydration. Physical examination should also focus on altered mental status, stupor, coma, Kussmaul respirations, fruity breath, signs of autonomic insufficiency, skin examination for diabetic dermopathy, furuncles, carbuncles, candidiasis, cataracts, retinopathy, glaucoma, peripheral neuropathy, corns and calluses, dermatophytosis, peripheral pulses, and/or any ulceration. In established T1DM, patients should be examined every 3 months for macrovascular and microvascular complications.[4] They should undergo funduscopic examination for retinopathy and monofilament testing for peripheral neuropathy.

Assessment of Vital Signs

Orthostatic hypotension may be present in patients with T1DM and autonomic neuropathy. Hence, assessment of orthostatic vital signs may be useful in determining the presence of an autonomic neuropathy. Relative tachycardia is a typical finding in autonomic neuropathy which can be determined by measuring pulse. If Kussmaul respiration is present, the appropriate test for diabetic ketoacidosis (DKA) should be done.

Blood Pressure

Blood pressure should be measured at each routine visit. Children found to have high-normal blood pressure [systolic blood pressure (SBP) or diastolic blood pressure (DBP) ≥90th percentile for age, sex, and height] or hypertension (SBP or DBP ≥95th percentile for age, sex, and height) should have blood pressure confirmed on three separate days.[5-7]

Funduscopic Examination

An initial dilated and comprehensive eye examination should be considered for the child at the start of puberty or at age 10 years or above, whichever is earlier, once the youth has had diabetes for 3–5 years. After the initial examination, annual routine follow-up is generally recommended, funduscopic examination can be done which includes a careful view of the retina. It is important to check both the optic disc and macula. Patients should be referred to an ophthalmologist in case hemorrhages or exudates are detected. Ophthalmologist may advise for less frequent examinations (every 2 years).[8,9]

Foot Examination

Patient's foot should be examined at every visit. In case of patients with wound at foot, the dorsalis pedis and posterior tibialis pulses should be palpated and their presence or absence should be noted. Generally, in these patients the healing of wound may be delayed due to infection, furthermore poor lower-extremity blood flow increases the risk of amputation.

Lower-extremity sensory neuropathy should be documented in these patients as these patients will have decreased sensitivity. Patients with peripheral neuropathy should be made aware about the importance of the prevention of foot ulcer which can lead to lower-extremity amputation. Hence, such patients should be educated to examine their feet every day.

Documenting lower-extremity sensory neuropathy is useful in patients who present with foot ulcers because decreased sensation limit the patient's ability to protect the feet and ankles. If peripheral neuropathy is found, patient should be made aware that foot care (including daily foot examination) is very important for the prevention of foot ulcers and lower-extremity amputation.

American Diabetes Association recommends considering an annual comprehensive foot examination for the child at the start of puberty or at age 10 years and above, whichever is earlier, once the youth has had T1DM for 5 years.[4]

Renal Assessment

At least an annual screening for albuminuria, with a random spot urine sample for albumin-to-creatinine ratio (UACR) should be considered once the child has had diabetes for 5 years. Measure creatinine clearance/estimated glomerular filtration rate at initial evaluation and then based on age, diabetes duration, and treatment.[10]

Infections

The hyperglycemic environment in T1DM patients leads to immune dysfunction and increases the susceptibility for infections, the most common being skin and urinary tract. The infections can reach to more severity and can affect all organs and systems. The most common infections being foot infections, malignant external otitis, rhinocerebral mucormycosis, gangrenous cholecystitis, emphysematous pyelonephritis, staphylococcal sepsis, and pneumococcal pneumonia. Immunization with antipneumococcal and influenza vaccines is recommended to reduce the morbidity and mortality in such situations.[11]

Diagnostic Criteria for Diabetic Ketoacidosis

Earlier the most widely used diagnostic criteria for DKA includes blood glucose level more than 250 mg/dL, a moderate degree of ketonemia, serum bicarbonate less than 15 mEq/L, arterial pH less than 7.3, and an increased anion gap metabolic acidosis. However, many patients have mild metabolic acidosis in spite of elevation of blood glucose level. Table 1 summarizes the criteria for diagnosis of DKD.[12]

Laboratory Tests

As appropriate, the various laboratory tests that should be done at the time of confirming the diagnosis and further follow-up include the following.

TABLE 1: Diagnostic criteria for diabetic ketoacidosis[12]

	Mild	Moderate	Severe
Plasma glucose (mg/dL)	>250	>250	>250
Arterial pH	7.25–7.30	7.00–<7.24	<7.00
Serum bicarbonate (mEq/L)	15–18	10–<15	<10
Urine ketones*	Positive	Positive	Positive
Serum ketones*	Positive	Positive	Positive
Effective serum osmolality (mOsm/kg)#	Variable	Variable	Variable
Anion gap£	>10	>12	>12
Mental status	Alert	Alert/drowsy	Stupor/coma

*Nitroprusside reaction method.
#Effective serum osmolality: 2 [measured Na+ (mEq/l)] + glucose (mg/dL)/18.
£Anion gap: (Na+) − [(Cl− + HCO3− (mEq/L)].

Plasma Glucose Concentration

For diagnosis, plasma glucose levels should be measured or a finger stick glucose test in case of emergency. All finger stick capillary glucose levels must be confirmed in serum or plasma to make the diagnosis. The diagnosis of diabetes mellitus can be confirmed with a random (nonfasting) plasma glucose concentration of 200 mg/dL or a fasting plasma glucose concentration of 126 mg/dL (6.99 mmol/L) or higher.[13,14]

Glycosylated Hemoglobin

Glycosylated hemoglobin (HbA1c) levels denote glycemic level status of last 3 months. Glycosylated hemoglobin levels of more than 6.5% is a diagnostic criterion for diagnosis of diabetes along with fasting plasma glucose more than 126 mg/dL and 2-hour plasma glucose more than 200 mg/dL during an oral glucose tolerance test. In a patient where classic symptoms of hyperglycemia are present or in case of hyperglycemic crisis, a random plasma glucose more than 200 mg/dL is diagnostic of diabetes. As recommended by American Diabetes Association (ADA), test should be repeated every 6 months in patients who are meeting their treatment goals and those who are not on glycemic target.[4]

Urine Ketones

It is not that reliable for diagnosing or monitoring DKA.[15]

Plasma Acetone Level

Specifically, the β-hydroxybutyrate level is a more reliable indicator of DKA, along with measurement of plasma bicarbonate or arterial pH as clinically required[15]

Insulin and C-peptide Levels[1]

The C-peptide and insulin hormone both are produced in the pancreas and released when proinsulin is converted to insulin. As per National Institutes of Health, the normal values of

C-peptide range between 0.5 and 2.0 ng/mL in blood. Level below the range is suggestive of T1DM and fasting C-peptide levels of 1 ng/dL in a patient of 1–2 years duration of disease suggest residual β function in T2DM. There can be exception where C-peptide levels are temporarily low in T2DM at the time of very high blood glucose levels, e.g., more than 300 mg/dL, but insulin production is recovered after normalization of glucose levels.[14,15]

Urine Albumin Creatinine Ratio

To diagnose and monitor kidney damage in patients with T1DM of duration 5 years and above or T2DM, the recommendations from ADA and National Kidney Disease Education Program are:
- Screen using a spot UACR (UACR estimates 24-h urine albumin excretion)
- Yearly assessment
- Frequency may be increased depending on clinical status or therapeutic interventions if any
- Urine albumin creatinine ratio is greater than 30 mg/g with or without decreased estimated glomerular filtration rate, suggestive of presence of kidney disease. Urine dipstick does not detect levels below 300 mg/g.[16]

Urine C-Peptide Creatinine Ratio

Insulin insufficiency is a hallmark of long-term T1DM. Urine C-peptide creatinine ratio (UCPCR) is used to identify insulin deficiency. More than 95% patients with T1DM of more than 5 years duration have shown UCPCR value less than 0.2 nmol/mmol in various studies. A cutoff value of 0.2 nmol/mmol also differentiates hepatocyte nuclear factor 1α and 4α (HNF1A/4A) maturity onset diabetes of the young (MODY) from of diabetes. In T1DM, UCPCR has shown a sensitivity of 97% and specificity of 96%. The test should be performed on a postprandial sample taken 2 hours postmeal stimulus.[17]

Immune Markers

Immune markers play an important role in diagnosis of T1DM and the key distinguishing feature of T1DM is the presence of autoantibodies against β-cell autoantigens. It includes autoantibodies reactive to insulin (IAA), glutamic acid decarboxylase (GADA), insulinoma-associated autoantigen 2, and zinc transporter 8.[18] Islet-cell (IA2), anti-GAD65, and anti-insulin autoantibodies can be present in early T1DM. Measurements of IA2 autoantibodies within 6 months of diagnosis can help differentiate between T1DM and T2DM, the titers decrease after 6 months. Anti-GAD65 antibodies can be present at diagnosis of T1DM and are persistently positive over time. Insulin autoantibodies concentration correlates with the rate of progression to overt T1DM in children followed from birth.[19,20]

Other Markers

For impending T1DM, some lipid and metabolite profiles can also serve as markers that include decreased phosphatidylcholine at birth, and reduced triglycerides. Reduced antioxidant ether phospholipids followed by increased lysophosphatidylcholine several months before seroconversion to autoantibody positivity.[21] Another study found higher concentrations of odd-chain triglycerides and polyunsaturated fatty acid-containing phospholipids, and lower concentrations of methionine, in those who developed T1DM-associated autoantibodies.

Genetic Testing

Type 1 diabetes mellitus is a polygenic disorder with more than 40 identified loci to affect disease susceptibility. The human leukocyte antigen (HLA) region on chromosome 6 (i.e., the *IDDM1* locus) provides perhaps one-half of the genetic susceptibility that leads to increased risk of T1DM. The HLA class II shows the strongest association with T1DM while class I can also influence the risk.[21] New deoxyribonucleic acid sequencing technology allows testing for mutations in all the known MODY genes (25 genes) in a single test rather than analyzing just one or two genes at a time. This targeted test identifies those genetic mutations that cause MODY or another monogenic form of young-onset diabetes such as maternally inherited diabetes and deafness or partial lipodystrophy.[22,23]

OTHER COMMON ASSOCIATED CONDITIONS

Celiac Disease

Children with T1DM should be screened for celiac disease by measuring tissue transglutaminase or deamidated gliadin antibodies, with documentation of normal total serum immunoglobulin A levels, soon after the diagnosis of diabetes. This screening is strongly recommended if in T1DM children with a positive family history of celiac disease, growth failure, failure to gain weight, weight loss, diarrhea, flatulence, abdominal pain, or signs of malabsorption or in children with frequent unexplained hypoglycemia or deterioration in glycemic control.[24]

Thyroid Disease

The children should be tested for antithyroidperoxidase and antithyroglobulin antibodies soon after diagnosis of T1DM. Measuring thyroid-stimulating hormone concentrations is important soon after diagnosis of T1DM. If normal, every 1–2 years or sooner should be checked, if the patient develops symptoms of thyroid dysfunction, thyromegaly, an abnormal growth rate or unusual glycemic variation.[25]

CONCLUSION

Clinical examination and approach to T1DM patients requires their complete evaluation from personal to family history, thorough general examination, screening for complications, and laboratory tests. As suggested by ADA guideline, T1DM patients should be on regular follow-up with periodic assessments. This will not only help them in maintaining their glycemic control but also change in therapy plan if required in timely manner.

CHAPTER 5: Clinical Examination of Type 1 Diabetes Mellitus

REFERENCES

1. Diagnosis and classification of diabetes mellitus. Diabetes Care. 2009;32(Suppl 1):S62-7.
2. Simmons KM, Michels AM. Type 1 diabetes: A predictable disease. World J Diabetes. 2015;6(3):380-90.
3. Gale EA. Type 1 diabetes in the young: the harvest of sorrow goes on. Diabetologia. 2005;48:1435-8.
4. Standards of medical care in Diabetes-2017. American Diabetes Association. Diabetes Care. 2017;40:Suppl 1.
5. Handelsman Y, Mechanick JI, Blonde L, et al. American Association of Clinical Endocrinologists Medical Guidelines for Clinical Practice for developing a diabetes mellitus comprehensive care plan. Endocr Pract. 2011;17 Suppl 2:1-53.
6. Chiang JL, Kirkman MS, Laffel LM, et al. Type 1 diabetes through the life span: A position statement of the American Diabetes Association. Diabetes Care. 2014;37(7):2034-54.
7. Orchard TJ, Forrest KY, Kuller LH, et al.; Pittsburgh Epidemiology of Diabetes Complications Study. Lipid and Blood Pressure Treatment Goals for Type 1 Diabetes. Diabetes Care. 2001;24(6):1053-9.
8. Lueder GT, Silverstein J; American Academy of Pediatrics Section on Ophthalmology and Section on Endocrinology. Screening for retinopathy in the pediatric patient with type 1 diabetes mellitus. Pediatrics. 2005;116(1):270-3.
9. Viswanathan V. Preventing microvascular complications in type 1 diabetes mellitus. Indian J Endocrinol Metab. 2015;19(Suppl 1):S36-8.
10. Perkins BA, Krolewski AS. Early nephropathy in type 1 diabetes: a new perspective on who will and who will not progress. Curr Diab Rep. 2005;5(6):455-63.
11. Casqueiro J, Casqueiro J, Alves C. Infections in patients with diabetes mellitus: A review of pathogenesis. Indian J Endocrinol Metab. 2012;16(Suppl1):S27-36.
12. Barski L, Kezerle L, Zeller L, et al. New approaches to the use of insulin in patients with diabetic ketoacidosis. Eur J Inter Med. 2013;24:213-6.
13. American Diabetes Association. Diagnosis and classification of diabetes mellitus. Diabetes Care. 2010;33 Suppl 1:S62-9.
14. Handelsman Y, Mechanick JI, Blonde L, et al. American Association of Clinical Endocrinologists Medical Guidelines for Clinical Practice for developing a diabetes mellitus comprehensive care plan. Endocr Pract. 2011;17 Suppl 2:1-53.
15. Khardori R. Type 1 diabetes mellitus workup. Available from: http://emedicine.medscape.com/article/117739-workup#c.
16. NKDEP. Urine Albumin-to-Creatinine Ratio (UACR) In Evaluating Patients with Diabetes for Kidney Disease. May 2008. NIH Publication No. 08-6286.
17. Besser REJ, Ludvigsson J, Jones AG, et al. Urine C–peptide creatinine ratio (UCPCR) is a non-invasive alternative to the mixed meal tolerance test in children and adults with type 1 diabetes. Diabetes Care. 2011;34(3):607-9.
18. Ziegler AG, Nepom GT. Prediction and pathogenesis in type 1 diabetes. Immunity. 2010;32:468-78.
19. Steck AK, Johnson K, Barriga KJ, et al. Age of islet autoantibody appearance and mean levels of insulin, but not GAD or IA-2 autoantibodies, predict age of diagnosis of type 1 diabetes: diabetes autoimmunity study in the young. Diabetes Care. 2011;34:1397-9.
20. Parikka V, Nanto-Salonen K, Saarinen M, et al. Early seroconversion and rapidly increasing autoantibody concentrations predict prepubertal manifestation of type 1 diabetes in children at genetic risk. Diabetologia. 2012;55:1926-36.
21. Oresic M, Simell S, Sysi-Aho M, et al. Dysregulation of lipid and amino acid metabolism precedes islet autoimmunity in children who later progress to type 1 diabetes. J Exp Med. 2008;205:2975-84.
22. Atkinson MA. Type 1 diabetes. Lancet. 2014;383(9911):69-82.
23. Ellard S, Lango Allen H, De Franco E, et al. Improved genetic testing for monogenic diabetes using targeted next-generation sequencing. Diabetologia. 2013;56:1958-63.
24. Umpierrez GE, Latif KA, Murphy MB, et al. Thyroid dysfunction in patients with type 1 diabetes. Diabetes Care. 2003;26(4):1181-5.
25. Volta U, Tovoli F, Caio G. Clinical and immunological features of celiac disease in patients with T1DM. Expert Rev Gastroenterol Hepatol. 2011;5(4):479-87.

CHAPTER 6

Initial and Annual Laboratory Investigations

Bipin K Sethi, V Sri Nagesh, Jayant V Kelwade, Harsh Y Parekh

INTRODUCTION

Type 1 diabetes mellitus (T1DM) in children is a complex disease that affects both the child and his/her family. The lives are transformed with some much-to-do in terms of learning to live with changed diet, monitoring of glucose, insulin shots, and modification of lifestyle. This entails lot of emotional trauma but firmness and compassion are needed in handling the family with what is a devastating situation for them. The tests that are conducted at diagnosis and later follow-up should reflect this and one should take care not to do any unnecessary workup at the same time not missing out on something critical.

Type 1 diabetes mellitus is an autoimmune disease characterized by absolute insulinopenia due to pancreatic β-cell destruction. Affected individuals require lifelong insulin therapy for survival. The disease manifests generally in youth but can occur at any age.

Type 1 diabetes mellitus is the end result of interplay of genetic, environmental, and autoimmune factors that finally destroy the pancreatic β-cells and leads to insulin deficiency.[1] The early presence of autoantibodies implicates a role for antibody-producing plasma B cells in the initial immunological events. Indeed, B cells clearly contribute to the pathogenesis of human T1DM. The T cells are considered to be the final executors of β-cell destruction as evidenced by the precipitation or prevention of diabetes by transfer or elimination of CD4 or CD8 T cells, respectively. The CD8 T cell-mediated β-cell killing is likely a major mechanism of β-cell destruction. Some individuals with phenotype of T1DM may lack these markers of autoimmunity.[1]

Diabetes is defined (World Health Organization Criteria)[2] by fasting plasma glucose more than or equal to 7.0 mmol/L (126 mg/dL) and/or 2-hour post glucose load more than or equal to 11.1 mmol/L (200 mg/dL), random plasma glucose more than 200 mg/dL in symptomatic patient, glycosylated hemoglobin (HbA1c) more than 6.5%. Glucose tolerance testing is rarely required, except in atypical cases or very early disease, in which most plasma glucose values are normal and the diagnosis of diabetes is uncertain. Also, it is not unusual for HbA1c to be normal in a case when the duration of diabetes is very short.

Initial approach to the patient includes case history data, the progress of the disease, and phenotype. Type 1 diabetes mellitus is characterized by the rapidity of symptoms, usually considerable hyperglycemia, ketoacidosis, weight loss, polyuria, polydipsia, and frequently no family history of diabetes.[3] Up till now, one believed that majority of children with diabetes has T1DM and diagnosis simply depended on phenotypical and clinical features. However, growing incidence of type 2 diabetes mellitus (T2DM) in children that parallels the incidence of obesity, has created new concern as well as confusion in diagnosis. Added to this, other types of diabetes like monogenic diabetes, latent autoimmune diabetes of adult further blur the picture. Hence, further investigations are needed to classify and diagnose the diabetes in children. Different tests which can be used to classify diabetes include serum insulin and C-peptide levels, autoantibodies, and genetic testing.

Very high fasting insulin and C-peptide levels can help in differential diagnosis of T1DM and early-onset T2DM.[4] However, low concentrations cannot exclude T2DM although serum insulin in T2DM usually does not reach a level as low to T1DM. Further, T1DM during honeymoon phase may show normal C-peptide and insulin levels. In that case, serum immunoglobulin considered as a 'gold standard'. The main autoantibodies in T1DM are reactive to four islet autoantigens (islet cell autoantibodies)—insulinoma-associated antigen-2 (IA2), insulin [micro-insulin autoantibody (IAA)], glutamic acid decarboxylase-65 (GAD65), and zinc transporter-8 (ZnT8); GAD65 is most specific.[5] In combination, these are likely to be present in 60-80% of children and adolescents with T1DM. Measurements of IA2 autoantibodies within 6 months of diagnosis can help differentiate between T1DM and T2DM. These titers decrease after 6 months. Anti- glutamic acid decarboxylase-65 antibodies can be present at diagnosis of T1DM and are persistently positive over time. The diagnostic sensitivity of GAD65, IA2, and insulin autoantibodies varies with age at onset and sex. The GAD65 antibodies are present in 70-80% of Caucasian subjects newly diagnosed with T1DM. The GAD65 antibodies are less frequent among boys developing diabetes before the age of 10 years, but in older children, teenagers, and young adults, the diagnostic sensitivity is 80% in both males and females. The GAD65 antibody titers are higher and more prevalent in patients with other associated autoimmune diseases such as thyroiditis. The IA2 antibodies have been reported in 32-75% of subjects with newly diagnosed T1DM. Insulinoma-associated antigen-2 antibodies decrease in frequency with increasing age at onset. Diagnostic sensitivity varies most with age in IAAs, decreasing from 50-60% in the very young (below age 10 years) to 10% among those diagnosed before 30 years of age. In addition, IAAs often may precede other autoimmune markers, which has led to the hypothesis that insulin may be an autoantigen in T1DM that plays a role early in the pathogenic process.[5] The mechanisms by which these islet autoantigen-specific antibodies show an age-dependent effect are not understood. The fact that the diagnostic sensitivity varies with age and sometimes with sex has important consequences when using diabetes autoantibodies to predict T1DM.

Testing for islet autoantibodies can substitute for expensive genetic testing in those patients suspected of having maturity-onset diabetes of the young (MODY). The prevalence of these antibodies is the same in patients with MODY as in the healthy population. A positive test for positive islet autoantibodies makes MODY highly unlikely. Genetic test for monogenic diabetes includes ABCC8 and KCNJ11.[6,7]

As the basic pathology of T1DM is autoimmune, it is commonly associated with other autoimmune disorders like thyroid dysfunction, celiac disease, pernicious anemia, Addison's disease, and APS; thyroid disorder being most common.[8] The intensity of screening however varies. While screening for thyroid dysfunction should be done routinely at baseline and annually thereafter, that for others should be done when clinically indicated.

TESTS AT DIAGNOSIS

Confirmation of Diabetes

This is seldom an issue what is lacking is the suspicion which lets the child go into metabolic decompensation and land with potentially serious complications like diabetic ketoacidosis (DKA).

Most children are symptomatic of polyuria, polydipsia, and weight loss, and a casual plasma glucose value of more than 200 mg/dL is sufficient for establishing the diagnosis. When symptoms are of very short duration, the HbA1c may not be high or in the range diagnostic of diabetes (>6.5%), hence, the latter is not necessary in such situations though the parents often want to know how long the malady could have been since. In less symptomatic cases, the likelihood of T1DM is lesser and one can go for the standard diagnostic criteria for diagnosis.

Markers of Decompensation

One of the most important things that needs to be done when child is first seen is to rule out the presence of DKA which is established if the pH is less than 7.3, bicarbonate is less than 18 mEq/L, and ketones are positive in urine or blood with a blood glucose more than 200 mg/dL.

Of these, urinary ketones is both easy to measure and universally available at least as dip stick tests, Rothera's and Gerhardt's tests are not as popular or widespread. If there is evidence of ketonuria, then one need to clinically assess the child and investigate further for features of full blown DKA and electrolytes, complete blood picture, investigations for (precipitating) infections.

Psychological Assessment

This is seldom needed and a caring healthcare team that has the time to spare for listening to the concerns and discussing treatment related issues is all that is necessary .The training for maintaining the home glucose measurement diaries and acting on them in conjunctions with treating unit is inculcated as also the training for hypoglycemic and hyperglycemic emergency recognition and first aid treatment.

CHAPTER 6: Initial and Annual Laboratory Investigations

TESTS AT FOLLOW-UP

Glycemic Parameter

Self-monitored Blood Glucose

The reading along with the meal and antecedent insulin dosage are keys to the fine tuning and the targets can be fixed with the parents.

Glycosylated Hemoglobin

Once the glucose values are getting better, this can be measured and the implications and also the reasons of a high value are discussed with the patient. A high HbA1c value often indicated the need for more frequent monitoring since many children just measure one or two values and many do not measure the postmeal values at all.

Hypertension

Hypertension can occur in any young adult with or without T1DM. In individuals with diabetes mellitus, hypertension is usually associated with nephropathy. Hence, evaluation of renal function with serum creatinine, blood urea nitrogen, urine albumin-creatinine ratio, and creatinine clearance are useful in the early detection of nephropathy. Other etiologies for hypertension and proteinuria should be ruled out as diabetic nephropathy is unusual within the first 10 years of onset of T1DM.

Baseline and annual lipid profile should be done in these individuals.

TESTS FOR MICROVASCULAR COMPLICATIONS

These are functions of duration of the disease and the degree of hyperglycemias. They are rare before 5 years of diagnosis and occur more frequently after the onset of puberty. The American Diabetes Association recommendations for these are as under:

Retinopathy: Detailed fundus examination should be done after age of 10 years or at puberty whichever is earlier; if the patient has diabetes of 3–5 years. Thereafter, annual examination is recommended.

Nephropathy: Annual screening for urinary albumin creatinine ratio is recommended after 5 years. Also, a basal creatinine should be done. This can be repeated depending on the age, duration, and treatment of patient.

CONCLUSION

Though the diagnosis of T1DM is clear cut in most instances, it must be remembered that it is solely based on clinical grounds and while one is usually correct, the question about the diagnosis being wrong does sometimes crop up. This could be at diagnosis or follow-up. While all cases need not go through this drill, instances when T1DM is wrongly diagnosed are most likely when the age at detection was less than 6 months or the patient was asymptomatic at diagnosis and has many relatives with diabetes(monogenic diabetes MODY).The former is easier to suspect but both need genetic testing for confirmation. Presence of markers of autoimmunity can confirm the diagnosis of T1DM but their absence cannot in anyway exclude it. Small subsets of T1DM patients do not demonstrate them even at diagnosis and this is also likely when the tests are conducted many years after the diagnosis.

The emerging epidemic of obesity means that T2DM is being encountered in younger subjects and this is another diagnosis to contend with specially when the patient is obese has features suggestive of insulin resistance like acanthosis nigricans, polycystic ovaries, etc.

The foregoing not withstanding clinical judgment though imperfect should be relied upon and no patient should be denied insulin, whenever in doubt, one should always err on the side of caution and administer insulin because in many instances, the other tests are either not easily available (genetic testing) or expensive, and more importantly, not giving it could lead to disastrous situation of ketoacidosis.

REFERENCES

1. Bluestone JA, Herold K, Eisenbarth G. Genetics, pathogenesis and clinical interventions in type 1 diabetes. Nature. 2010;464(7293):1293-300.
2. Definition and diagnosis of diabetes mellitus and intermediate hyperglycemia: report of a WHO/IDF consultation. Geneva: World Health Organization. 2006; p. 21.
3. Diabetes Fact sheet N312. WHO. October 2013. Accessed March, 2014.
4. Wolfsdorf JI. Can biochemical markers discriminate between new-onset type 1 and type 2 diabetes mellitus in children. Nat Clin Pract Endocrinol Metab. 2007;3:800-1.
5. Gilliam LK, Palmer JP, Lernmark Å. Autoantibodies and the disease process of type 1 diabetes mellitus. In: LeRoith D, Taylor SI, Olefsky JM (Editors). Diabetes Mellitus: A Fundamental and Clinical Text, 3rd edition. Philadelphia: Lippincott; 2004. pp. 499-518.
6. McDonald TJ, Colclough K, Brown R, Shields B, Shepherd M, Bingley P, et al. Islet autoantibodies can discriminate maturity-onset diabetes of the young (MODY) from type 1 diabetes. Diabet Med. 2011;28(9):1028-33.
7. Hattersley A, Bruining J, Shield J, Njolstad P, Donaghue KC. The diagnosis and management of monogenic diabetes in children and adolescents. Pediatr Diabetes. 2009;10 Suppl 12:33-42.
8. Van den Driessche A, Eenkhoorn V, Van Gaal L, De Block C. Type 1 diabetes and autoimmune polyglandular syndrome: a clinical review. Neth J Med. 2009;67(11):376-87.

CHAPTER 7

Glycemic Monitoring in Children

Meha Sharma, Deep Dutta, Sanjay Kalra

INTRODUCTION

India is the diabetes capital of the world. As of 2017, the current prevalence of diabetes in India is 9–10% with an additional 14–15% people having prediabetes.[1] The majority of these cases are type 2 diabetes mellitus (T2DM). There has been an exponential increase in T2DM in Indians of all age groups, from young children to adults. The problem is compounded by the increased prevalence of childhood obesity. Apart from T2DM, the incidence of type 1 diabetes mellitus (T1DM) has also been increasing globally (3–4% per year), especially in younger children.[2,3] Despite the significant advancement and options available with insulin therapy, improvement in insulin pharmacodynamics and kinetics, and insulin delivery techniques, a large majority of children with T1DM, especially in developing countries like India, fail to achieve the optimal glycemic targets, and hence are exposed to increased risk of end organ damage, morbidity, and mortality. Glycemic monitoring, an important spoke in the wheel of diabetes management, is perhaps the most neglected aspect of diabetes management, especially in children. Lack of glycemic monitoring, or inappropriate glycemic monitoring, leads to loss of valuable information needed by treating doctors for modulation of insulin therapy, thus exposing the child to increased glycemic variability, hypoglycemia, and hyperglycemic spikes.

The Diabetes Control and Complications Trial (DCCT) also gave us the concept of glycemic memory, viz., a good glycemic control in the early years of T1DM during childhood and adolescence leads to a lower burden of microvascular and macrovascular complication decades later, when the glycemic control may not be as intensive as during the initial years of diagnosis of diabetes. This highlights the increased importance of near-normal glycemic control of diabetes in the early years of diagnosis. This chapter intends to highlight the importance and options available for optimal glycemic monitoring in children with diabetes, focusing on T1DM.

GLYCEMIC MONITORING OPTIONS

Self-monitoring of Blood Glucose

Self-monitoring of blood glucose, is an excellent tool for home monitoring of blood glucose. It is cheap, cost-effective, and provides immediate documentation of hyperglycemia, hypoglycemia, and glycemic variability at a particular point of time allowing for timely modulation of antidiabetic medications including insulin therapy.

Self-monitoring of blood glucose charting helps a lot in fine-tuning insulin therapy, make small adjustments to basal and bolus insulin doses, which helps in ensuring a good glycemic control with lesser glycemic variability. Patients who SMBG in general have a better sense of well-being, are more confident in life, have a feeling they have a better control over their disease and life, and have lesser incidence of depression.[4-6]

Self-monitoring of blood glucose frequency per day may vary from 2–7 times per day. In younger children, a SMBG 4–6 times per day is usually recommended, especially in those with poor glycemic control. A more liberal SMBG of 2–3 times per day can be done in older children with a better glycemic control. A greater frequency of SMBG has been directly associated with a better glycemic control in children with T1DM.[7] The use of SMBG during exercise may also allow improved insulin management and a decreased risk for hypoglycemia during and following exercise.

Rotation of sites for testing apart from the traditionally used and most validated site, the fingertips, has an important role in ensuring long-term compliance to SMBG practices. Alternative sites for SMBG include the palm of the hand or the forearm. In the fasting state, glucose readings from the forearm are similar to the fingertip.[8] Alternate sites for SMBG sometimes have limitations of being slower in reflecting falling blood glucose levels, and hence in the setting of suspected hypoglycemia, it is always advised that fingertips are used for crosschecking the diagnosis.

A large variety of glucometers are available in the market for SMBG testing. Impedance-based glucometers are in general believed to be more accurate than colorimetric-based glucometers. Glucometers measure capillary blood glucose, which is then extrapolated to venous blood glucose using complex inbuilt algorithms. It must be remembered that glucometer readings are most accurate in the blood glucose ranges of 60–160 mg/dL. For blood glucose values, both above and below these ranges, the deviation from venous blood glucose values increases. Hence, whenever in doubt, the SMBG reading should be crosschecked with a simultaneous venous blood glucose value measurement.

Self-monitoring of Blood Glucose Logs and Record Keeping of Blood Glucose Charting

Another important, and perhaps the most neglected aspect of glycemic monitoring in diabetes, is the gross inadequacy in maintaining of blood glucose charting and glucometer SMBG logs. It is not uncommon to see, in clinical practice, patients coming with glucometer reading values jotted down on bits and pieces of paper. The caregiver, often, finds it difficult to interpret such values as often the factors, like the day of blood glucose checking, the timing of the day of blood glucose checking, and its relation to meals, are missing, thus hampering optimal treatment modulation.

Honesty and frankness are key components in the patient-doctor relationship with regards to diabetes management. It is important for the medical health professional to ensure that he/she does not appear intimidating to the patients and their relatives. Inaccurate blood glucose charting, malingering, missing, checking blood glucose values in the glucometers but failing to enter them in the SMBG logs (especially when the glucose readings are too high or low) are some of the problems encountered by the authors during interpretation of blood glucose logs in children with T1DM. In a large cohort of children with T1DM, errors in blood glucose logs have been demonstrated to have an adverse impact on long-term glycemic control by the authors (accepted, in press). Proper storage of SMBG logs are important as they can then be traced back several months later and the trend in glycemic control in the child can be traced over long periods of time, which can further help in modulating therapy.

The onus is on the treating doctor to ensure that the children as well as the parents are properly taught 7-point blood glucose charting system at the time of diagnosis of diabetes itself. It is a good practice to always share with the patients, printouts of blood glucose logs, which can be used by them. Because of the significant financial burden associated with regular 7-point blood glucose charting, options of less frequent glucose charting, with rotation of timings of blood glucose charting should be discussed with the patients and their caregivers, especially in a stable patient with T1DM.

Frequent home review of records to identify patterns in glycemic levels and subsequent adjustment in diabetes management are required for successful intensified diabetes management. In some instances, especially among young children and teenagers, maintaining written monitoring records may be difficult. In such scenarios, a computerized blood glucose monitoring data for review can be maintained, e.g., in Microsoft Excel spreadsheets; this may substitute for a manual record, although details of management may be lost with this method. Such sheets can easily be shared with the treating physician through mails or smartphones. Applications are available in smartphones now, which can be used for the same purpose.

Sick-day Guidelines

It is important to train the patients and their caregivers regarding the sick-day guidelines in T1DM. They should be sensitized the importance of more frequent blood glucose charting in a sick child with T1DM, and the need for serum/urine ketone monitoring if the SMBG values are persistently higher than 250 mg/dL. Lack of eating by the child should be associated with cessation of insulin therapy, as this would predispose the child to ketosis, both due to starvation as well as diabetic ketoacidosis. They should not hesitate in contacting the treating doctor in case of any doubts. These small steps are critical to avoid serious life-threatening hypoglycemic as well as hyperglycemic crisis in the child.

Glycosylated Hemoglobin

Glycosylated hemoglobin (HbA1c) is a measure of long-term glycemic control as well as glycemic variability. It gives a glycemic history of previous 3 months usually, unless the patient has some disorder affecting the half-life of red blood cells. Elevated HbA1c also predicts long-term microvascular and macrovascular outcomes.[4,5] Variations in HbA1c explained 96% of the complications in the DCCT, which involved children and adults with T1DM.[6]

Every child should have a minimum of one measurement of HbA1c per year. Ideally, there should be 4–6 measurements per year in younger children and 3–4 measurements per year in older children.[7] Patients with poorer glycemic control need more frequent measurements, and the measurements can be delayed in children who have achieved the glycemic target range. A target range for all age-groups of less than 7.5% is recommended as per most of the guidelines. Each child should have their targets individually determined with the goal of achieving a value as close to normal as possible while avoiding severe hypoglycemia as well as frequent mild-to-moderate hypoglycemia. The goal is to avoid the long-term microvascular and macrovascular complications of diabetes while also avoiding sequelae of acute hypoglycemia and the central nervous system changes associated with both hypoglycemia and hyperglycemia.

The youngest children (<6 years) are at increased risk for adverse neurologic outcomes from severe hypoglycemia, as the first 6 years are crucial for the neurodevelopment and cognitive development of a child. Since the brain axis is still maturing in these children, they have a form of physiologic hypoglycemic awareness, and have no symptoms when blood glucose values are less than 70 mg/dL. This exposes them to silent brain injury and hypoglycemic brain damage, which can have severe long-term outcomes. Hence, we should be really cautious about hypoglycemia while managing diabetes in children less than 6 years of age.

As teens approach adulthood, the hypothalamic brain axis is more matured, and hence, these children can more robustly detect hypoglycemia, hence a glycemic target of less than 7 mg/dL should be targeted in these children like that in adults. However, it is important to recognize the hormonal alterations and psychological changes in adolescence, their rebellious and independent streak, often have an adverse effect on medication compliance, which may have a bad impact on glycemic control. Of all age-groups, adolescents are currently the farthest from achieving HbA1c of less than 7.5 mg/dL, reflecting the diabetes mismanagement that frequently accompanies the increased independence in diabetes care during the adolescent years, as well as the effect of psychological and hormonal challenges of adolescence.

Facilities for the measurement of HbA1c should be available to all centers caring for young people with diabetes. Frequency of measurement will depend on local facilities and availability.

Fructosamine and Other Glycated Products

Fructosamine measures the glycation of serum proteins predominantly albumin and is a measure of glycemic control and variability over the previous 21–28 days, which is much shorter than that of HbA1c (3 months). Fructosamine is a useful tool for monitoring glycemia in individuals with abnormal red cell survival time like hemoglobinopathies, sickle cell anemia, patients with recent transfusion, or severe anemia.

Continuous Glucose Monitoring Systems

For children with diabetes, a good quality of life (QOL) includes enjoying meals at one's own terms, freedom of choosing what to eat, feeling safe in school, and with support and encouragement from parents, teachers in schools, siblings, and friends. Diabetes management imposes considerable lifestyle demands that are difficult and often frustrating for children to negotiate at a young age, especially when they do not have a full understanding of the disease pathophysiology and long-term outcomes. Insulin pump and continuous glucose monitoring systems provide patients with more flexibility in their daily life and information about glucose fluctuations. Several studies report improvements in glycemic control in children with T1DM using the insulin pump or sensor-augmented pump therapy.[9] Further, emerging closed loop and web- and phone-based technologies have great potential for supporting diabetes self-management and perhaps QOL.[9]

Digital Monitoring

In recent years, interest has grown in fields such as e-health and m-health, which have used modern communication platforms to provide better diabetes care.[10] Digital health, an all-embracing term, takes this movement forward.[11] The United States Food and Drug Administration defines digital health as including mobile health, health information technology, wearable devices, tele-health and telemedicine, and personalized medicine.[12] The aim is to reduce inefficiencies, improve access, reduce costs, increase quality, and make medicine more personalized for patients. Glycemic monitoring is increasingly being done though digital technology platforms, which provide more efficient glucose monitoring and management systems.

For example, transfer of data from a blood glucose-monitoring device, coupled with electronic food, physical activity, and lifestyle daily entries, should be able to prompt insulin dose adjustment and lifestyle modification. If required, a change in insulin regimes may be suggested as well. Seamless transmission of data to automated algorithms facilitates accurate, timely, and appropriate decision-making.

PARENTAL ROLE IN GLYCEMIC MONITORING AND CONTROL

Managing and monitoring diabetes in children is a team effort of the patient and the caregivers. Parents should develop confidence in their wards and should progressively shift the responsibility of glycemic monitoring and insulin administration to their children. This will make the children more autonomous, more confident of their disease state, which will have a positive impact on their larger life as a whole. Parents and children can work as a team and the tasks shared may include meal planning, SMBG and sharing and discussing glucose logs for fine-tuning of insulin dose to be administered, setting goals, as well as giving positive feedback when possible.[13] The role of the parents should be to be available to offer guidance or advice when any problems occur.[13,14]

Studies have shown that parents who give time to their children, are warm and affectionate and have positive discussion with the children, these children tend to have a better glycemic control and were better oriented to diabetes self-care and management (e.g., home blood glucose monitoring, giving insulin shots, not skipping meals).[15,16] A key to a good glycemic control among children with diabetes is a fine balance of freedom along with supervision by the parents over their wards.[17]

CONCLUSION

Glycemic monitoring in children is a team effort involving the patient, caregivers (parents), and healthcare professionals. With the advent of technology, a great variety of options are available now. Optimal use of these options can play a great role in improving QOL and long-term outcomes in children with diabetes.

REFERENCES

1. Dutta D, Mukhopadhyay S. Intervening at prediabetes stage is critical to controlling the diabetes epidemic among Asian Indians. Indian J Med Res. 2016;143:23-26.
2. Patterson CC, Gyurus E, Rosenbauer J, Cinek O, Neu A, Schober E, et al. Trends in childhood type 1 diabeetes incidence in Europe during 19892008: evidence of nonuniformity over time in rates of increase. Diabetologia. 2012;55(8):21427.
3. Bell RA, MayerDavis EJ, Beyer JW, D'Agostino RB Jr, Lawrence JM, Linder B, et al. Diabetes in nonHispanic white youth: prevalence, incidence, and clinical characteristics: the SEARCH for Diabetes in Youth Study. Diabetes Care. 2009;32 Suppl 2:S10211.
4. Effect of intensive diabetes treatment on the development and progression of long-term complications in adolescents with insulin-dependent diabetes mellitus: Diabetes Control and Complications Trial. Diabetes Control and Complications Trial Research Group. J Pediatr. 1994;125:177-88.
5. The effect of intensive treatment of diabetes on the development and progression of long-term complications in insulin-dependent diabetes mellitus. The Diabetes Control and Complications Trial Research Group. N Engl J Med. 1993;329: 977-86.
6. Lachin JM, Genuth S, Nathan DM, Zinman B, Rutledge BN, DCCT/EDIC Research Group. Effect of glycemic exposure on the risk of microvascular complications in the diabetes control and complications trial–revisited. Diabetes. 2008;57:995-1001.
7. Rewers MJ, Pillay K, de Beaufort C, Craig ME, Hanas R, Acerini CL, et al. ISPAD Clinical Practice Consensus Guidelines 2014. Assessment and monitoring of glycemic control in children and adolescents with diabetes. Pediatr Diabetes. 2014;15 Suppl 20:102-14.
8. Lucidarme N, Alberti C, Zaccaria I, Claude E, Tubiana-Rufi N. Alternate-site testing is reliable in children and adolescents with type 1 diabetes, except at the forearm for hypoglycemia detection. Diabetes Care. 2005;28:710-1.
9. Hirose M, Beverly EA, Weinger K. Quality of life and technology: impact on children and families with diabetes. Curr Diab Rep. 2012;12(6):711-20.
10. Eysenbach G. What is e-health? J Med Internet Res. 2001;3(2):e20.
11. Nicholas D, Huntington P, Williams P, Blackburn P. Digital health information provision and health outcomes. Journal of Information Science. 2001;27(4):265-76.
12. US Food and Drug Administration (2017). Digital health. [online] Available from www.fda.gov/medicaldevices/digitalhealth/default.htm. [Accessed February, 2017].
13. Young MT, Lord JH, Patel NJ, Gruhn MA, Jaser SS. Good cop, bad cop: quality of parental involvement in type 1 diabetes management in youth. Curr Diab Rep. 2014;14(11):546.
14. Vesco AT, Anderson BJ, Laffel LM, Dolan LM, Ingerski LM, Hood KK. Responsibility sharing between adolescents with type 1 diabetes and their caregivers: importance of adolescent perceptions on diabetes management and control. J Pediatr Psychol. 2010;35(10):1168-77.
15. Shorer M, David R, Schoenberg-Taz M, Levavi-Lavi I, Phillip M, Meyerovitch J. Role of parenting style in achieving metabolic control in adolescents with type 1 diabetes. Diabetes Care. 2011;34(8):1735-7.
16. Greene MS, Mandleco B, Roper SO, Marshall ES, Dyches T. Metabolic control, self-care behaviors, and parenting in adolescents with type 1 diabetes a correlational study. Diabetes Educ. 2010;36(2):326-36.
17. Céspedes-Knadle YM, Munoz CE. Development of a group intervention for teens with type 1 diabetes. J Specialists Group Work. 2011;36(4):278-95.

CHAPTER 8

Childhood Diabetes: Common Pitfalls in Diagnosis and Management

Sweety Agrawal, Nikhil Tandon

INTRODUCTION

Childhood diabetes comprises type 1, type 2, fibrocalculous pancreatic diabetes, and rare genetic causes like maturity onset diabetes in the young, neonatal diabetes, and mitochondrial diabetes. Type 1 diabetes mellitus (T1DM) is the most common form, however, type 2 diabetes mellitus (T2DM) is increasingly being reported in children and adolescents. An attempt at appropriate diagnosis and classification of youth onset diabetes must be made in view of the varying treatment options, prognosis, complication rates, and disease associations which have to be screened for. For instance, patients with some genetic forms of diabetes, like hepatocyte nuclear factor (HNF)-1α mutation, show remarkable sensitivity to sulfonylureas and do not require insulin therapy at onset. In view of the spectrum of childhood diabetes, specifically with implications for therapy, we attempt to look at the various pitfalls in the diagnosis and management of childhood diabetes.

PITFALLS IN DIAGNOSIS OF CHILDHOOD DIABETES

Diagnosis of diabetes in childhood is made using the American Diabetes Association (ADA) criteria. As per the National Institute for Health and Care Excellence (NICE) guidelines on diagnosis and management of diabetes in children and young people (2015), while diagnosing diabetes in a child or young person, assume T1DM unless there are strong indications of T2DM, monogenic or mitochondrial diabetes. But at the same time, the physician should be alert towards the possibility of other types of diabetes. Incidence of T2DM in youth is increasing and should be suspected in appropriate situations like childhood obesity, strong family history of T2DM, acanthosis nigricans, and presence of associated comorbidities such as polycystic ovarian syndrome. However, prepubertal children are unlikely to have T2DM even if obese and antibodies are useful in making the diagnosis. In an infant or toddler, classical symptoms of diabetes are often overlooked or ascribed to other causes until the disease has progressed to frank diabetic ketoacidosis (DKA). The hyperventilation of DKA may be misdiagnosed as pneumonia or asthma, abdominal pain may simulate an acute abdomen and polyuria may be mistaken for a urinary tract infection thereby delaying the diagnosis. Efforts should be made to categorize the patient into one of the various forms of diabetes on the basis of clinical signs, symptoms, and investigations as described below.

Type 1 Diabetes Mellitus

Type 1 diabetes mellitus usually presents with abrupt onset of symptoms including polyuria, polydipsia, weight loss, and excessive tiredness. About 15–70% of the patients have DKA at presentation[1] and glycosylated hemoglobin (HbA1c) levels are markedly elevated. These patients are usually lean and family history of diabetes is often lacking. They usually show presence of islet cell antibodies and have absent or very low pancreatic β-cell reserve on the C-peptide test. These patients require lifelong insulin for control of hyperglycemia and prevention of ketoacidosis.

Type 2 Diabetes Mellitus

Consider type 2 diabetes in the following scenario:[2]
- Strong family history of T2DM
- Presence of obesity
- Age above 10 years
- Evidence of insulin resistance in the form of acanthosis nigricans
- High risk racial or ethnic group
- Absent islet autoantibodies
- Elevated C-peptide
- No insulin requirement, or an insulin requirement of less than 0.5 units/kg body weight/day after the partial remission phase (honeymoon phase).

UNCERTAINTIES IN CLASSIFICATION OF YOUTH ONSET TYPE 1 AND TYPE 2 DIABETES MELLITUS

Often the distinction between T1DM and T2DM is not clear because of the following reasons:
- Due to increasing prevalence of childhood obesity, as many as 30% of newly diagnosed T1DM are obese
- A significant proportion of pediatric T2DM patients present with ketoacidosis[3]
- There is considerable overlap in insulin or C-peptide levels between T1DM and T2DM at onset and over the first year. This is due to the honeymoon phase and the effects of glucotoxicity and lipotoxicity to impair insulin secretion at the time of testing in both T1DM and T2DM. Hence, C-peptide measurements are not recommended in the acute phase. However, persistence of C-peptide above normal level for age is unusual in T1DM after 12–14 months[4]
- Insulin resistance exists in both T1DM and T2DM, although it is more severe in T2DM[5]
- Measurement of antibodies helps in diagnosis, however, it may be limited by lack of ready availability of assays, cost, and varying rates of antibody positivity in different ethnic groups.

CHAPTER 8: Childhood Diabetes: Common Pitfalls in Diagnosis and Management

Pancreatic Diabetes

Fibrocalculous pancreatic diabetes (FCPD) is seen in tropical countries secondary to nonalcoholic chronic calcific pancreatitis. Patients are usually lean and from a poor socioeconomic class. Diagnosis should be considered in patients with:[6]

- Evidence of chronic pancreatitis in the form of pancreatic calculi on X-ray abdomen or unequivocal ductal dilatation on ultrasonography/computed tomography or at least three of the following:
  - Recurrent abdominal pain since childhood
  - Steatorrhea
  - Altered pancreatic morphology, e.g., increased echogenicity
  - Abnormal pancreatic function tests
- Absence of other causes of chronic pancreatitis, i.e., alcoholism, hepatobiliary disease, primary hyperparathyroidism, etc.

Monogenic and Other Types of Diabetes in the Young

Maturity Onset Diabetes of the Young

Maturity onset diabetes of the young (MODY) should be considered in the following scenario:[7]

- Autosomal dominant inheritance with at least three generations involved
- Onset of diabetes below 25 years of age
- Absence of ketosis
- Insulin independence (although insulin may be needed for optimal control).

Diagnosis and subtyping can be confirmed by genetic testing. Specific features can suggest subtypes of MODY such as renal cysts in HNF-1β and macrosomia or neonatal hypoglycemia in HNF-4α mutations.

Neonatal Diabetes Mellitus

One should think about the possibility of neonatal diabetes in the following situations:
- Onset of diabetes in the first 6 months of life—T1DM being rare in this age group
- Absence of ketosis
- Absence of antibodies.

Mitochondrial Diabetes

Mostly present in young adulthood or middle age with diabetes, onset in pediatric age group is rare. Diabetes onset is usually insidious. It should be suspected in patients with diabetes and sensorineural hearing loss inherited from the mother's side.

Syndromic Diabetes

Consider in patients with associated features like deafness, retinitis pigmentosa, or optic atrophy or features specific for a particular syndrome like Wolfram syndrome, Down's syndrome, Turner syndrome, Klinefelter syndrome, Bardet-Biedl syndrome, and Friedreich ataxia.

Monogenic Insulin Resistance Syndromes

These are associated with severe acanthosis nigricans with increased insulin requirements. Consider congenital lipodystrophies in patients with typical physical features, i.e., muscular appearance with absence of subcutaneous fat.

Genetic testing should be performed in this group—molecular diagnosis of neonatal diabetes mellitus and MODY gives information on which patients can be treated with sulfonylureas and which patients have transient neonatal diabetes mellitus which will resolve but may relapse later. Identification of children with syndromic and monogenic diabetes helps to predict the expected clinical course of disease and guide the most appropriate management. It also enables genetic counseling and triggers genetic testing in other members of the family.

PITFALLS IN MANAGEMENT OF CHILDHOOD DIABETES

Management of Type 1 and Type 2 Diabetes Mellitus

The main features in T1DM management are nutrition management, physical activity, insulin therapy, and self-monitoring of blood glucose. Lifestyle modification is the cornerstone of management of T2DM. As per the ADA 2016 guidelines, metformin is the only oral hypoglycemic agent currently approved for use in children with T2DM. Insulin therapy is initiated if the child presents with ketosis or ketoacidosis. Moreover, insulin is also preferred when the distinction between T1DM and T2DM is unclear and in patients who have random blood glucose concentrations of more than or equal to 250 mg/dL and/or HbA1c >9%. Treatment goals are similar in T1DM and T2DM with target HbA1c in all pediatric age groups being <7.5%.

Lifestyle changes including dietary advice and regular physical activity with an emphasis on maintaining proper meal and exercise timings must be emphasized. A major pitfall in management in this group of patients is a lack of diabetes education including knowledge about insulin injection technique, rotation, and proper blood glucose monitoring. Without adequate blood glucose monitoring, achievement of good glycemic control is difficult and the risk of acute hyperglycemic crises as well as hypoglycemic episodes rises. Regular HbA1c monitoring is also essential. Frequent review of home records for adjustment in diabetes management is also required for successful treatment. Education about symptoms of hypoglycemia and corrective measures to be taken for them is essential. Failure to educate the patient regarding sick day guidelines also contributes to increased risk of acute emergencies. Another major pitfall is an inability to address the rising rates of obesity in T1DM patients and evaluate for the presence of comorbidities including hypertension, dyslipidemia, and metabolic syndrome and take corrective measures for treatment. Finally, regular monitoring for diabetes related complications is essential and helps in timely detection and treatment of the same.

Treatment of Monogenic Forms of Diabetes

If genetic testing for the various forms of MODY is available, and diagnosis can be confirmed, sulfonylureas are recommended as the first line treatment for HNF-4α and HNF-1α mutations as these patients are sensitive to this class of drugs. Good control may be maintained for many years, although eventually most patients progress to insulin. Patients with glucokinase mutations have mild hyperglycemia and antidiabetic agents are not needed in most patients.

CHAPTER 8: Childhood Diabetes: Common Pitfalls in Diagnosis and Management

Some forms of neonatal diabetes mellitus also respond to sulfonylureas while others are transient and are likely to resolve, but may relapse. In partial lipodystrophy, insulin sensitizers like metformin and glitazones may be effective initially but glitazones can cause further accumulation of fat in face and neck. Patients with congenital severe lipodystrophy benefit from treatment with recombinant leptin. Patients with mitochondrial diabetes may respond to diet or oral hypoglycemic agents initially but often require insulin within months or years. Metformin has to be avoided as it may trigger episodes of lactic acidosis.

Management of Comorbidities

Comorbidities may already be present at the time of diagnosis in youth with T2DM and these should not be overlooked. Hence, blood pressure measurement, fasting lipid profile, assessment for proteinuria, and dilated eye examination is to be performed at diagnosis and periodically thereafter. Moreover, additional problems which should be addressed are polycystic ovary disease, sleep apnea, hepatic steatosis, and psychosocial issues. Similarly, patients with T1DM must be screened for coexistent diseases including hypothyroidism and celiac disease. Those with FCPD and evidence of exocrine insufficiency need replacement of pancreatic enzymes. This might contribute towards better glycemic control as well. Moreover, FCPD is associated with a higher risk of pancreatic cancer later in life, with one series reporting a relative risk 100 times higher than the general population.[8] Therefore, screening for pancreatic adenocarcinoma should be done if there is a history of weight loss or jaundice.

CONCLUSION

All youth onset diabetes is not T1DM. A detailed history, physical examination, and appropriate investigations help to classify diabetes and initiate appropriate treatment. One needs to have a high index of suspicion to detect the rare forms of diabetes which may benefit from a different management strategy and needs care of associated conditions. Finally, treatment needs to be individualized and the best treatment regimen for an individual patient must be determined.

REFERENCES

1. Wolfsdorf JI, Allgrove J, Craig ME, , Edge J, Glaser N, Jain V, et al; International Society for Pediatric and Adolescent Diabetes. ISPAD Clinical Practice Consensus Guidelines 2014. Diabetic ketoacidosis and hyperglycemic hyperosmolar state. Pediatr Diabetes. 2014;15(Suppl. 20):154-79.
2. Couper JJ, Haller MJ, Ziegler A-G, Knip M, Ludvigsson J, Craig ME. Phases of type 1 diabetes in children and adolescents. Pediatric Diabetes. 2014:15(Suppl. 20):18-25.
3. American Diabetes Association. Type 2 diabetes in children and adolescents: consensus conference report. Diabetes Care. 2000:23:381-9.
4. The Epidemiology of Diabetes Interventions and Complications Study Group. Sustained effect of intensive treatment of type 1 diabetes mellitus on development and progression of diabetic nephropathy: the Epidemiology of Diabetes Interventions and Complications (EDIC) study. JAMA. 2003:290:2159-67.
5. Nadeau KJ, Regensteiner JG, Bauer TA, Brown MS, Dorosz JL, Hull A, et al. Insulin resistance in adolescents with type 1 diabetes and its relationship to cardiovascular function. J Clin Endocrinol Metab. 2010:95:513-21.
6. Mohan V, Nagalotimath SJ, Yajnik CS, Tripathy BB. Fibrocalculous pancreatic diabetes. Diabetes Metab Rev. 1998;14(2):153-70.
7. Fajans SS. Maturity-onset diabetes of the young (MODY). Diabetes Metab Rev. 1989;5:579-606.
8. Chari ST, Mohan V, Pitchumoni CS, Viswanathan M, Madanagopalan N, Lowenfels AB. Risk of pancreatic carcinoma in tropical calcifying pancreatitis: an epidemiologic study. Pancreas. 1994;9(1):62-6.

SECTION 3

Nonpharmacological Management

Editor
PV Rao

CHAPTER 9

Medical Nutrition Therapy in Children with Type 1 Diabetes Mellitus

Anjana Hulse, KM Prasanna Kumar

INTRODUCTION

According to Diabetes Control and Complications Trial (DCCT), United Kingdom Prospective Diabetes Study (UKPDS), and other existing literature, optimal glycemic control is extremely important in order to prevent microvascular complications of diabetes.[1,2] Medical nutrition therapy (MNT) was an important aspect of diabetes management in DCCT.[1] Medical nutrition therapy is an integral part of disease management and self-management in children with diabetes.[3] In practice, as the literature is scanty on nutritional management in diabetes in children, many nutritional recommendations and the information given to the patients are not based on scientific evidence.

Nutritional aspect of diabetes management in children has gone through a revolutionary change in the past few years. Recent nutrition recommendations for children and adolescents with type 1 diabetes mellitus (T1DM) focus on achieving optimal glycemic control without compromising on growth and without excessive hypoglycemia.[4] One should keep in mind the type of food available, socioeconomic status of the family, ethnic, and cultural diversity within the country, while planning a nutritional plan for a child with diabetes. Dietary recommendations should be such that it should meet not only the nutritional requirements and psychological needs of the individual child but also that of the whole family. In short, affordability, accessibility, and acceptability are crucial before planning a nutritional advice. This is achievable through personalized meal planning, flexible insulin regimens, self-monitoring of blood glucose, dose adjustments as needed, and diabetes education. Nutritional therapy when used with other components of diabetes care, can further improve clinical and metabolic outcome.

The American Diabetes Association (ADA) 2009 clinical practice recommendations state that "individuals who have diabetes should receive individualized MNT as needed to achieve treatment goals, preferably provided by a registered dietician familiar with the components of diabetes MNT".[5,6] International Society for Paediatric and Adolescent Diabetes (ISPAD) recommends that a specialist pediatric dietician with experience in childhood diabetes should be part of the interdisciplinary pediatric diabetes team, be available at diagnosis, and in the first year thereafter to provide a minimum of two to four follow-up sessions.[4,6,7]

WHAT IS MEDICAL NUTRITION THERAPY?

Medical nutrition therapy is defined as "nutritional diagnostic therapy and counseling services for the purpose of disease management, which are furnished by a registered dietician or nutrition professional."[6,7] The American Dietetic Association defines the nutrition counseling component of MNT as "a supportive process to set priorities, establish goals, and create individualized action plans which acknowledge and foster responsibility for self-care."[8]

GOALS OF MEDICAL NUTRITION THERAPY IN CHILDREN WITH TYPE 1 DIABETES

- To provide adequate calorie to ensure optimal growth and development
- To maintain optimal metabolic status in the form of normal or near normal glycemic status, lipid profile, and blood pressure
- To address individual nutritional needs taking into consideration personal and ethnic background
- To achieve and maintain an appropriate body mass index (BMI) and waist circumference. This includes the strong recommendation for children and young people to undertake regular physical activity
- To provide flexible dietary regimen so that the psychological well-being of the child is preserved
- To integrate insulin regimen in the lifestyle of the child or adolescent
- To prevent and treat acute complications of diabetes such as hypoglycemia, hyperglycemic episodes, illness, and exercise-related problems.

ENERGY REQUIREMENTS, CARBOHYDRATES AND TYPE 1 DIABETES MELLITUS

When a child is diagnosed with diabetes and started on insulin, appetite and energy requirements will be very high. This is in order to replenish the catabolic weight loss. The energy requirement gradually decreases when appropriate weight gain is achieved. This may take about 6 weeks.[9] Energy requirement of a child depends on various factors such as age and size of the child, physical activity, associated illnesses, type, and availability of food. During puberty, energy requirement, as well as insulin requirement increases significantly. Therefore, dietary requirement of children with T1DM should be reviewed regularly.[10] In general, overweight and obesity is increasing in children. Hence regular monitoring in the form of height weight, BMI and waist circumference is essential for early detection or prevention of obesity and related complications.[11]

TABLE 1: Estimated daily calorie requirement for children

Age	1 year	2–3 years	4-8 years	9–13 years	14–18 years
Calorie (kcal)	900	1,000	–	–	–
Female	–	–	1,200	1,600	1,800
Male	–	–	1,400	1,800	2,200

Unlike in adults, total daily energy requirement varies in children based on their age, pubertal status, and physical activity. American Academy of Pediatrics recommends daily calorie requirement for a sedentary child as mentioned in table 1. Increased physical activity will require additional calories: up to 200 kcal/day if moderately physically active and 200–400 kcal/day if physically very active.[12]

National guidelines for adults and children with diabetes in Australia and Canada recommend a carbohydrate intake to provide 45–60% energy.[13,14] Similar recommendations have come from other scientific bodies.[15] In patients with T1DM, it is the total number of calories than the type of carbohydrates that affects the glycemic response.

The usefulness of low glycemic diet in children with T1DM is debatable. Studies comparing low glycemic index diet to high glycemic diet for longer than one day have not shown any benefit when premeal insulin doses were adjusted to the calorie intake.[16,17] There is a strong relationship between premeal insulin dose and post meal glycemic response to carbohydrate content in the meal. In individuals who were on intensive insulin therapy who used insulin carbohydrate ratio, the total carbohydrate in the meal did not change glycemic response.[17] This view is further supported by the DCCT in which the subjects who adjusted their premeal insulin based on the carbohydrate content of their meal had their glycosylated hemoglobin (HbA1c) 0.5% (p <0.03) lower than those who did not alter their insulin doses.[1] For individuals who are on fixed dose of regular and intermediate acting (NPH) insulin, consistency in daily carbohydrate intake in terms of amount and type of carbohydrate is essential to optimize glycemic control.[17]

FOOD COMPONENTS

Carbohydrates

It is universally recommended that carbohydrates should not be restricted in children so that their growth is not compromised. According to ISPAD Clinical Practice Consensus Guidelines 2014 Compendium, caregivers should encourage healthy sources of carbohydrate foods such as whole grain breads and cereals, legumes (peas, beans, and lentils), fruit, vegetables, and low-fat dairy products (full fat in children under 2 years).[4] Sucrose can be substituted in moderation for other carbohydrate sources without causing hyperglycemia. If added, sucrose should be appropriately balanced against insulin doses.[18]

Fiber

Intake of a variety of fiber-containing foods such as legumes, fruit, vegetables, and whole grain cereals should be encouraged. Soluble fiber in vegetables, legumes, and fruit may be particularly useful in helping to reduce lipid levels. Insoluble fiber found in grains and cereals promotes healthy bowel function. Higher fiber foods may help to improve satiety and replace more energy dense foods. Processed foods tend to be lower in fiber. Therefore, unprocessed, fresh foods should be encouraged. Children should be encouraged to consume water along with food rich in fiber. Daily recommendation for fiber in grams for children older than 2 years is "age in years plus five".[4,19]

Proteins

Intake decreases during childhood from approximately 2 g/kg/day in early infancy to 1 g/kg/day for a 10 years old and to 0.8–0.9 g/kg/day in later adolescence.[20] High protein drink and food supplements are generally unnecessary for children with diabetes. Sources of vegetable protein such as legumes should be encouraged. Sources of animal protein also recommended include fish, lean cuts of meat, and low-fat dairy products. Protein intake should be at the lower limit of normal in children with T1DM with persistent microalbuminuria or nephropathy. However, there is insufficient evidence to restrict protein intake.[4]

Fat

The primary goal regarding dietary fat in clinical practice is usually to decrease the intake of total fat, saturated fat, and trans-fatty acids. Monounsaturated fatty acids (MUFA) and polyunsaturated fatty acids (PUFA) can be used as substitutes to improve the lipid. About 10–20% energy from MUFA is recommended.[21] Monounsaturated fatty acids is found in olive, sesame, and rapeseed oils, and also in nuts and peanut butter may be beneficial in controlling lipid levels and convey some protection against cardiovascular disease. Less than 10% energy from PUFA is recommended.[21] Polyunsaturated fatty acids derived from vegetable origins such as corn, sunflower, safflower, and soybean or from oily marine fish may assist in the reduction of lipid levels when substituted for saturated fat. Advice for children is to eat oily fish once or twice weekly in amounts of 80–120 g.[3] Medical nutrition therapy should be tailored to reduce saturated fat intake to less than 7%, and increase dietary sources of both soluble fiber and antioxidants. Only if glucose control and/or lifestyle cannot be optimized, or hyperlipidemia persists despite these measures, pharmacological treatment should be considered.[4]

Micronutrients

Children with T1DM require the same amount of micronutrients as normal healthy children. They do not need routine supplementation of vitamins or minerals in the form of drugs. They should be encouraged to consume fresh fruits and vegetables which are rich in micronutrients. According to some studies, the incidence of vitamin D deficiency in children with T1DM seems to be higher than the general population.[22] When vitamin D deficiency is diagnosed, the child should be treated in line with normal vitamin D deficiency treatment recommendations.

Children with diabetes should limit their salt intake to at least that of recommendations for the general population. A guide is 1,500 mg/day (3.8 g of salt/day) for children aged greater than equal to 9 years. Guidelines for salt intake in younger children are 1–3 years: 1,000 mg/day (2.5 g salt/day); 4–8 years: 1,200 mg/day (3 g salt/day).[4]

Artificial Sweeteners

Water should be encouraged instead of sugary drinks. Sugary drinks are not encouraged as they lead to weight gain and may cause hyperglycemia as the insulin dose is commonly not matched to the carbohydrate quantity. Saccharin, neotame, aspartame, and sucralose are commonly used in low sugar, "light" or "diet" products to improve sweetness and palatability. Acceptable daily intakes (ADI) have been established in some countries. There are no published scientific reports documenting harm from an intake of artificial sweeteners in doses not exceeding ADI.[4]

TOOLS FOR DIETARY COUNSELING IN CHILDREN WITH TYPE 1 DIABETES MELLITUS

Considerable time should be spent on educating the child and the family about carbohydrate containing food and balanced diet at the time of diagnosis as well as during the follow-up visits. Food pyramid and recently food plate methods are used to educate the families about healthy eating. The visual display of food varieties and portion sizes is a good way to educate children and their parents. There is no international consensus on the most appropriate tools and method/s for education, that can be made easily understandable for the child and his/her family.

Carbohydrate Counting

Carbohydrate counting is a meal planning approach that focuses on carbohydrate as the primary nutrient affecting postprandial glycemic response. It aims to improve glycemic control and allow flexibility of food choices. Various studies have demonstrated improved glycemic control in terms of reduction of HbA1c by 0.4–0.8% in subjects using carbohydrate counting method.[23,24] The DCCT too used carbohydrate counting as one of its tools in the intensive group.[1] Three levels of carbohydrate counting have been identified by the American Academy of Nutrition and Dietetics.[25]

Level 1

Consistent carbohydrate intake. This level introduces the basic concept of carbohydrate as the food component that raises blood glucose. A consistent intake of carbohydrate is encouraged using exchange or portion lists of measured quantities of food. This is appropriate for those on twice daily insulin doses where a consistent carbohydrate intake from day-to-day is required.

SECTION 3: Nonpharmacological Management

Level 2

Pattern management principles. This level is an intermediate step in which patients continue to eat regular carbohydrate, use a consistent baseline insulin dose and frequently monitor blood glucose levels. They learn to recognize patterns of blood glucose response to carbohydrate intake modified by insulin and exercise. With this understanding and team support they make adjustments to their insulin dose for food and exercise to achieve blood glucose goals.

Level 3

Insulin carbohydrate ratio (ICR): This level of carbohydrate counting is appropriate for people using multiple daily injections or insulin pump therapy. It involves the calculation of ICR that is individualized for each child according to age, sex, pubertal status, duration of diagnosis, and activity. This enables young people with diabetes to adjust their prandial insulin dose according to carbohydrate consumption.

There are different ways of counting carbohydrates:
- Weighing and measuring to determine carbohydrates using a gram scale or a computer scale: It is convenient for measuring carbohydrates in odd sized foods like fruits, unsliced bread, etc. The weight of the food should be multiplied by carbohydrates percentages (carb percentages of various foods are available in various nutrition books)
- Nutrition books, software give carbohydrates counts: Books give carbohydrates count per serving. Soft-wares provide carb count for various brands and standard foods. It is a feature in newer insulin pumps too
- Food labels: For packaged foods label gives how many grams of carbohydrates are there in each serving.

Methods of quantification of carbohydrates may vary from center to center. It is mentioned as one of the following:
- Gram increments of carbohydrate
- 10–12 g carbohydrate portions
- 15 g carbohydrate exchanges.

Carbohydrate portions or exchanges should be distributed throughout the day as at least 3 main meals and 2–3 smaller meals. Exchange list for various Indian foods is available from diabetes centers across the country and various associations such as ADA and American Dietetic Association.[26] Accurate estimation of carbohydrates is essential for good glycemic control using ICR. Overestimation and underestimation of carbohydrates is common and is a challenge for the family and the child. Constant education and follow-up by dietician with expertise in carbohydrate counting is needed. With team support and education, a child with T1DM can do well and could have a flexible lifestyle by using carbohydrate counting.

Nutritional Management of Physical Activity

For a child with T1DM, regular physical activity is essential for maintaining good glycemic control and to maintain weight. However, occasionally unplanned physical activity may lead

CHAPTER 9: Medical Nutrition Therapy in Children with Type 1 Diabetes Mellitus

to hypoglycemic episodes. Excess physical activity may also lead to hyperglycemia followed by delayed hypoglycemia. The amount of carbohydrate required for exercise is dependent on the blood glucose level at the start of exercise, the intensity of the exercise, the frequency of routine exercise, the prevailing insulin level, the insulin regimen, and the age and weight of the child. The following points could be noted:[4]

- Routine physical activity such as playing in the evening does not require extra carbohydrates
- If extra carbohydrate is necessary for a short duration activity then quick acting carbohydrate as a beverage (e.g., an isotonic sports drink) is usually most useful
- For a planned physical activity or a competitive sport, a carbohydrate based, low-fat meal should be eaten 1–3 hours prior to sport to ensure adequacy of glycogen stores and availability of carbohydrate for exercise. It may be preferable to have a meal 4 hours prior to activity to maximize glycogen stores and to help ensure only basal insulin is acting.

NUTRITIONAL MANAGEMENT OF ASSOCIATED CONDITIONS

Type 1 diabetes mellitus is often associated with various eating disorders and other autoimmune disease such as celiac disease. Celiac disease is more common in children with T1DM than in the general population. According to international studies prevalence ranges from 0.6 to 16.4% of children with diabetes.[4] Studies done in India have quoted a prevalence of 7–11.1%.[27,28] Children with celiac disease can often be asymptomatic. When they present with symptoms, common symptoms they come with are poor growth, delayed puberty, nutritional deficiencies, hypoglycemia, and hyperglycemia. A gluten-free diet (GFD) is the only accepted treatment for celiac disease.

Adhering to gluten free diet would not be easy for these children with celiac disease. It is now generally accepted in Europe and some other countries such as Canada and the United States that foods containing less than 20 parts per million (ppm) gluten are suitable for a GFD (even if gluten is detectable) in accordance with Codex Alimentarius (International Food Standards).[4] Children with T1DM and celiac disease, should eliminate wheat, rye, barley, and products derived from these grains from their diet. Food rich in starchy carbohydrate such as potato, rice, and maize and products derived from these and other gluten-free grains must be used as substitutes. Use of oats and wheat starch in celiac disease is controversial. According to some researchers, gluten-free oats is acceptable as gluten-free diet. Children with celiac disease require close monitoring of their growth and nutrition.

Various eating disorders are common in diabetic children. Eating disorders that met DSM-IV criteria were more prevalent in diabetic subjects (10%) than in nondiabetic controls (4%).[29] Omitting insulin dose is also common in teenage girls to avoid weight gain. Clinicians should have a low index of suspicion while evaluating these children and adolescents with T1DM. An interdisciplinary approach to treatment is considered the standard of care for both eating disorders and diabetes. Close liaison with the specialist eating disorder team may be required.[4] Emphasis on diet may sometimes negatively influence glycemic control in youth with T1DM. Perceived restriction of diet in T1DM among the adolescents could be abolished by emphasizing on carbohydrate quantity rather than quality.[30]

CONCLUSION

Optimal management of T1DM in children requires multidisciplinary approach. The role of trained pediatric dieticians in diabetes team is invaluable. Medical nutrition therapy is an integral part of diabetes management in children. It is important for all the team members of diabetes team to be familiar with MNT in T1DM. Success of MNT in T1DM depends on involvement of not only the child but also the whole family.

REFERENCES

1. The Diabetes Control and Complications Trial Research Group. The effect of intensive treatment of diabetes on the development and progression of long-term complications in insulin-dependent diabetes mellitus New Engl J Med. 1993;329.977-86.
2. UK Prospective Diabetes Study Group. UK prospective diabetes study (UKPDS). Diabetologia. 1991;34(12):877-90.
3. Smart C, Aslander-van Vliet E, Waldron S. Nutritional management in children and adolescents with diabetes. Pediatr Diabetes. 2009;10(Suppl. 12):100-17.
4. Smart CE, Annan F, Bruno LP, Higgins LA, Acerini CL. Nutritional management in children and adolescents with diabetes. Paediatric Diabetes. 2014;15(Suppl. 20):135-53.
5. Evert AB, Boucher JL, Cypress M, Dunbar SA, Franz MJ, Mayer-Davis EJ, et al. Nutrition therapy recommendations for the management of adults with diabetes. Diabetes Care. 2014;37 Suppl 1:S120-43.
6. U.S. Department of Health and Human Services: Final MNT regulations.CMS-1169-FC. Federal Register, 1 November 2001. 42 CFR Parts 405, 410, 411, 414, and 415.
7. Morris SF, Wylie-Rosett J. Medical nutrition therapy: a key to diabetes management and prevention. Clinical Diabetes. 2010;28(1):12.
8. American Dietetic Association: Comparison of the American Dietetic Association (ADA) Nutrition Care Process for nutrition education services and the ADA Nutrition Care Process for medical nutrition therapy (MNT) services. Available from: www.eatright.org/advocacy/mnt.
9. Davis NL, Bursell JD, Evans WD, Warner JT, Gregory JW. Body composition in children with type 1 diabetes in the first year after diagnosis: relationship to glycaemic control and cardiovascular risk. Arch Dis Child. 2012;97:312-5.
10. Silverstein J, Klingensmith G, Copeland K, Plotnick L, Kaufman F, Laffel L, et al. Care of children and adolescents with type 1 diabetes: a statement of the American Diabetes Association. Diabetes Care. 2005;28:186-12.
11. American Diabetes Association. "Standards of medical care in diabetes—2009. Diabetes Care. 2009;32 Suppl 1:S13-61.
12. Gidding SS, Dennison BA, Birch LL, Daniels SR, Gillman MW, Lichtenstein AH, et al. Dietary recommendations for children and adolescents: a guide for practitioners. Pediatrics. 2006;117(2):544-59.
13. Canadian Diabetes Association Clinical Practice Guidelines Expert Committee. Clinical practice guidelines. Nutrition therapy. Can J Diabetes. 2013;37:S45-55.
14. Craig ME, Twigg SM, Donaghue K, Cheung NW, et al, for the Australian Type 1 Diabetes Guidelines Expert Advisory Group. National Evidence-Based Clinical Care Guidelines for Type 1 Diabetes in Children, Adolescents and Adults. Canberra: Australian Government, Department of Health and Aging; 2011.
15. Franz MJ, Horton ES Sr, Bantle JP, Beebe CA, Brunzell JD, Coulston AM, et al. Nutrition Principles for the Management of Diabetes and Related Complications. Diabetes Care. 1994;17(5);490-518.
16. Fontvieille AM, Rizkalla SW, Penfornis A, Acosta M, Bornet FR, Slama G. The use of low glycaemic index foods improves metabolic control of diabetic patients over five weeks. Diabetic Medicine. 1992;9(5):444-50.
17. Wolever TM, Hamad S, Chiasson JL, Josse RG, Leiter LA, Rodger NW, et al. Day-to-day consistency in amount and source of carbohydrate intake associated with improved blood glucose control in type 1 diabetes. J Am Coll Nutrition. 1999;18(3):242-7.
18. Silverstein J, Klingensmith G, Copeland K, Plotnick L, Kaufman F, Laffel L, et al. Care of children and adolescents with type 1 diabetes: a statement of the American Diabetes Association. Diabetes Care. 2005;28:186-212.
19. Williams CL. Dietary fiber in childhood. J Pediatr. 2006:149:S121-30.
20. Dewey K, Beaton G, Fjeld C, Lonnerdal B, Reeds P. Protein requirements of infants and children. Eur J Clin Nutr. 1996;50:S119-50.

21. Dyson PA, Kelly T, Deakin T, Duncan A, Frost G, Harrison Z, et al. Diabetes UK evidence based nutrition guidelines for the prevention and management of diabetes. Diabet Med. 2011:28:1282-8.
22. Svoren BM, Volkening LK, Wood JR, Laffel LM. Significant vitamin D deficiency in youth with type 1 diabetes mellitus. J Paediatr. 2009;154(1):132-4.
23. Scavone G, Manto A, Pitocco D, Gagliardi L, Caputo S, Mancini L, et al. Effect of carbohydrate counting and medical nutritional therapy on glycaemic control in type 1 diabetic subjects: a pilot study. Diabet Med. 2010;27(4):477-9.
24. Mehta SN, Quinn N, Volkening LK, Laffel LM. Impact of carbohydrate counting on glycaemic control in children with type 1 diabetes. Diabetes Care. 2009;32(6):1014-16.
25. Gillespie SJ, Kulkarni KD, Daly AE. Using carbohydrate counting in diabetes clinical practice. J Am Diet Assoc. 1998;98:897-905.
26. Exchange Lists for Meal Planning. American Diabetes Association, Inc. and the American Dietetic Association; 2008.
27. Kota SK, Meher LK, Jammula S, Kota SK, Modi KD. Clinical profile of coexisting conditions in type 1 diabetes mellitus patients. J Gastroenterol Hepatol. 2011;26(2):378-81.
28. Bhadada SK, Kochhar R, Bhansali A, Dutta U, Kumar PR, Poornachandra KS, et al. Prevalence and clinical profile of celiac disease in type 1 diabetes mellitus in north India. J Gastroenterology Hepatology. 2011;26(2):378-81.
29. Jones JM, Lawson ML, Daneman D, Olmsted MP, Rodin G. Eating disorders in adolescent females with and without type 1 diabetes: cross sectional study. BMJ. 2000;320(7249):1563-6.
30. Mehta SN, Haynie DL, Higgins LA, Bucey NN, Rovner AJ, Volkening LK, et al. Emphasis on carbohydrates may negatively influence dietary patterns in youth with type 1 diabetes. Diabetes Care. 2009;32(12):2174-6.

CHAPTER 10

Exercise in Children and Adolescents with Type 1 Diabetes Mellitus

Rajesh R Joshi

INTRODUCTION

Exercise is as important as taking insulin and healthy eating in managing diabetes because all three affect each other. If any one of these change, another may need to be adjusted for good glycemic control.

Children and adolescents with type 1 diabetes mellitus (T1DM) should not be restricted to do any form of physical activity. However participation in activities which may endanger life—like parachuting, scuba diving, or rock climbing should be restricted/carefully monitored. A diabetes care plan containing written advice about exercise and sports should be provided to parents early after diagnosis of diabetes.

When one's heart rate is above normal for 20 minutes or if one is breathing heavily, this equals to exercise. Exercise has following benefits for a person with diabetes:
- Makes insulin work better and reduces its dose
- Controls blood pressure
- Improves lipid profile
- Decreases cardiovascular mortality
- Improves overall physical fitness, flexibility, and strength
- Improves mental well-being and self-esteem and helps cope with stress
- May help maintain normal blood circulation to the feet later in life.

As hypoglycemia is common with exercise, it becomes important to understand metabolic changes associated with physical activity and change insulin therapy (for preplanned activity) and/or diet accordingly.

WHAT HAPPENS TO GLUCOSE HOMEOSTASIS DURING EXERCISE?

Glucose homeostasis in people with type 1 diabetes is extremely challenging. There is impaired glucose counter-regulation resulting frequently in hypo- or hyperglycemia. Glucose production in moderately controlled diabetics is by gluconeogenesis. Glucose disposal due to exercise was found to be increased immediately after end of exercise and then 7–11 hours later, a biphasic response to muscle and liver glycogen deposition.

Effect of Mild to Moderate Exercise (E.g., Jogging, Cycling)

This type of exercise (≤60% VO_2 max) is aerobic. The requirement of glucose by body is approximately 2–3 mg/kg/min of exercise. This activity causes noninsulin mediated glucose utilization by muscles. Exercise has been shown to increase noninsulin dependent glucose uptake by muscle by the translocation of glucose transporter type-4 receptors to the cell surface.

Fuel source is based initially on muscle glycogen, then on nonesterified fatty acids and later on by hepatic glucose production. Arterial glucose levels change little because of tight matching and regulation between glucose uptake and utilization. Gluconeogenesis due to 2–4-fold rise of catecholamines occurs only after prolonged exercise of more than 2 hours.

Children with T1DM have different milieu dependent on poor/moderate control or overinsulinized state. Due to unavailability of changes of endogenous insulin during muscle contraction and oxygen consumption, they may have hypoglycemia or ketosis. There is risk for ketosis and hyperglycemia during exercise when initial blood glucose (BG) is >300 mg/dL and ketones >0.74 mmol/L. The significant predictive factor for hypoglycemia during and after exercise is baseline glucose during initiation of exercise with majority occurring when starting BG was <120 mg/dL. Blood glucose level was also found to be lower overnight on exercise days compared to sedentary days. This was more likely with bedtime BG <130 mg/dL.

Effect of Intensive Exercise (E.g., Sprint, Basketball, Hockey)

This exercise (>80% VO_2 max) is anaerobic as it involves short bouts of intense activity with brief rest intervals. Childhood games or field sports are mainly of this type where body requirement of glucose increases by 5–6 mg/kg/min of exercise. Fuel source is mainly glucose and glycogen. Glucose from muscle and liver forms lactate by anaerobic oxidation. There may be hyperglycemia due to 14–18-fold increase in catecholamines at end of exercise if glucose production exceeds glucose utilization. During anaerobic exercise, there is little change in plasma insulin (constant level/ minimal decline) but increases during recovery period during which muscle glycogen is restored and plasma glucose normalizes.

In T1DM, vigorous exercise may cause post exercise hyperglycemia if insulin replacement is suboptimal. However, these children may have late post exercise hypoglycemia due to abnormal adaptive counterregulatory hormone response or due to loss of glucose store release. Guidelines to be followed during exercise:
- FIT:
    o Frequency—exercise 5–7 times a week
    o Intensity—increase heart rate and maintain for at least 20 minutes
    o Time—30–60 minutes, plus 5–10 minutes warm up and cool down.

SECTION 3: Nonpharmacological Management

Exercise is any movement of the body. Walking, jumping rope, playing with other children, riding a bicycle, doing aerobics, playing sports, dancing, and many other activities are forms of exercise. The type and duration of exercise should fit into family's lifestyle and can change on a daily basis.

Things that affect blood sugar response to exercise in T1DM:
- Control of diabetes and level of BG before exercise
- Exercising when insulin is peaking or before meals puts a diabetic at more risk of hypoglycemia [especially if one takes neutral protamine hagedorn (NPH)]
- Longer the exercise more chances of low BG
- Injecting insulin over the muscles one uses while exercising absorbs insulin more rapidly leading to hypoglycemia
- Nonfamiliarity with exercise requiring more energy expenditure than in a trained state—can cause low BG
- Hyperglycemia during physical activity can be due to hypoinsulinemic states before and during exercise, emotion of competing causing adrenaline surge or excessive carbohydrate consumed during exercise
- Weight bearing aerobic exercise decrease BG while nonweight bearing anaerobic exercise increase BG.

WAYS TO PREVENT EXERCISE INDUCED HYPOGLYCEMIA

- Preplanned exercise—insulin dose reduction and dietary modification
- Unplanned exercise—dietary modification (extra carbohydrates).

Extra BG monitoring during and after physical activity and if the exercise is unaccustomed then BG testing at bedtime and 3 AM is also warranted.

Use of detailed records of physical activity, insulin, food, and glucose results is important for good diabetes control during physical activity. Alcohol should be avoided as it inhibits gluconeogenesis which leads to hypoglycemia.

Diet during Exercise

Carbohydrate (CHO) intake up to 1.5 g/kg/h of strenuous exercise preferably complex carbohydrates to increase liver and muscle glycogen stores. Prolonged exercise may require CHO before during and after exercise. Additional snacks at bed time (complex CHO or protein foods with CHO) if BG ≤125 mg/dL especially if NPH insulin is used. With basal analogs, the bedtime glucose level can be slightly lower without a substantial risk of night-time hypoglycemia but no specific value is a guarantee that hypoglycemia will be avoided. Guideline for carbohydrate replacement is given in table 1.

Insulin Adjustments with Exercise

Dosing of insulin should be individualized as there are numerous factors affecting insulin levels like the dose and type of insulin, timing of the injection, site of injection, duration, and intensity of physical exercise, emotional stress, and fitness status.

TABLE 1: Pre-exercise carbohydrate replacement

Plasma blood glucose	Simple carbohydrate (CHO)
<80 mg/dL	Withhold physical activity, ingest 15 g CHO
80–140 mg/dL	Ingest 1–1.5 g/kg of CHO prior to activity
140–250	Within safety range, ingest 15–30 g of CHO after activity
>250 mg/dL no ketonuria	Begin activity. No CHO ingestion
>250 mg/dL with ketonuria	Postpone activity till no ketones. Give small dose of insulin. Drink plenty of fluids

- Preplanned activity—reduce premeal insulin by approximately 30–50% or delay activity during peak of insulin action
- Prolonged exercise—reduce evening NPH/long-acting insulin by 20–30% to prevent nocturnal hypoglycemia
- Short sprints added to aerobic training can minimize the risk of hypoglycemia
- Those on insulin pump for short period of unplanned exercise may stop the basal insulin for duration of exercise
- If preplanned activity, then reduce the basal insulin by 50%, 60 minutes before the exercise
- If there is concern of late onset hypoglycemia, overnight basal can be reduced by 10–30%
- New pump technologies such as low-glucose suspend and programmed low-glucose management may also be useful in the future.

Exercise Hyperglycemia

- Blood glucose >250 mg/dL and no ketones—insulin supplementation (0.05 µ/kg) before exercise
- Blood glucose >250 mg/dL and ketones are present—give insulin and delay exercise till ketones are cleared.

The rise in blood glucose after intense exercise may be prevented by giving a small additional dose of rapid-acting insulin at half-time or immediately after the exercise is finished—for example, a 50% correction bolus when levels are >270 mg/dL.

Checklist to Be Given to People with Diabetes while Exercising

- Know BG before starting any significant activity or exercise
  - Care should be taken that the BG meter and test strips chosen are suitable for the environment where they will be used
  - If BG low, eat a rapidly acting CHO snack
  - If high (over 250 mg/dL), delay exercise specially if there are ketones as it may drive blood glucose even higher if one exercises during hyperglycemia
- Check the blood sugar level as needed throughout exercise
- Know signs of low BG and pay attention to how you feel (Table 2)
- Carry an easy-to-consume source of fast-acting sugar (such as juice, hard candy, or glucose) when you exercise. This will be used to treat hypoglycemia, should it occur

SECTION 3: Nonpharmacological Management

TABLE 2: Clinical features of low blood glucose

Early symptoms	Late symptoms
• Headache • Dizzy • Shakiness • Weak • Sweatiness • Tired • Hunger • Pale skin • Abdominal pain • Unconsciousness • Nervousness • Seizures	• Personality change • Confusion • Blurred vision • Irritability

- Plan for exercise by increasing food intake or decreasing insulin—be prepared to snack
  - Monitor BG during and after exercise as you need to learn how exercise affects you
  - Snack as needed to prevent low blood sugars during exercise (about 15 g carbohydrates for every hour of exercise)
  - When deciding how many carbohydrates to eat, take into account the type, duration, and intensity of the exercise, as well as your pre-exercise blood sugar reading
  - To know how much insulin is still active from the last injection
- If the activity is prolonged, carbohydrate snacks are periodically required. Remember that you may get a low BG up to 24 hours after exercise
- Always wear a diabetes identity card and carry phone money with you
- Tell someone where you are going or exercise with a friend—it is important that your coach/friend knows you have diabetes and how to treat a low BG
- Drink plenty of fluids to prevent dehydration
- Have fun during exercise. Find exercise you enjoy and incorporate in your daily life

Warning: Do not take insulin to cover exercise-related snacks or snacks used to prevent or treat a low blood sugar!

Rarely, exercise may adversely affect diabetes related complications like:
- Increase proteinuria
- Increase risk of retinal and vitreal hemorrhages possibly due to increased blood pressure during exercise
- Increased risk of foot ulcers and tissue injury due to diabetic neuropathy.

Age and Exercise

Adults are advised to discuss plan to begin new exercise program with their diabetes care providers. Starting slowly and gradually increasing amount of exercise is important. Having a medical check-up before starting new exercise program is recommended if one has T1DM for more than 15 years, or having additional risk factor for myocardial infarction, eye disease, kidney disease or neuropathies.

Strenuous activities like weight lifting and jogging are discouraged with proliferative retinopathy. Weight-bearing exercises should be limited with severe peripheral neuropathy.

Continuous Glucose Monitoring

A number of relatively small studies have examined the utility of using continuous glucose monitoring (CGM) with exercise. In most studies, CGM has been demonstrated to accurately track the change in glycemia during exercise in patients with T1DM. However, real-time CGM tends to overestimate blood glucose levels if hypoglycemia is developing, likely because of the 10–20 minutes time delay in equilibrium between interstitial fluid and capillary glucose.

Real-time CGM use may help reduce the fear of exercise-associated hypoglycemia if directional arrows and alerts are used. Continuous glucose monitoring may be very useful in situations in which self-monitoring blood glucose is impractical (e.g., cycling road racing) or impossible, such as with scuba diving and when subjects are sleeping, to help reveal nocturnal hypoglycemia. Continuous glucose monitoring may hold the promise of preventing hypoglycemia altogether during sports by keeping users more aware of their glucose concentrations and thus better prepared to take preventative actions.

CONCLUSION

Regular physical activity is important for children and adolescents with T1DM to improve fitness, insulin sensitivity, mental well being and decrease cardiovascular morbidity. Blood glucose should be checked before, during and after exercise. Anaerobic high intensity activity is likely to produce hyperglycemia while continuous moderate physical activity produces hypoglycemia which can last up to 6–24 hours after exercise due to liver glycogen depletion. Hence checking bed time and 3 am BG is important. For planned exercise reducing insulin dose before exercise and for unplanned physical activity taking 15 g of carbohydrates for every 30 minute of exercise is a general recommendation. Exercise is not recommended if the BG is above 250 mg/dL especially in presence of ketones.

REFERENCES

1. Type 1 diabetes mellitus in children and adolescents in India. Clinical Practice Guidelines 2011. Indian Society for Pediatric and adolescent endocrinology.
2. ISPAD Clinical Practice Consensus Guidelines.
3. Pivovarov JA, Taplin CE, Riddell MC. Current perspectives on physical activity and exercise for youth with diabetes. Pediatric Diabetes. 2015;16:242-55.

CHAPTER 11

Diabetes Education

Archana S Sarda

INTRODUCTION

Diabetes in children is a lifelong journey. The treatment and skills needed by a child with diabetes and his/her family to control and cope change as a child grows into an adult. As a result, success in diabetes care is more than treatment by a healthcare provider and is rooted in patient empowerment. Empowerment has been defined as "ability of a person affected by a disease to be an active member of his or her management plan".[1] Way back in 1989, the St. Vincent declaration[2] declared that reducing the burden of diabetes could only be achieved through an active partnership between people with diabetes and service providers, particularly in the areas of disease management and education. Diabetes education is today accepted as an integral part of diabetes management. The following definition of diabetes education has been proposed: "the process of providing the person with knowledge and skills needed to perform diabetes self-care, manage crisis, and to make lifestyle changes to successfully manage the disease".[3] Diabetes education includes "appropriate to age" self-management designs, tools to impart education, trained team of caregivers, adaptability of education module to individual cultural/socioeconomic needs, and lastly a warmth that infuses hope and happiness along with knowledge. Not a simple task, yet treatment and life of a child with diabetes are inadequate without it.

THE NECESSITY

Education is the cornerstone of successful management of diabetes. There is evidence that educational interventions in childhood and adolescent diabetes have a beneficial effect on glycemic control and psychosocial outcomes. Education optimizes both conventional diabetes treatment as well as advanced treatment with technology effectively.

Let us look at the basic pillars of treatment of a child with type 1 diabetes mellitus (T1DM) and how they fare with/without education.

CHAPTER 11: Diabetes Education

Modality—Insulin Therapy

Insulin therapy forms the foundation of diabetes treatment in a child. Options of vials with syringes (40 IU/100 IU), devices with cartridges, insulin pump are today available to be individualized as per age, affordability, and availability. Insulin needs to be stored at recommended temperatures. Injection sites need to be carefully chosen and rotated. Mixing insulin, changing needle, replacing reusable bits, disposal of used needles, carrying to school/trip, etc., are part and parcel of daily insulin therapy.

Outcomes

The best of insulin prescription can go haywire when appropriate insulin education is missing. The vial and syringe strength mismatch can lead to life threatening outcomes especially in a case where one can buy without a written prescription from a pharmacy. Inappropriate site of insulin injections and nonrotation presents with lipohypertrophy so often. In the rural areas without electricity we find erratic insulin responses due to inability to maintain storage temperature unless taught to do so. Non-delivery from a device is a known reason for uncontrolled blood sugar levels in an unaware person. This basic education needs reinforcement from time to time at different stages of growth and treatment. The best insulin therapy is futile without accompanying education at regular interval.

Modality—Self-monitoring Blood Glucose

Self-monitoring of blood glucose (SMBG) is a vital component of treatment of T1DM in a child. A child is given a glucometer and strips and asked to monitor the blood sugar levels daily. The child is also asked to keep a log of the same. The insulin dose depends on these readings and the diet, both of which change all the time.

Outcomes

Glucometers give numbers to the child and his/her family. What one does with those numbers can come only with related education. In a country like India, where strips are fairly expensive, often a family will have to limit the number of checks per day. How does a child manage that unless taught and trained for optimum usage of monitoring? Again these requirements change as the child grows or goes to school/college. Hence, education is a continuous and individualized process.

Modality—Nutrition

Nutrition therapy forms a pillar of T1DM therapy. A child needs to eat healthy, at regular intervals, balance the carbohydrates, protein, and fiber in his/her diet, know what to avoid and how to adjust the insulin dose for each meal.

Outcomes

The growth and development of a child with T1DM is largely dependent on good control of blood sugar levels. Blood sugar levels are dependent mainly on the triad of nutrition, monitoring, and insulin dose adjustments amongst all other aspects of self-management. Food is different in every household, every culture. Unless carbohydrate counting and nutrition management is taught in a localized scenario, it is almost impossible to adjust the insulin doses to reach target blood sugar levels.

This role of diabetes education is a necessity and applies to all aspects of diabetes care including emergency management and psychosocial growth. Education makes treatment cost effective and has a direct positive impact on the child's/family's/ community's well-being. The outcomes fall short of expectations in absence of structured and appropriate diabetes education.

THE CONTENT

It is widely accepted that diabetes cannot be successfully managed without behavioral modification.[4,5] Hence, the diabetes care team needs to develop counseling techniques that can go hand in hand with subject teaching. The content of teaching topics should aim at comprehensive care of successful therapy with positive coping for the child and his/her family. The topics for early and essential education:

- Explanation of diagnosis and symptoms. To eliminate any guilt or misconceptions
- The immediate need for insulin and its action
- Insulin related practical skills including:
    - Injection/pump technique
    - Site rotation
    - Insulin storage
- Normal blood glucose levels and targets at various times appropriate to age
- Self-monitoring of blood glucose and why it is needed
- Self-monitoring of blood glucose related practical skills
    - Handling a glucometer
    - Frequency of monitoring
    - Possible errors in a glucometer
- Dietary advice including carbohydrate counting
- Exercise and its possible effects
- Hypoglycemia
    - To recognize symptoms
    - Its prevention
    - Its management
- Sick day management
    - Not stopping insulin
    - Monitoring ketones
    - Diabetic ketoacidosis prevention
- Care plan for school and home
- Identity card
- Psychological counseling to parent and child
- Integration of the plan with social activities
- Identifying emergency contacts and resources.

The topics for continuing education at higher level:
- Insulin secretion, action, and physiology
- Insulin types, the absorption, action profiles
- Nutrition—food plans, eating out, coping with special events, sweeteners
- Monitoring effectively—glucose, ketone, and glycosylated hemoglobin
- Use of continuous glucose monitoring
- Hypoglycemia—reinforcement
- Hyperglycemia
- Ketosis
- Sick day
- Weight gain and growth
- Complications—their prevention and assessment
- Exercise
- Holiday planning
- Smoking, alcohol, and drugs
- Sexuality
- Preconception counseling
- Postconception counseling
- Employment
- Driving vehicles
- Goal setting
- Problem solving in day to day unexpected situations
- Self-esteem building
- Updates of latest research.

These topics need to be taught in an age-appropriate, structured manner over time.

This opportunity can be effectively used for psychosocial development of the child and family. Diabetes education given effectively goes a long way in creating harmony in lives of children with diabetes and positive outcomes.

THE METHOD

The content of diabetes education can be presented in different ways depending on the patient's age, literacy, choice of learning method, and cultural context. A variety of techniques can be used to teach, adapted to meet the different needs.

THE PHILOSOPHY

Table 1 summarizes the philosophy of education in children, adolescents, and parents with diabetes.[6] Health professionals should learn to incorporate and deliver the education using behavioral approaches which are learner centered and not didactic.[7,8] All the team members should follow a common philosophy and common goals in diabetes education.[9]

SECTION 3: Nonpharmacological Management

TABLE 1: Principles and practice of education in children, adolescents, and their parents/primary care givers[6]

Motivation	The learners needs to and/or have a desire to learn
Context	Where is the learner now?
	Where does the learner want to be later?
Environment	Learner centered, comfortable, trusting
	Enjoyable/entertaining/interesting/open
Significance	Meaningful, important links or joins up
	Reward or gain
Concepts	Simple to complex in gentle steps (short attention span)
Activity	Constantly interacted, practical (fitting into real life)
	Goal setting and problem solving
Reinforcement	Repetition, review, summarize
Reassess	Evaluate, audit
Move forward	Continuing education

THE BARRIERS

The method used for imparting diabetes education has to be individualized based on assessable factors before undertaking the task.

- Literacy: Health literacy, or ability to read, understand, and implement medical directions, has been linked to glycemic control. In a study of 200 families with a child who had T1DM, a lower level of literacy and numerical skills of the care giver predicted worse glycemic control in the child.[10] Training an illiterate family would involve a lot of verbal communication and pictorial presentation. Using tools such as pictures (for insulin site rotation for example), can be effective. It is often found that an older sibling is going to school and can be trained to be part of the care giving team. In extreme cases, a neighbor might be of use or a nearest chemist/school teacher till a member of family gets trained
- Emotional barrier to learn: Many families are in a state of denial, nonacceptance, or shock with the diagnosis of T1DM in the child. The thought of insulin injections and multiple pricks is unbelievable and a nightmare to them. The other members of family add to this by being critical and dramatic. The educator needs to let the diagnosis sink in and acceptance set in without which learning cannot happen. A group program with peer interaction is an effective way to do this as "why only my child" is the usual mental block
- Misconceptions: Hearsays and myths about diabetes and its treatment are often a hurdle to effective learning by the family. They are convinced by "people whom they know" and have heard so many "horror stories" about diabetes, that they are not receptive. This needs to be addressed before teaching starts. A gentle personal session and a meeting with a few "success stories" usually does the trick
- Superstitions: In a country like India, there are many belief systems where alternate therapies to medical conditions are popular. Ranging from religious ceremonies to a

CHAPTER 11: Diabetes Education

certain leaf which cures diabetes, these can have serious repercussions on a child as insulin is withheld. These situations have to be addressed without ridiculing the family's faith
- Support system: Often, with the parents out to work or single parent, it becomes essential to specify who the care giver will be for a child with diabetes. A grandparent, a relative, a nanny, a neighbor, or a teacher might become the main recipient in such cases. Individualization of teaching methods to suit the available support in family becomes essential.

THE PROCESS

Time

The actual process of diabetes education requires a few hours of contact with the child and family initially. Many shorter sessions are necessary, spread over time.

Team

These sessions can be conducted by a trained team of endocrinologist, pediatrician, general practitioner, a diabetologist, nurse, nutritionist, diabetes educator, a psychologist, and/or a trained volunteer. It is important that all members of the team are on the same track so as to have nonconflicting teaching. Training should include teaching methodology as well as psychology in addition to the medical knowledge.

Location

It should be accessible to patient and family. It can be a hospital or a community center.

Structure

In many countries, a recommended structured education program exists. In countries like India where it does not, it is recommended that one's own outline is created based on the principles and curriculum so as to have a system in place. Innovative and localized processes are more effective when added on to the structured education.

Primary Sessions

- One to one with treating physician: The first session is best time to create a positive motivation towards self-management by the treating physician in whom they have faith. Often, the first doctor they meet is the pediatrician who has treated the child in ketosis.
  - The quality time spent by the first contact physician paves the way for a successful journey ahead. This session is personal with no tools. The doctor's explanation of diagnosis and reassurance of a good life forms the basis of this session. Answering the family's questions honestly and gently go a long way in allaying fears. Any scare set in at this time takes roots and inhibits progress. The patient is then referred to an education team for a structured training program
- Individualized planning: The educator now sets the goals for a child and family explaining to them the things they will now need to learn at first level. Insulin care, nutrition,

emergency, and monitoring features in this primary list. Leaflets, posters, handbooks, and videos of the subject concerned are good tools at this stage to be used while waiting or to reinforce after training. These sessions are, however, individual or in small groups of similar in age and skill children. It is of utmost importance here to know the cultural and socioeconomic background of the family to be able to give suitable practical guidelines

- Medical nutrition therapy: This forms the foundation of care and needs to be handled by a trained dietician. Affordability, availability, and acceptability of what is recommended are essential. Healthy age appropriate diet, carbohydrate counting, and clearing misconceptions about "sweets" are part of the first training. Tools ranging from books to mobile apps are useful for nutrition care
- Technical knowledge: The use of pump, devices, insulin vials, glucometer, CGM, etc., can be given in groups. Hands on training with live demonstration takes place at first level. Tools, such as videos and manuals in local language, are useful here to educate and reinforce. Not to be missed here are the special situations such as nonavailability of refrigerator to store insulin. These issues have to be tackled with innovative alternatives
- Counseling: The first time of diagnosis and primary teaching can be quite overwhelming for a family. Confidence to carry out so many unfamiliar tasks and the needed skills is low at this moment. Counseling the family that this is natural and they will be able to do the needful is essential. Reassuring that this gets better with time gives them courage to face an unfamiliar situation
- Emergency care and contact: Knowing what to do in an emergency, who to contact and how to take care of the first time diagnosed child and family till they get empowered with subsequent training. This is a good time to give an identity card, a hypo-kit, and tools such as leaflets and manual. A reference to a good website can be used.

THE ADVANCED ONGOING SESSIONS

These sessions are initially needed frequently (say fortnightly), for reinforcement and to crosscheck that the child and family are on a suitable self-management path. Initial hurdles in learning and technique are smoothened out. Individual variations are addressed by the concerned expert.

These sessions later are to be continued at regular intervals (say monthly), with specific topics by their experts at a specified day and time. A child and family can attend the topic of choice as per need. Each session would consist of a revision with new information and advanced updates.

Various methods of teaching individually and in groups can be used and many more created as one goes along. It is important to remember that participants in a group must be similar in age, skill level, and socioeconomic background. The educational program should utilize appropriate patient centered, interactive teaching methods for all people involved in the management of diabetes, particularly the child or adolescent.[11-23]

Some methods are:
- One to one: Here an expert teaches a family the topic and answers their personal queries. It is useful in individual planning and specialized needs
- One to small group: An expert teaches families of similar needs in a group. This session is usually interactive and the participants get motivated by seeing others like them
- Small group discussion: Here an expert moderates but does not teach. The learning arises out of the questions, answers, and sharing that everyone does. The direction is carefully but casually led by the expert. A very effective method, especially in adolescents
- Peer group interaction: Here there is no expert present. Parents and/or children discuss, share and resolve between themselves. This is a great method to shed inhibitions and set participants at ease
- Role model session: A child/parent who has successfully gone through the turmoil of diagnosis, education, and treatment of T1DM, shares the ups and downs and the success achieved. This session creates an instant connect and hope
- A quiz: It is a fun way to teach and learn. Group is divided into two and asked questions. A scoreboard is kept and keeps everyone active
- A lecture: A formal way of teaching with teaching aids. Advantage is that a large heterogeneous group can be addressed at the same time. Audio-visual aids are useful tools here. A good method for giving information based teaching. It is followed by question answer session
- Demonstration: Formal hands on demonstration by an expert. Technology is best taught this way to a large group. Audio visual aids enhance understanding. A question answer session at the end is essential to resolve any issues
- Play way methods: A number of games are available and can be designed to involve children and adults alike to beat the stress of learning
- Summer camps: An indirect but strong way of teaching self-management, instilling self-confidence, and independence to young ones with diabetes
- Day trips, treks, etc.: A powerful and subtle way of inculcating life skill needed by a person with diabetes.

Teaching and learning is an interactive ongoing process. Making it age and culture appropriate goes a long way in creating impact. Group education may be more cost effective and its experience enhanced by peer group.[24-25] There is some evidence that benefits may be gained from participation in organized meetings or camping experiences.[26] A structured education program, localized methods of delivery, a trained and motivated team, and suitable education tools are the vital components of effective diabetes education.

Team

The team that participates in diabetes education involves the givers and the recipients. The recipients can often be empowered to become givers at some stage.

Qualified Team

This interdisciplinary team decides the structure and the method to deliver diabetes education. This team trains the extended team to become capable of imparting education. The goal of this team is to empower the child and family with self-care and self-esteem.

The team should consist of:
- A pediatric endocrinologist/diabetologist or a physician trained in care of children
- A diabetes specialist nurse/diabetes educator
- A nutritionist
- A psychologist
- Social worker.

Extended Team

This team is created over time by the qualified team by choosing motivated persons who are part of diabetes education at some stage. The extended team is empathetic and sensitive. They are essential to reach out to community in large numbers. At times they are more effective as they are part of the learner's community. Especially in places where qualified sources are limited, extended team forms the backbone of diabetes educators.

The team should consist of:
- Trained volunteers
- Trained mothers
- Trained older children with T1DM
- Trained school teacher
- Trained general practitioner
- Trained sibling.

Core Team

This team is the center of the diabetes education program and success depends on their involvement and empowerment. They are also future members of extended team.

The team should consist of:
- The child/adolescent with diabetes
- The parents
- The siblings.

Community Team

Every person in the community can participate in spreading awareness and education for detection and treatment of diabetes. Community participation builds a positive ecosystem for children in schools and society. Exhibitions and walks on world diabetes day are some ways of community participation.

The local, national, and international politicians and policy makers in health and education are a major part of diabetes education team. Their sensitivity and knowledge of the topic can create mass awareness, funds, and facilities.

Organizations

Organizations like the International Diabetes Federation and International Society for Pediatric and Adolescent Diabetes set the standards, guidelines, create education material, and work globally for welfare of children with diabetes. Many such local, national, and international organizations definitely are part of the team imparting diabetes education. Non-governmental organizations across the globe have taken up the cause of T1DM and become part of the team.

Today, with the help of and access to all the above sources, it is possible to create an effective trained team to impart diabetes education in the remotest of areas and minimal of resources.

THE EDUCATION TOOLS

Learning should be reinforced using education materials appropriate to the child's and adolescent's age and maturity.[27] All materials should follow the same principles and have same goals. The tools can range from a simple chalk and board to a complex app. The aim is to impart diabetes education effectively and simply with a medium best suited to the learner. Making learning fun breaks the barriers to learn and is step towards effective empowerment. Some of the tools used in diabetes education are leaflets, brochures, handbooks, videos, presentations, websites, apps, online games, puzzles, quizzes, chats, puppets, models, role plays, skits, rotation grids, food plates, conversation maps, playing cards, board games, and flash cards. It is the educator's creativity and urge to teach that leads to innovative tools appropriate to local needs.

CONCLUSION

The Diabetes Control and Complications trial provided unequivocal evidence that intensification of management reduces microvascular complications and that intensification requires effective diabetes self-management. Effective self-management requires frequent and high levels of educational input and continuing support to young patients as their parents and other care givers.[28-29] In contrast, those people who do not receive education or do not continue to have educational contacts are more likely to suffer from diabetes related complication.[30-31]

Diabetes education needs to be structured, delivered by a trained multidisciplinary team, using educational tools and innovative methods to teach to all young people with diabetes and their care givers. In resource constraint settings, it is possible to create a diabetes education program using the basic principles in a local language, simple tools, and an extended trained team. Diabetes education empowers a child or adolescent and family with self-management skills and a positive attitude to live a normal and meaningful life.

REFERENCES

1. Santurri LE. Patient Empowerment: improving the outcomes of chronic diseases through self-management education. The MPHP 439 Online Text Book, Case Western Reserve University; 2006. Available from: http//www.cwru.edu/med/epdbio/mphp439/patient_empowerment.htm

SECTION 3: Nonpharmacological Management

2. World Health Organisation Europe/IDF Europe: Diabetes Care and Research in Europe: the St. Vincent declaration 1989. Available from: http://www.codex.vr.se/texts/SVD.pdf.
3. Murphy HR, Raymann G, Skinner TC. Psycho-educational interventions for children and young people with type 1 diabetes. Diabet Med. 2006:23:935-43.
4. Doherty Y, James P, Roberts S. Stage of change counselling. In: Snoek FJ, Skinner TC, editors. Psychology in Diabetes Care. 2nd ed. Chichester: John Wiley; 2007.
5. Prochaska JO, Diclemente CC. Towards a comprehensive model of change. In: Miller WR, Heather N, editors. Treating Addictive Behaviors: Process of Change. New York: Plenum; 1986. pp. 1007-30.
6. Lange K, Swift P, Pankowska E, Danne T. ISPAD Clinical Practice Consensus Guidelines 2014 Compendium. Diabetes education in children and adolescents. Pediatric Diabetes.2014;15(Suppl 20):77-85.
7. Anderson RM, Funnell M, Carlson A, Salehstatin N, Cradock S, Skinner TC. Facilitating self care through empowerment. In: Snoek FJ, Skinner TC, editors. Psychology in Diabetes Care. 2nd ed. Chichester: John Wiley; 2007.
8. Anderson RM, Funnell M, Butler P, Arnold MS, Fitzgerald JT, Feste C. Patient empowerment: results of a randomized control trial. Diabetes Care. 1995:18:943-9.
9. Cameron F, de Beaufort C, Aanstoot HJ, Hoey H, Lange K, Castano L, et al. International Study Group. Lessons from the Hvidoere International Study Group on childhood diabetes: be dogmatic about outcome and flexible in approach. Pediatr Diabetes. 2013;14:473-80.
10. Hassan K, Heptulla RA. Glycaemic control in paediatric type1 diabetes: role of caregiver literacy. Pediatrics. 2010;125:e1104.
11. Haas L, Maryniuk M, Beck J, Cox CE, Duker P, Edwards L, et al; 2012 Standards Revision Task Force. National standards for diabetes self-management education and support. Diabetes Care. 2012:37(Suppl. 1):S144-S153.
12. Silverstein J, Klingensmith G, Copeland K, Plotnick L, Kaufman F, Laffel L, et al. American Diabetes Association. CARE of children and adolescents with type 1 diabetes: a statement of the American Diabetes Association (ADA Statement). Diabetes Care. 2005;28:186-212.
13. Canadian Diabetes Association Clinical Practice Guidelines Expert Committee. Canadian Diabetes Association 2013 Clinical Practice Guidelines for the Prevention and Management of Diabetes in Canada. Can J Diabetes. 2013;37(Suppl. 1):S1-S212.
14. Craig ME, Twigg SM, Donaghue KC, et al.; Australian Type Diabetes Guidelines Expert Advisory Group. National Evidence-based Clinical Care Guidelines for Type 1 Diabetes in Children, Adolescents and Adults. Canberra: Australian Government Department of Health and Ageing; 2011. Available from: http://www.diabetessociety. com.au/position-statements.asp).
15. National Institute for Clinical Excellence UK (NICE). Type 1 diabetes: Diagnosis and management of type 1 diabetes in children, young people and adults; 2004. Available from: http://www.nice.org.uk/pdf/ CG015NICEguideline.pdf).
16. DH Diabetes Policy Team. Making Every Young Person with Diabetes Matter: Report of the Children and Young People with Diabetes Working Group. UK Department of Health, London; 2007. Available from: http://www.dh.gov.uk/prod_consum_dh/groups/dh_digitalassets/@dh/@en/documents/digitalasset/dh_073 675.pdf).
17. Holterhus PM, Beyer P, B¨urger-B¨using J, et al. Diagnostik, Therapie und Verlaufskontrolle des Diabetes mellitus im Kindes- und Jugendalter. S3 Leitlinie der Deutschen Diabetes Gesellschaft. [Diagnosis, Therapy and Long Term Care of Diabetes in Childhood and Adolescence – S3 Guideline]. Mainz: Kirchheim. 2009:1-306.
18. Kulzer B, Albus C, Herpertz S, Kruse J, Lange K, Lederbogen F, et al. Evidenzbasierte Leitlinie - Psychosoziales und Diabetes mellitus S2-Leitlinie Psychosozialesund Diabetes. Herausgeber: S.Matthaei, M. Kellerer. Diabetologie und Stoffwechsel (2013) Teil 1. (2013) 8:198-242. [S2-Guidelines: Diabetes and psychosocial aspects]
19. Diabetes UK and Department of Health. Structured Patient Education in Diabetes. Report from the Patient Education Working Group. Diabetes UK and Department of Health; 2005. Available from: http://www.dh.gov.uk/publications.
20. IDF Consultative Section on Diabetes Education (DECS). International Curriculum for Diabetes Health Professional Education. 2nd ed. Brussels: International Diabetes Federation. 2008. Available from: http://www. idf.org.
21. Martin D, Lange K, Sima A, Kownatka D, Skovlund S, Danne T, Robert JJ; SWEET group. Recommendations for age-appropriate education of children and adolescents with diabetes and their parents in the European Union. Pediatr Diabetes. 2012;13 Suppl 16:20-8.
22. Waldron S, Rurik I, Madacsy L, Donnasson-Eudes S, Rosu M, Skovlund SE, et; SWEET group. Good practice recommendations on paediatric training programmes for healthcare professionals in the EU. Pediatr Diabetes. 2012;13(Suppl. 16):29-38.
23. Lange K, Klotmann S, Saßmann H, Aschemeier B, Wintergerst E, Gerhardsson P, et al; SWEET group. A pediatric diabetes toolbox for creating centres of reference. Pediatr Diabetes. 2012;13 (Suppl. 16):49-61.

24. uhlhauser I, Bruckner I, Berger M et al. Evaluation of an intensified insulin treatment and teaching programme as routine management of type 1 diabetes (insulin-dependent) diabetes. The BucharestD¨usseldorf Study Diabetologia. 1987;30:681-90.
25. DAFNE Study Group. Training in flexible, intensive insulin management to enable dietary freedom in people with type 1 diabetes: dose adjustment for normal eating (DAFNE) randomized controlled trial. Br Med J. 2002;325:746-9.
26. Carlson KT, Carlson GW Jr, Tolbert L, Demma LJ. Blood glucose levels in children with type1 diabetes attending a residential diabetes camp: a 2-year review. Diabet Med. 2013;30:e123-6.
27. García-P´erez L, Perestelo-P´erez L, Serrano Aguilar P, Del Mar Trujillo-Martín M. Effectiveness of a psycho educative intervention in a summer camp for children with type 1 diabetes mellitus. Diabetes Educ. 2010;36:310-7.
28. Diabetes Control and Complications Research Group. Effect of intensive diabetes treatment on the development and progression of long-term complications in adolescents with insulin-dependent diabetes mellitus. J Pediatr. 1994;125:177-88.
29. Implications of the Diabetes Control and Complications Trial. ADA Position Statement. Diabetes Care. 2003;26:S25-7.
30. Haas L, Maryniuk M, Beck J, Cox CE, Duker P, Edwards L, et al; 2012 Standards Revision Task Force. National standards for diabetes self-management education and support. Diabetes Care. 2012;37(Suppl. 1):S144-53.
31. Craig ME, Twigg SM, Donaghue KC, et al; Australian Type Diabetes Guidelines Expert Advisory Group. National Evidence-based Clinical Care Guidelines for Type 1 Diabetes in Children, Adolescents and Adults. Canberra: Australian Government Department of Health and Ageing; 2011. Available from: http://www.diabetessociety.com.au/position-statements.asp.

CHAPTER 12

Biopsychosocial Dimensions in Diabetes: A Brief Outline

Sangeeta Das

INTRODUCTION

Diabetes is a lifelong disease. Taking the insulin injection same time everyday for the entire life in type 1 diabetes mellitus (T1DM) is a challenging task. In addition, the burden of optimal regular monitoring, constant fear of hypoglycemia, and apprehension regarding complications puts the person with diabetes in a disadvantageous situation. The story is similar about type 2 diabetes mellitus (T2DM) in children, adolescents, adults, as well as other types of diabetes. Therefore, psychological interventions and patient education become as important as "biomedical" care, if one has to achieve optimal outcomes.

As India moves from a high prevalence of acute to chronic disease, T1DM, T2DM in general and in children in particular, is becoming a major health concern. Certainly, a purely pharmacological approach to successfully contain and, perhaps, even reverse the effects of diabetes, is insufficient; factors beyond the pale of pharmacological interventions, which dwell upon the holistic approach of supporting the patient psychologically, socially, and emotionally through the treatment process must be given due consideration.

DIABETES IS MULTIDIMENSIONAL

It has been emphasized that there is more to diabetes than just glucose control, and emotions play an important role in diabetes. The emotional and psychological needs of people living with diabetes are complex. Indian patients also showed a significantly higher perception of burden of social and personal distress associated with diabetes. These not only impact the patients' ability to adhere to therapy but also their psychosocial wellbeing.

The concept of health and disease is undergoing a change. It is no more only a biological entity. Today, it includes ample and essential psychosocial factors. This biopsychosocial factors are of paramount importance in integral management of a chronic disease like diabetes mellitus with many comorbidities. The biopsychosocial construct knowledge that disease results from a dynamic interaction among biological, psychosocial, developmental, sociocultural, and ecological factors.

PSYCHOLOGY, SOCIOLOGY, AND DIABETES

The relationship of diabetes and psychosocial factors has been known since long. "Sorrow" was postulated to be a precipitating factor for diabetes in the 17th century. Efforts to pinpoint a diabetes personality "or" psycho-type', however, proved unsuccessful.

The link between diabetes and psychosocial stress is based upon strong biological foundations. Stress increases concentration of interleukin-6, and this may lead to insulin resistance. An understanding of social psychology also helps suggest coping skills and mechanisms, which can be utilized to prevent and manage diabetes, as well as promote healthy living with the condition. Mental and emotional well-being improves quality of life, and also contributes to better biomedical health. Interventions, such as spirituality, meditation, and yoga, can be used to achieve such wellbeing.[1]

RESPONSIBILITY FOR SELF-CARE

Living with diabetes carries certain responsibilities with it. One must learn how to prevent, limit, and manage both hyper- and hypoglycemia. This has to be done lifelong on a 24 × 7 × 365 basis. While diabetes self-care is difficult, it is not impossible. Though the demands of self-management are challenging, they can be mastered by diligence and habit. In T1DM, however, the large number of behavioral and practical changes required, may appear daunting. This sometimes create apprehension and concern, and is termed as diabetes distress.

Diabetes is managed by a complicated regime of self-care behavior. Diabetes self-care is difficult because of number of reasons. Further, the demands of diabetes self-management can be overwhelming. Ideally, when people learn new and complicated routines, they try out new behaviors in a gradual way eventually making them part of the new routine. Yet, with diabetes, the individual must quickly learn a large number of new behaviors and they must begin performing them all immediately and at once (e.g., the newly diagnosed individual is instructed in self-testing, dietary modifications, medication/insulin usage, and exercise at a short span).

In general, research has shown behavior changes occur best when simple changes are made first and change occurs gradually over time. However, the individual with diabetes has to try to manage all of the factors simultaneously and right away.

Another principle of successful behavior management is the opportunity to take breaks or "time out" from difficult tasks. However, there are no weekends off, no vacations, and no retirement from diabetes. The demands of diabetes self-care are constant.[2,3]

SECTION 3: Nonpharmacological Management

EMOTION, PSYCHOLOGY, AND DIABETES

Psychological, emotional, and social issues in diabetes manifest as coping and adjustment difficulties, a sense of non-wellbeing and decreased quality of life. Modern researchers and healthcare providers in diabetes have now realized the importance of psychosocial issues. In coming years, psychosocial issues will be considered important aspects affecting diabetes management by patients themselves, so as to establish good control and avoid the sequelae and complications of diabetes.

The adjustment, wellbeing, and quality of life issues in diabetes have been termed as "substantial and unremitting", because of the demanding regimens of diabetes management. It has been correctly described that a person with diabetes has to think about diabetes at least every 15 minutes. The regimens of diabetes management are very demanding.[2] There is the demand for controlling blood glucose as close to normal as possible, unpleasant pricking of the body even, at times, five to six occasions a day to control blood glucose. Hence, the psychosocial aspect of diabetes has been termed as "diabetes overwhelms us."

Positive psychology is an important aspect of diabetes care. It has to be emphasized to the patient with diabetes that "a known and well-controlled diabetes is much better than a nondiabetic." This is because a diabetic undergoes constant monitoring testing by the healthcare providers as regular check-ups and good glycemic and blood pressure control achieved through this may prevent or at least postpone the complication.

PSYCHOLOGICAL REACTIONS TO DIABETES[4]

When someone has diabetes, physical health is often his main focus. However, diabetes is about more than one's physical health. It affects every aspect of one's life including one's emotional health, one's feeling, attitude, and mental state. Diabetes can also affect the emotional health of family and friends. A variety of psychological reactions may occur at the time of diagnosis of diabetes.

Denial

As a defense measure, one may believe there could be a mistake in the test or the report. It is a reaction against some restrictive or uncomfortable situations. Up to a point, denial is a normal reaction but it can keep from taking proactive measures to overcome ill health.

Anger

Anger at the time of diagnosis is expected but unwanted or uncontrollable anger maybe pathological. However, the expression of anger should not be hurting to oneself or others.

Guilt

Guilt may occur in a realistic on unrealistic situation. The child may ask, "why me?" It may be an example of feeling guilty about one's behavior and not taking control of events and correcting them.

Depression[5]

This may result from unpleasant, uncorrectable situations. It may be similar to denial, but should not become overwhelming or long-lasting. It may be countered by becoming involved in distracting activity. Depression is two to three times more prevalent among patients with diabetes mellitus than in general population affecting 15–20% of the diabetic population. Diabetes patients are more prone to suffer from recurrent episodes of depression requiring repeated treatment. If depression is persistent, professional help is needed.

Fear of Hypoglycemia

Hypoglycemia is generally considered to be major complication of intensive insulin therapy, with serious adverse effects on the emotional and social functioning of patients and their social environment. Fear of hypoglycemia is strongly related to the threat of losing control over one's physical and mental abilities, along with feeling of embarrassment. Many worry about losing consciousness and possible damage to the brain.

With the increasing awareness of the risks of persistent poor glycemic control, it should come as no surprise that many persons with diabetes worry about their health and future. Health worries of diabetic patients appear to pertain predominantly to loss of eyesight, amputation of a foot or leg, and more generally becoming dependent on others.

Anxiety

Many people call themselves "high strong" or declare themselves that they have always been a worrier. Dealing with a chronic illness, like diabetes, may make a person more likely to develop an anxiety disorder. This happens because of experiencing a situation that may last for the whole life. Some people are born with a tendency to become more anxious than others. Fear is the main issue with anxiety. It can be the fear of injection, fear of complications, or even a general fear. Sometimes, children and young people have social anxiety. They are afraid that if they do something when they are with other people, it may be embarrassing. Rarely, anxiety in diabetes can take a very severe stress disorder termed as "posttraumatic stress disorder." This can arise if one happens to experience a situation which is life-threatening and traumatic.

Acceptance

Acceptance and resolution may be delayed and take up to 12 months after the diagnosis of diabetes. It requires an understanding of diabetes and is consolidated when successful glycemic control is established with optimal lifestyle parameters.

Adjustment to Diabetes

The ATT39 is a measure of psychological adjustment to diabetes that was developed in response to the need for more specific measurement tools for the assessment of psychosocial issues in diabetes. Specific instruments were expected to provide more sensitive measurement of the dynamic psychological processes unique to diabetes and greater predictive validity that was available from the broad personality measures than in use. Many children have adjustment problems soon after the diagnosis of diabetes.

Eating Disorders

Eating disorders are frequently observed in young women and adolescent females with T1DM and are associated with poorer glycemic control and an increased risk of long-term complications. Therefore, these individuals should be regularly screened for eating disorders. Those with an identified or suspected eating disorder should be referred to a medical team or to a knowledgeable professional in treating such disorders.

ASSESSMENT OF PSYCHOLOGICAL PROBLEMS

The psychological problems have impact on quality of life, perception of health, adjustments, and wellbeing of a diabetic patient. Therefore, it is of paramount importance to assess the following parameters:[2,6]

- Quality of life
- Treatment satisfaction
- Fear of hypoglycemia
- Depression and anxiety
- Eating disorders
- Adjustments
- Wellbeing.

Wellbeing

It was used in a World Health Organization study evaluating new treatments for the management of diabetes. The wellbeing scales were developed from a questionnaire originally designed for use with adults was insulin-treated diabetes but have also been developed with a population of people with tablet treated diabetes and are probably equally suitable for people with diabetes treated with diet alone.

Quality of Life

The Diabetes Quality of Life (DQOL) was developed in the early 1980s for use in the Diabetes Control and Complications Trial (DCCT). The DQOL was designed to evaluate the relative burden of an intensive diabetes treatment regimen, with the goal of maintaining blood glucose levels as close possible to those of people without diabetes in comparison to standard diabetes therapy.

CHAPTER 12: Biopsychosocial Dimensions in Diabetes: A Brief Outline

DIABETES TREATMENT SATISFACTION

The Diabetes Treatment Satisfaction Questionnaire (DTSQ) has been specifically designed to measure satisfaction with diabetes. The DTSQ has evolved through three stages. The earliest version of the measure was designed to evaluate changes in satisfaction after 1 year in a feasibility study of continuous subcutaneous insulin infusion pumps conducted in Sheffield. The change in treatment satisfaction was used to evaluate improvements in satisfaction with treatment in that study where baseline reports of satisfaction were not available and a retrospective comparison was needed. The change in the treatment satisfaction questionnaire was used an evaluate improvements in satisfaction with treatment in that study where baseline reports of satisfaction were not available and a retrospective comparison was needed.

In the second stage of development of satisfaction with treatment scales, the measures of absolute levels of satisfaction with treatment were development first on a sample of patients with T2DM table treated diabetes and subsequently on a sample of T1DM. In the third stage, the DTSQ has been designed to be appropriate for people with all types of diabetes regardless of the form of treatment used.

NEED FOR PSYCHOSOCIAL ASSESSMENT

There are few special situation to which a healthcare provider has to be attentive, especially for children and T1DM in a psychological angle. The following are indications for referral to a psychologist:
- Poor glycemic control without any clear reason
- Problems at school
- Obvious psychological distress
- Repeated admission to the hospital
- Eating disorders and changes in the attitudes.

BIOPSYCHOSOCIAL INTERVENTIONS[7,8]

All the above calls for an in depth biopsychosocial factor analysis and one may provide relief through approaches based on:
- Analysis of behavior
- Behavior modification therapy
- Working of parent—teenage child relationship
- By repeated goal setting and positive reinforcement.

Following are the biopsychosocial interventions for the diabetic patient:
- Routine case assessment
- Empowerment
- Family interventions
- Cognitive behavioral therapy
- Motivational interviewing
- Problem solving.

Biopsychosocial Factors Responsible For Heterogeneity in Management

The following must be considered while planning interventions:
- Monetary issues
- Cultural and religious factors
- Alternative systems of medicine
- Educational qualification
- Place of residence (whether rural or urban).

RECOMMENDATIONS FOR INTEGRATED BIOPSYCHOSOCIAL MANAGEMENT[1]

- Physicians trained in the skills of communication, counseling, and focused advice on coping with the disease and its complications
- Healthcare professionals must be made aware of the biopsychosocial model of managing diabetes and obtain basic grounding in psychosocial aspects of diabetes. Familiarity with biopsychosocial models of diabetes where psychosocial factors are not forgotten
- Proficiency in teaching skills
- Appropriate patient education skills keeping in mind India's low general literacy and "diabetes literacy"
- Empowering patients to learn from the peers, adapt to diabetes dynamics and enthusing motivation, zeal, and tenacity of purpose to conquer diabetes
- Biopsychosocial strengthening at the level of one's family, school, workplace, and community
- All involved (family, school, healthcare providers, and community) in the patient management must be conscious of psychiatric comorbidities in diabetes such as depression and anxiety
- To adopt a definite patient centered approach which is defined as an approach to "providing care that is respectful of and responsive to individual patient preferences, needs, and values, and ensuring that patient values guide all clinical decisions."

MODERN TECHNOLOGY IN IMPROVING BIOPSYCHOSOCIAL CARE

The modern technologies include automated phone, text, email, videoconferencing, and websites. Videoconferencing via Skype seems to allow the patient-caregiver relationship to be maintained. A program of telemedicine case management improved self-efficacy and glycosylated hemoglobin in older diabetic patients with comorbid depression.[5] Web-based intervention have been found useful in improving the psychosocial wellbeing of patients aged over 60. Thus, the internet can not only be an educational resource but also be an emotional resource for patients. Professionally, moderated web-based discussion forums covering nutrition, motivation, and family relationships were reported as improving participants' ability to cope with their diabetes.

There is ample proof that psychosocial interventions improve various facets of diabetes. One recent paper describes significant improvement of depression by psychosocial interventions done by the nurses.[2]

CONCLUSION

Diabetes cannot be managed without understanding, and addressing, both psychosocial and biomedical domains of health. Living with diabetes carries responsibilities which have to be fulfilled by the person, family and health care provider. Self-care behavior, motivation, wellbeing and quality of life must be promoted during all interactions between person and provider. One also needs to identify, and correct, the various psychological reactions to diabetes, such as denial, anger, quilt, depression, and anxiety.

Validated tools can be used to assess wellbeing, quality of life, fear of hypoglycemia, and satisfaction with treatment.

Until diabetes distress is handled, optimal outcomes cannot be achieved. Appropriate biopsychosocial interventions are available for use in children who need them. Such interventions should be presented only after a comprehensive assessment. Focus on integrated bio psychosocial management of diabetes will definitely help improve the quality of care, and quality of life of children living with diabetes.

REFERENCES

1. Kalra S, Sridhar GR, Balhara YP, Sahay RK, Bantwal G, Baruah MP, et al. National recommendations: Psychosocial management of diabetes in India. Indian J Endocrinol Metab. 2013;17(3):376.
2. Harvey JN. Psychosocial interventions for the diabetic patient. Diabetes Metab Syndr Obes. 2015;8:29-43.
3. Knight KM, Dornan T, Bundy C. The diabetes educator: trying hard, but must concentrate more on behaviour. Diabet Med. 2006;23(5):485-501.
4. Boon-How Chew, Sazlina Shariff-Ghazali, and Aaron Fernandez. Psychological aspects of diabetes care: Effecting behavioral change in patients. World J Diabetes. 2014;5(6):796-808.
5. Kok JL, Williams A, Zhao L. Psychosocial interventions for people with diabetes and co-morbid depression. A systematic review. International journal of nursing studies. 2015;52(10):1625-39.
6. Iraklis Avramopoulos, Alexandros Moulis, and Nikos Nikas. Glycaemic control, treatment satisfaction and quality of life in type 2 diabetes patients in Greece: The PANORAMA study Greek results. World J Diabetes. 2015;6(1):208-16.
7. Kahana S, Drotar D, Frazier T. Meta-analysis of psychological interventions to promote adherence to treatment in pediatric chronic health conditions. J Pediatr Psychol. 2008;33(6):590-611.
8. Hampson SE, Skinner TC, Hart J, Storey L, Gage H, Foxcroft D, et al. Effects of educational and psychosocial interventions for adolescents with diabetes mellitus: a systematic review. Health Technol Assess. 2001;5(10):1-79.

SECTION 4

Pharmacological Management

Editor
Subhankar Chowdhury

CHAPTER 13

Insulin Therapy

Ashok K Das

INTRODUCTION

As an autoimmune disorder, type 1 diabetes mellitus (T1DM) destroys pancreatic β-cells, which causes children to present typically with complete β-cell failure and acute, severe hyperglycemia. Eventually, however, complete insulin deficiency requires insulin replacement therapy with the dual goal of normalizing blood glucose levels while avoiding hypoglycemic episodes. Thus, insulin replacement represents a cornerstone of management for patients with T1DM.[1]

The Diabetes Control and Complications Trial highlighted the critical importance of precise insulin dosing to achieve these goals.[2] Long-term follow-up of these subjects for an additional 27 years, reported in the Epidemiology of Diabetes Interventions and Complications trial, confirmed that an improvement in long-term glucose control, as obtained with early intensified insulin therapy including heavy support and education, can reduce the incidence of complications, delay the progression of existing complications in T1DM, and reduce mortality, also in pediatric patients.[3-5]

MANAGEMENT FRAMEWORK[1]

Essential components of care provide a framework for developing a management strategy and a shared understanding for physicians and patients with T1DM. These include:
- A combination of basal and bolus insulin, either as a part of multiple daily injections (MDI) or continuous subcutaneous insulin infusion (CSII)
- Monitoring, including self-monitoring of blood glucose (SMBG) with or without continuous glucose monitoring or ambulatory glucose profile and glycosylated hemoglobin (HbA1c) with individualized glucose targets that balance effectiveness and the risk of hypoglycemia
- Patient education around the relationship between insulin, SMBG, activity, and food, specifically carbohydrates; risks with insulin therapy also needs to be discussed

SECTION 4: Pharmacological Management

- An experienced interdisciplinary team that can facilitate overall management, insulin adjustments, goal setting, safety, education, and support.

INSULIN THERAPY

The goal of treatment in T1DM is to provide insulin in as physiological manner as possible. To mimic physiologic insulin secretion, both long- and short-acting insulins are used. Long-acting insulin suppresses glucose output from the liver overnight and provides basal insulin between meals; bolus doses of short-acting insulin modulate glucose excursions associated with carbohydrate consumption.[1]

Daily insulin dosage depends on many factors:
- Age of child
- Body weight
- Stage of puberty
- Duration of diabetes
- Injection sites: Any lipodystrophy
- Food intake and nutritional distribution
- Exercise regimes and daily routines
- Self-monitoring of blood glucose and HbA1c values
- Intercurrent illness.

Types of Insulins

Conventional Insulins

- Short-acting insulin—regular human insulin:[6] Short-acting regular "human" insulin (RHI) was a result of the development of recombinant DNA technology, which finally allowed for the large-scale synthesis of human origin insulin. However, the pharmacokinetic (PK)/pharmacodynamic (PD) properties of RHI do not accurately match the insulin secretion pattern of a healthy person without diabetes, due to its slow rate of absorption (Table 1). This pattern of slow onset and long duration of action of RHI exacerbates the risk of developing early postprandial hyperglycemia, and the subsequent risk of hypoglycemia before the next meal
- Intermediate acting insulin—Neutral protamine Hagedorn/Isophane insulin:[7] Neutral protamine Hagedorn (NPH) is an intermediate acting insulin (Table 1), which gave the flexibility to inject fewer doses of insulin; thus increasing patient convenience. The aim of NPH development was to introduce the first slow-release insulins using the animal protein protamine, from fish sperm that reduced the solubility of insulin and zinc. It reduced, but did not eliminate, the incidence of hypoglycemic episodes. A high level of hypoglycemia, particularly nocturnal hypoglycemia, was and still is one of the major limitations of NPH
- Biphasic human insulin:[8,9] Biphasic human insulin (BHI) is a premixed insulin containing short-acting insulin and NPH in different proportions. For example, BHI 30 contains 30% short-acting insulin and 70% NPH or BHI 50 contains 50% short-acting insulin and 50%

CHAPTER 13: Insulin Therapy

TABLE 1: Key pharmacokinetic/pharmacodynamic data of available insulins[22]

Name	Type	Onset (min)	Peak (h)	Duration (h)
Human insulins				
RHI	Short-acting (bolus)	30–60	2–3	5–8
BHI 30/70	Premixed	30–60	Dual	10–16
BHI 50/50	Premixed	30–60	Dual	10–16
NPH	Intermediate-acting (basal)	120–240	4–10	10–16
Modern insulins				
Aspart	Rapid-acting (bolus)	5–15	0.5–1.5	<5
Lispro	Rapid-acting (bolus)	5–15	0.5–1.5	<5
Glulisine	Rapid-acting (bolus)	20	1.5	5.3
BIAsp 30/70	Premixed	5–15	Dual	10–16
BIAsp 50/50	Premixed	5–15	Dual	10–16
LM 25/75	Premixed	5–15	Dual	10–16
LM 50/50	Premixed	5–15	Dual	10–16
Glargine	Long-acting (basal)	120–240	No pronounced peak	Up to 24
Detemir	Long-acting (basal)	48–120		Up to 24
Degludec	Ultra long-acting (basal)	30–90	Peakless	>42
Degludec/aspart	Co-formulation	5–15	0.5–1.5	>24

RHI, regular human insulin; BHI, biphasic human insulin; NPH, neutral protamine Hagedorn; BIAsp, biphasic insulin aspart; LM, lispro mix.

NPH (Table 1). It allows the patient to administer fewer daily injections than the classic basal-bolus therapy, which requires injections of rapid-acting insulin before meals and intermediate or long-acting insulin in the morning or at bedtime. However, it fails to recreate the physiological insulin profile and shows periods of unwanted hyper- and hypoglycemia

- Limitations of conventional insulins:[10]
  o Onset: delayed
  o Advised to inject 30 minutes before meals
  o Peak: 2–3 hours
  o Less insulin increase in early phase of glucose absorption → excessive rise in glucose at 1–2 hours after meal
  o Duration: 8 hours
  o At 4–5 hours after subcutaneous injection, inappropriate hyperinsulinemia → hypoglycemia
  o Snack in between meals to counter hypoglycemia
  o Glycemic variability
  o Dose has a profound effect on time action profile.

SECTION 4: Pharmacological Management

Modern Insulins

- Rapid-acting insulin analogs—aspart, lispro, and glulisine:[11-13] Rapid acting analogs of human insulin have been developed that can dissociate rapidly from hexamers, thus allowing faster absorption and rapid onset of action (Table 1). They are used as meal time insulins. Currently, three rapid-acting bolus insulin analogs are available: (i) insulin glulisine, (ii) insulin lispro, and (iii) insulin aspart. While RHI is recommended 30 minutes before meals, rapid-acting insulin analogs have the flexibility of being administered just before a meal or even after the meal has begun. These rapid-acting analogs show low intrapatient variability, while demonstrating similar PK/PD properties. Compared to equivalent doses of RHI, all rapid-acting analogs reach twice the maximal concentration within half the time. Figures 1A and B show the action of RHI and rapid acting insulin analogs
- Long-acting insulin analogs—detemir and glargine:[14,15] Basal analogs provide consistent, flat, long-acting insulin levels to mimic the constant release of insulin that regulates endogenous glucose output. Currently, two basal insulin analogs, insulin glargine, and insulin detemir are available. Insulin glargine has an acidic pH (pH 4) in solution which forms microprecipitates, due to neutralization, after being injected subcutaneously, resulting in its slow release into the circulation. Insulin detemir is acylated leading to high binding affinity for albumin, which in turn results in delayed absorption. This delayed absorption, along with its hexamer-forming abilities, gives it a prolonged action. In comparison with NPH, both insulin detemir and insulin glargine show prolonged duration of action and little peak activity. Duration of action is dose-dependent and similar for both insulin glargine and insulin detemir suggesting that a majority of patients with type 2 diabetes mellitus can administer these basal analogs once daily.

Figures 2A and B show the action of NPH and basal insulin analogs:

- Premixed insulin analogs:[16,17] Fixed ratio combinations of bolus and intermediate acting insulin analogs were designed to enhance convenience of insulin therapy and to minimize patient self-mixing error. Currently available insulin analog premixes include:

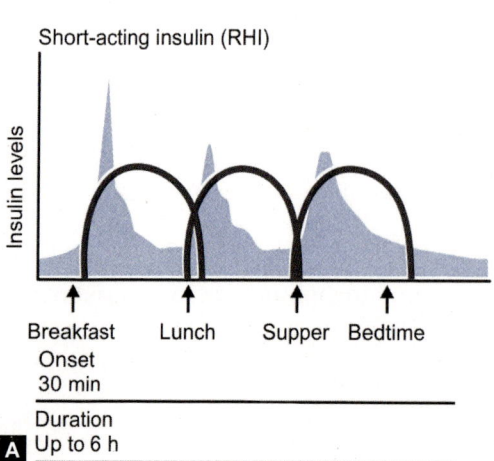 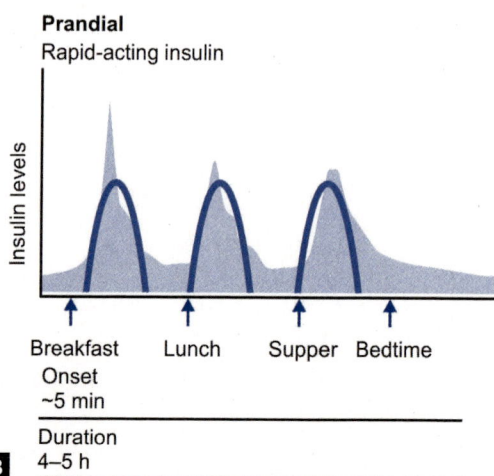

Figs 1A and B: Action of **(A)** regular human insulin; **(B)** rapid acting insulin analogs

CHAPTER 13: Insulin Therapy

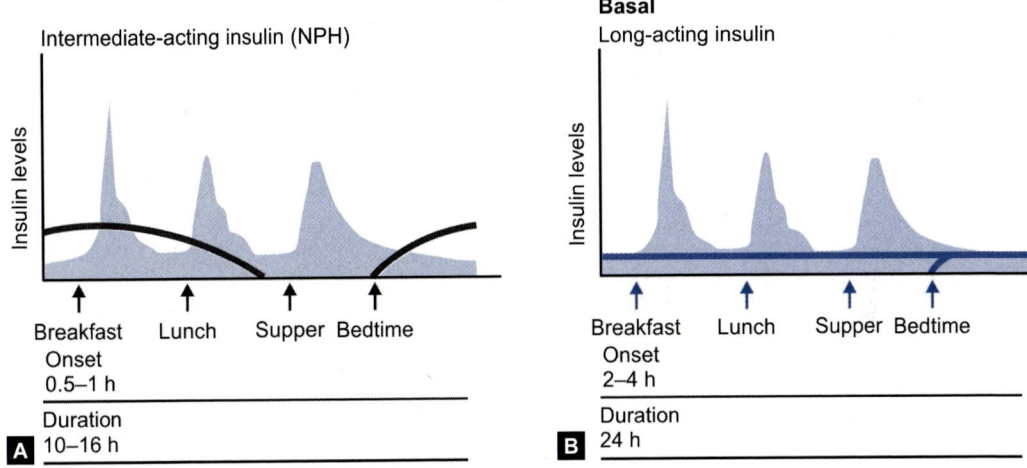

Figs 2A and B: Action of **(A)** Neutral protamine Hagedorn (NPH); **(B)** basal insulin analogs. Note the slight peak in the NPH plot

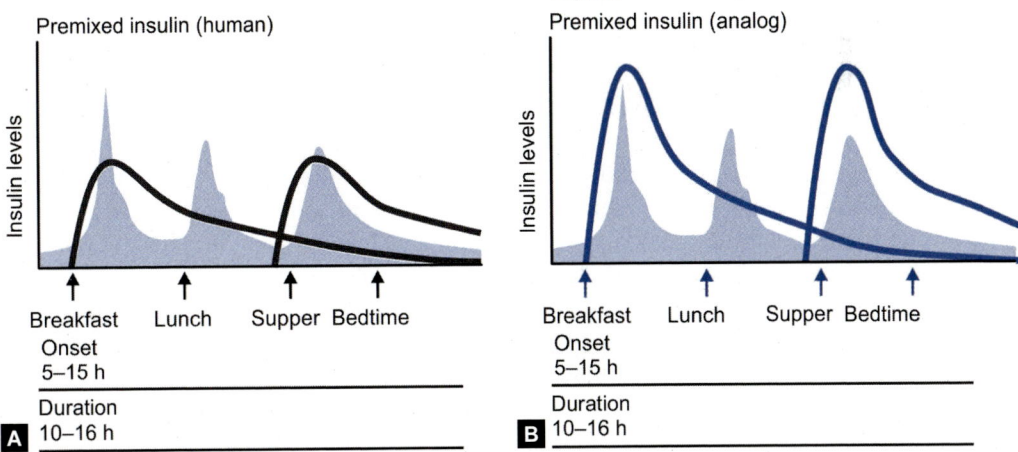

Figs 3A and B: Action of **(A)** biphasic human insulin (BHI); **(B)** premixed insulin analogs

- Biphasic insulin aspart 30 (BIAsp 30): A 30/70 mixture of insulin aspart/protaminated insulin aspart
- Lispro mix 25 (LM 25): A 25/75 mixture of insulin lispro/protaminated insulin lispro
- Biphasic insulin aspart 50 (BIAsp 50): A 50/50 mixture of insulin aspart/protaminated insulin aspart
- Lispro mix 50 (LM 50): A 50/50 mixture of insulin lispro/protaminated insulin lispro.
- In comparison to BHI 30, which also contains a mixture of intermediate and short-acting insulins, analog premixes have more physiologic PK profiles and provide better postprandial plasma glucose control.

SECTION 4: Pharmacological Management

TABLE 2: Advantages of analog premix over human premix[18]

Parameters	Premix human insulin	Premix insulin analog
Postprandial glucose control	+	+++
Fasting glucose control	++	++
HbA1c control	+	++
Less hypoglycemia	+	++
Meal-time flexibility	+	+++

HbA1c, glycosylated hemoglobin.

Figures 3A and B show the action of BHI and premixed insulin analogs:
- Insulin analog premixes also have more convenient injection schedules (can be injected immediately before eating or even after the start of a meal) compared to an injection-meal interval of at least 30 minutes, for conventional human premixed insulin (Table 2)[19]
- There is no clear evidence that premixed insulins in young children are less effective, but there is some evidence of poorer metabolic control when used in adolescents. They may be useful to reduce the number of injections when compliance (or adherence) to the regimen is a problem[20]
- Ultra-long acting insulin analog:[21] Insulin degludec is the only available ultra-long acting basal insulin analogs currently available. It self-associates to form large multihexamer assemblies at the site of injection leading to a half-life longer than 25.4 hours (twice as long as that of insulin glargine) and detection in circulation for at least 96 hours after injection with a possibility of a flexible dosing regimen. The low insulin-like growth factor 1 receptor binding affinity and the low mitogenic/metabolic potency ratio ensure molecular safety. Furthermore, binding of the fatty acid moiety of insulin degludec (IDeg) to albumin contributes to some extent to the protraction mechanism
- Co-formulation of long-acting insulin with rapid-acting insulin:[22] Co-formulation of long-acting insulin analogs with rapid acting insulin analogs was not possible in the past due to the physicochemical incompatibilities.

Insulin degludec/insulin aspart (IDegIAsp) is the first soluble co-formulation of two different insulin analogs (70% IDeg, as basal insulin and 30% IAsp, as prandial insulin). In the formulation, IDeg exists as stable dihexamers, and IAsp as hexamers. Whereas, under conditions mimicking the subcutaneous environment, IDeg forms very large multi-hexamers that are slowly absorbed and IAsp hexamer is dissociated into monomers, that are rapidly absorbed. This allows the co-formulation to maintain distinct PK/PD profiles of basal and prandial components in a single injection, in one pen.

INSULIN REGIMES[20]

The choice of insulin regimen will depend on many factors including: age, duration of diabetes, lifestyle (dietary patterns, exercise schedules, school, work commitments, etc.), targets of metabolic control, and particularly individual patient/family preferences.

- Split or mixed: Two injections per day, of NPH with rapid-acting or regular insulin before breakfast and dinner
- Premixed: Two injections per day, before breakfast and dinner
- Split or mixed variant: Three injections daily using a mixture of short or rapid- and NPH before breakfast; rapid or regular insulin alone before lunch or dinner (the main meal); NPH before bed or variations of this (the idea is to reduce fasting hypoglycemia by giving the NPH later in the evening)
- Basal-bolus with MDI: A long-acting insulin once a day in the morning or evening and a rapid-acting insulin before meals or snacks (with the dose adjusted according to the carbohydrate intake and the blood glucose level)
- Basal bolus with continuous subcutaneous insulin infusion: Rapid-acting insulin infused continuously 24 hours a day through an insulin pump at 1 or more basal rates, with additional boluses given before each meal, and correction doses administered if blood glucose levels exceed target levels.

Of the total daily insulin requirements, 40–60% should be basal insulin, the rest preprandial rapid-acting or regular insulin.

When a mixture of two insulins is drawn up (e.g., regular with NPH), it is prudent to ensure that there is no contamination between insulins in the vials. To prevent this, follow the given points:

- Draw regular (clear insulin) into the syringe before drawing the cloudy insulin (intermediate/long-acting)
- Gently roll (do not shake) the vial of cloudy insulin 10–20 times, to mix the insulin suspension before drawing it up into the clear insulin (Figs 4A to C)
- Use insulins from different manufacturers with caution, as there may be an interaction between the buffering agents
- If rapid-acting insulin analogs are being used, they may be mixed in the same syringe as NPH, immediately before injections.

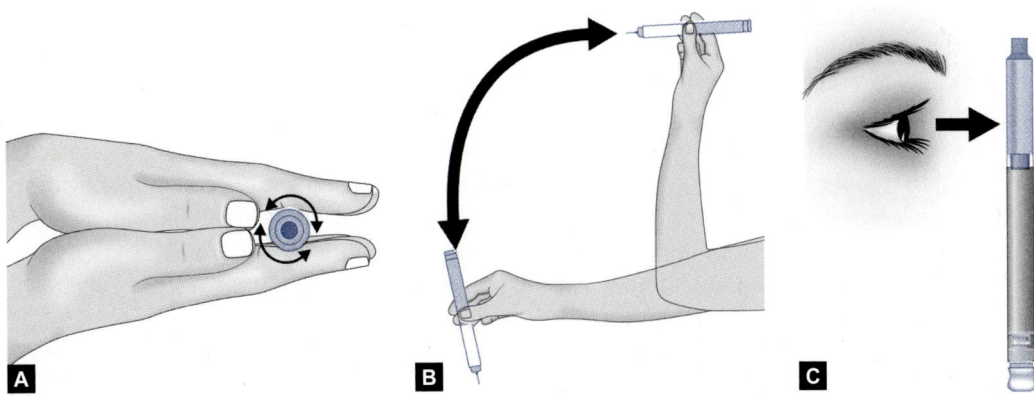

Figs 4A to C: Mixing/resuspension of cloudy insulin. **(A)** Roll 10 times; **(B)** Tip 10 times; **(C)** Visual check

STORING AND MIXING OF INSULIN[23]

Storage

- Follow the specific storage guidelines provided by the manufacturer
- Insulin should be stored in a cool and dark place
- Insulin pens and vials, which are not being used, should be refrigerated but not frozen. If frozen, insulin should be discarded
- Insulin being used can be kept at room temperature (15–25°C) to limit local irritation at the injection site which may occur when cold insulin is used
- Discard 30 days after initial use or follow manufacturer's instructions
- Insulin vial and pens stored in a refrigerator should be taken out and kept at room temperature for at least 30 minutes before use
- Pens should never be stored with needles on because of higher risk of air entering through the needles which may block them and affect the dose delivery
- In areas where refrigerators are not available (i.e., rural areas): Put the vial in a plastic bag, tie a rubber band, and keep in a wide-mouthed bottle or earthen pitcher filled with water
- Keep the vial or pen out of reach of children
- Physician should be consulted if travelling to a place with a time zone difference of two or more hours because it may require a change in insulin injection schedule
- Insulin should not be placed in the baggage hold of the plane due to the risk of exposure to extreme temperatures
- Never use insulin beyond its expiry date
- Avoid extremes of temperatures such as direct sunlight, kitchen, leaving vials in a car, on top of a radiator, on top of a television, etc. as it will make the medication less effective.

INSULIN INJECTION TECHNIQUE[23]

Proper insulin absorption occurs when it is delivered to subcutaneous tissue. Insulin must be injected after properly locating an appropriate site for subcutaneous fat deposit by lightly raising the skin by pinching the site. Only the thumb, index, and middle finger must be used to perform a correct lifted skin fold (Figs 5A to C). Skin of a very thin person may have to be gently pinched.

Needle can be inserted at an incident angle, between 45° and 90°, with 45° being appropriate for very thin people and 90° for overweight people or when using short needle. Sterilization with alcohol swabbing is not necessary, as there are bactericidal agents in the insulin vial and as such injection site infections are very rare. However, if antiseptic cleaning agent is used then it should be allowed to evaporate before injecting insulin.

The recommended insulin injection sites are:
- Abdomen: Fastest and most consistent rate
- Arms: Medium rate
- Thighs: Slowest rate
- Buttocks: Slowest rate

CHAPTER 13: Insulin Therapy

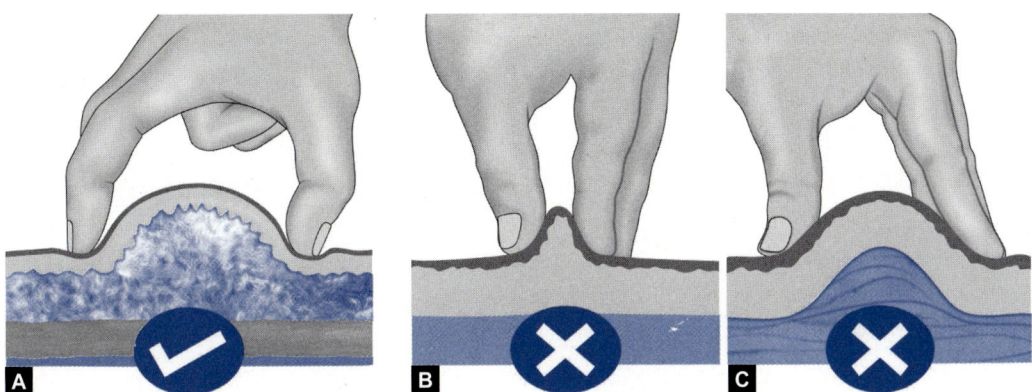

Figs 5A to C: Representation of correct and incorrect way of insulin injection

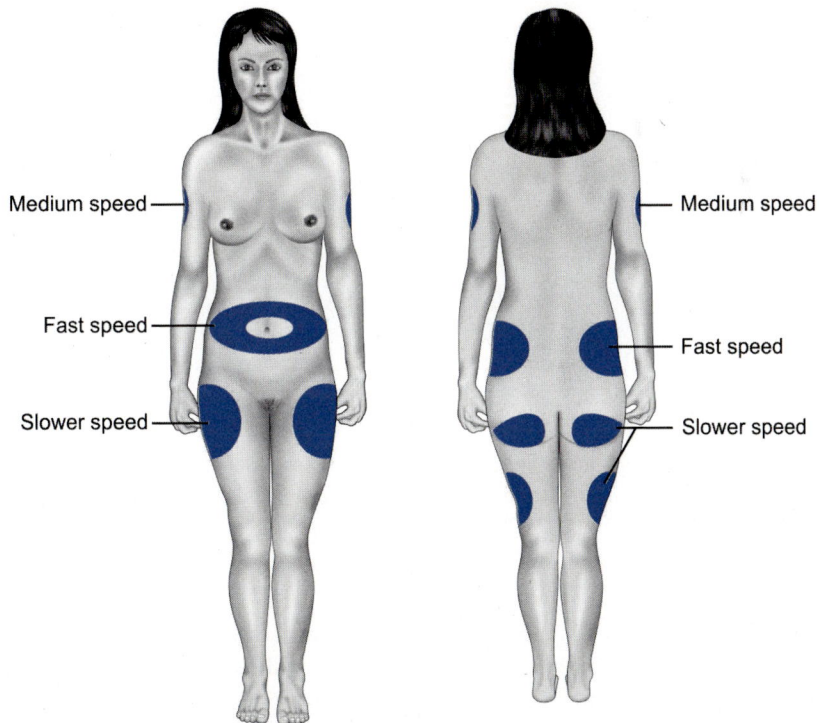

Fig. 6: Recommended sites of insulin injection

Due to the ease of performing a pinch up and abundant fat deposit, the abdomen is usually the most preferred site. Additionally, insulin shows fastest absorption when injected in abdominal sites. Once an appropriate site has been located and the skin fold is raised, the syringe must be held like a pencil using the other hand and the needle should be positioned to make sure it is angled correctly for injection. The needle should be gently inserted under the skin at the correct angle and the plunger should be pressed with the thumb in a gentle, steady

SECTION 4: Pharmacological Management

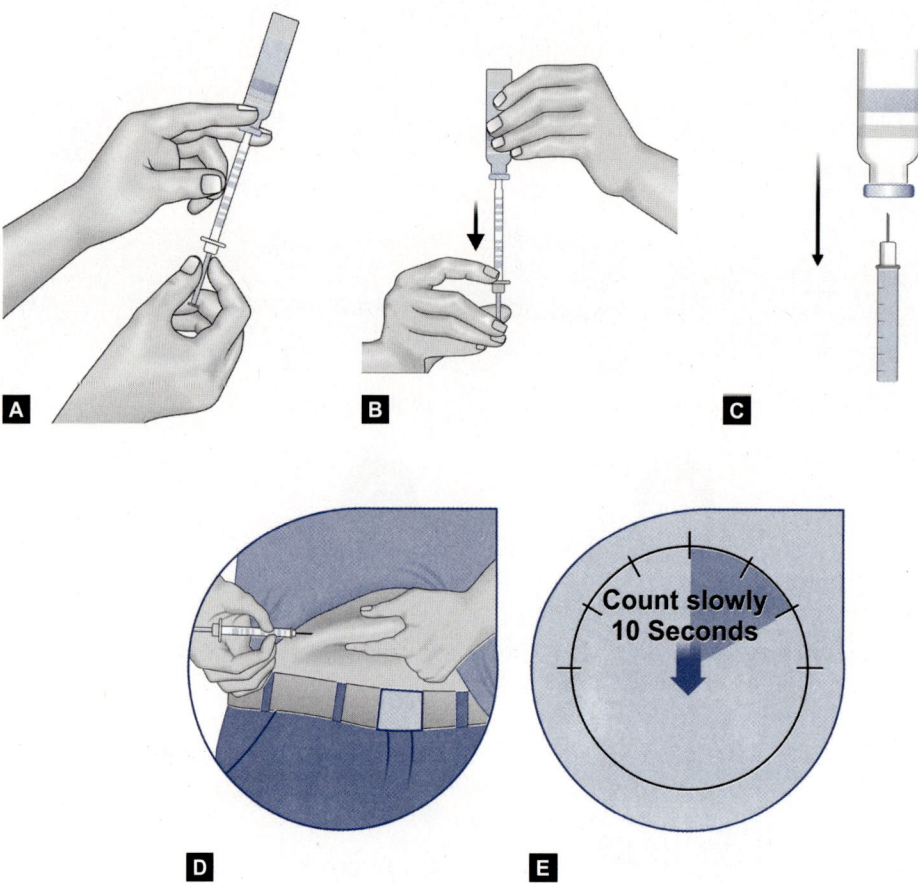

Figs 7A to E: Correct process of injecting the insulin. **(A)** Turn the insulin bottle and syringe upside down; **(B)** Pull the plunger down slowly, to get the insulin into the syringe; **(C)** Pull the syringe out of the bottle; **(D)** Make a skin fold using two fingers. Hold the syringe at 90° and inject; **(E)** Count for 10 seconds and release the pinch-up

motion until the insulin is gone. After injecting the insulin, the needle should be pulled out at the same angle it was inserted in and the injection site should be pressed gently for a few seconds to prevent the insulin from leaking (Figs 6 and 7A to E).

How to Use a Pen to Give an Injection (Figs 8A to F)[23]

To avoid issues of variability due to self-measurement by patients, pen devices are advocated whenever possible. The sequence of steps involved in the proper use of pens for injecting insulin involves the following:
- Wash hands
- Check expiry date on cartridge and amount of insulin left

CHAPTER 13: Insulin Therapy

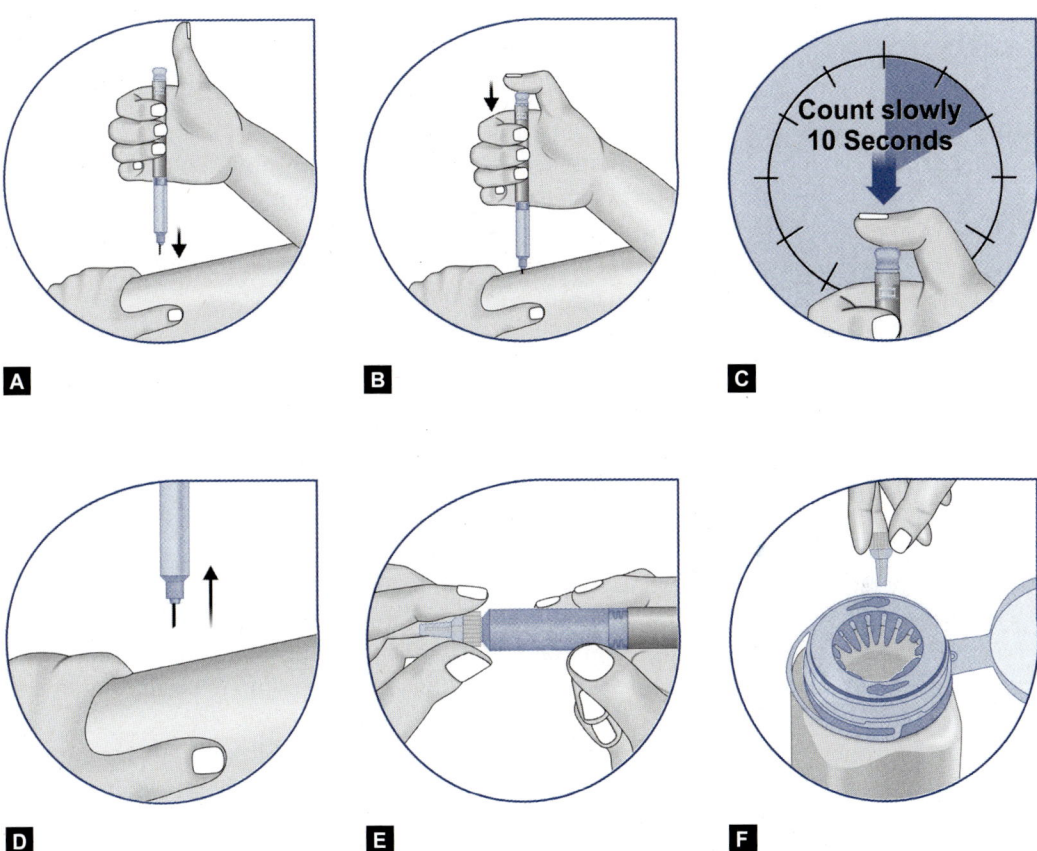

Figs 8A to F: How to use a pen to give an injection. **(A)** Choose the appropriate site for injection; **(B)** Push the needle through the skin at 90° keeping thumb away from dosage button; **(C)** Push thumb button down completely and count to 10 or follow manufactures recommendations; **(D)** Remove needle from subcutaneous tissue; **(E)** Remove needle from pen; **(F)** Dispose of needle safely

- Fit a new pen needle
- Turn pen up and down (4–5 times) few times
- Remove outer cover and inner cap of needle
- Dial two to four units to perform air shot, repeat until insulin drop is seen
- Dial required dose
- Stretch skin taut/lift skin fold (whichever appropriate)
- Insert needle smoothly into skin and press plunger
- When dose is given, count to ten before removing needle from skin
- Remove needle from pen and dispose in sharps box
- Store pen in its case at room temperature, away from heat or sun.

SECTION 4: Pharmacological Management

INSULIN ABSORPTION[20]

Insulin activity profiles show substantial variability, both day-to-day in the same individual and between individuals, particularly in children. The onset, peak effect, and duration of action depend upon many factors which can affect the speed and consistency of absorption. Faster absorption usually results in a shorter duration of action.

- Age: Younger children with less subcutaneous fat → faster absorption
- Fat mass: Large subcutaneous fat thickness and/or lipohypertrophy → slower absorption
- Dose of injection: Larger dose → slower absorption
- Site and depth of subcutaneous injection: Abdomen → faster absorption than thigh
- Intramuscular injection → faster absorption in thigh
- Exercise: Leg injection followed by exercise of same leg → faster absorption
- Insulin concentration, type, and formulation: Lower concentration → faster absorption
- Ambient and body temperature: Higher temperatures → faster absorption
- In general, the absorption speed of rapid-acting analogs is less affected by the above mentioned factors.

Problems with Insulin Injection[20]

- Local hypersensitivity reactions to insulin injections are uncommon but when they do occur, it would be essential to identify the insulin (or, more rarely, preservative) responsible. A trial of an alternative insulin preparation may solve the problem. If true allergy is suspected, desensitization can be performed. Adding a small amount of corticosteroids to the insulin may help
- Lipohypertrophy, with the accumulation of fat in lumps underneath the skin, is common in children. Lipoatrophy has become uncommon since the introduction of highly purified insulins and analogs
- Painful injections are a common problem. It is important to check angle, length of the needle, and depth of injection to ensure injections are not being given intramuscularly and that the needle is sharp. Reused needles can cause more pain
- Leakage of insulin is also common and cannot be totally avoided. Encourage slower withdrawal of needle from skin, stretching of the skin after the needle is withdrawn, or pressure with clean finger over the injection site
- Bruising and bleeding are more common after intramuscular injection or tight squeezing of the skin. Use of thinner needles has shown significantly less bleeding at the injection site. Bubbles in insulin should be removed whenever possible. When using insulin pens, air in the cartridge can cause drops of insulin appearing on the tip of the pen needle, if withdrawn too quickly.

Insulin use in Continuous Subcutaneous Insulin Infusion Pumps

Continuous subcutaneous insulin infusion is a sophisticated and precise insulin delivery method which uses a small programmable pump with a fine tube connected to a soft plastic cannula (introduced by needle), that goes into the subcutaneous tissue under the skin, often in the abdomen.[24] The aim of CSII is to try to mimic endogenous insulin delivery profile more closely to the pattern of insulin delivery from pancreas, by providing continuously infused, low-volume basal insulin for fasting periods and delivery of increased rate boluses to cover meals.[25,26]

The insulin pump allows the user to program many different basal rates of infusion depending on individual lifestyle. In addition, the user can program the pump to deliver a bolus insulin dose during meals to cover the excess demands of carbohydrate ingestion. New insulin pumps allow applying this bolus in four different ways:[27]
1. Infusion of the total dose at once or
2. Splitting the dose into two boluses
3. Infusion of a part of the bolus in the usual manner plus infusion of the other part over a prolonged period of time (with a higher infusion rate than the basal rate) or
4. Infusion of the total dose in the form of an elevated basal rate.

Most pumps use rapid-acting insulin analogs (RAIAs), i.e., lispro, aspart, and glulisine. The PD and PK features of RAIAs (instant absorption, quick peak, and fast withdrawal) make them the best choice, because of better mimicking of the physiological secretion of insulin from the β-cells. Furthermore, insulin analogs have fewer tendencies to form crystals inside the plastic tubes of pump which can lead to obstruction.[28]

Current data suggest that insulin glulisine is least compatible and insulin aspart is most compatible in insulin pumps.[29]

Indications for Insulin Pump Therapy in Type 1 Dibetes Mellitus[1]

1. Persistent elevation in HbA1c despite adjustments in MDI and ongoing patient education
2. Continued hypoglycemia despite adjustments in MDI and ongoing patient education
3. Significant insulin sensitivity, where 0.5–1 U dosing amounts often result in significant glucose excursions/hypoglycemia
4. To get to glucose/HbA1c goal in those attempting pregnancy, who are unable with MDI.

Advantages of Continuous Subcutaneous Insulin Infusion over Multiple Daily Injections[29]

- More consistent and precise in providing patient's individual insulin requirements
- Low risk of severe hypoglycemia
- Equal or better glycemic control
    - Reduces the risk of long-term complications
    - Possibly prevents cognitive impairment in young children
- Improved psychosocial functioning
- More flexibility with lifestyle which will improve health-related quality of life
- In patients with poor adherence associated with fear of MDI, CSII is an effective alternative.

SELF-MONITORING OF BLOOD GLUCOSE[30]

Self-monitoring of blood glucose has been found to be effective for patients with T1DM. Self-monitoring of blood glucose allows patients to evaluate their individual response to therapy and assess whether glycemic targets are being achieved. The SMBG results are useful in preventing hypoglycemia, adjusting medications (particularly prandial insulin doses), and understanding the impact of appropriate nutrition therapy and physical activity.

Self-monitoring of blood glucose frequency and timing should be dictated by the patient's specific needs and goals. When prescribing SMBG, providers must ensure that patients receive ongoing instruction and regular evaluation of their SMBG technique, and their ability to use SMBG data to adjust therapy (insulin and/or food) (Tables 3 and 4).

INTERNATIONAL RECOMMENDATIONS[30]

- Patients with T1DM should perform SMBG, at least before meals and snacks. Self-monitoring of blood glucose performed at other times, including post-meal, helps to assess insulin-to-carbohydrate ratios. The SMBG should also be performed at bedtime; mid-sleep; before, during and after exercise; during suspected hypoglycemia; after treating a hypoglycemic episode (to check if normoglycemia has been restored); when correcting high blood glucose levels; prior to driving and other critical tasks; and more frequently during stress or illness (Tables 3 and 4)
- Individuals with T1DM need to have unrestricted access to glucose test strips. These individuals may require more than or equal to 10 strips per day to monitor for hypoglycemia, assess insulin requirements before eating and to check if the blood glucose level is safe for sleeping overnight
- Regardless of age, individuals may require 10 or more strips daily to monitor for hypoglycemia, assess insulin needs prior to eating, and determine if their blood glucose level is safe enough for overnight sleeping

TABLE 3: Some extensive self-monitoring of blood glucose profiles

Pre-breakfast	Post-breakfast	Prelunch	Post-lunch	Predinner	Postdinner	Bed-time	4 AM	
X	x		X	x	x			5-point
X	x	X	X	x	x	X		7-point
X	x	X	X	x	x	X	x	8-point

TABLE 4: Some commonly used self-monitoring of blood glucose profiles

Pre-breakfast	Post-breakfast	Prelunch	Post-lunch	Predinner	Postdinner	Bed-time	Commonly used in
X		X		x		X	Basal-bolus regimen
X				x			Premixed regimen

- Continuous glucose monitoring is useful to reduce HbA1c levels without increasing the risk or episodes of hypoglycemia. Continuous glucose monitoring can also help reduce glycemic excursions in children.

FUTURE INSULINS AND DELIVERY SYSTEMS

Despite improvements in both basal and prandial insulin, there remain a number of challenges for individuals with T1DM (Table 5). Hypoglycemia is still the greatest challenge; it prevents many from achieving optimal glycemic control, and nocturnal hypoglycemia is most feared by patients and physicians alike. Missed injections and mistimed injections due to less flexible regimens are also limitations that many face regularly.

A better basal insulin would have a flat-time action profile with minimal day-to-day variability. A more ideal rapid-acting insulin would further improve postprandial levels and have a shorter time action profile to avoid late hypoglycemia but long enough so that the between-meal glucose levels do not rise too high.

The concept of a smart insulin involves an insulin that would be responsive to the existing plasma glucose levels and would work more effectively when glucose levels are high and less effectively when glucose levels are lower.[31]

TABLE 5: Newer insulins in the pipeline[31]

Basal insulin	Prandial insulin
Glargine U 300	Insulin PH20
	Linjeta
	Faster-acting insulin aspart

TABLE 6: Alternative routes of insulin administration[32,33]

Route	Advantage	Disadvantage
Pulmonary/inhaled	<ul><li>High permeability</li><li>Large surface area</li><li>Rich vasculature</li><li>Lack of mucociliary clearance</li><li>Immunotolerance</li></ul>	<ul><li>Low bioavailability (9–22%)</li><li>Variation in absorption</li><li>Large quantity insulin required</li><li>Cannot be used by smokers</li><li>Mild-to-moderate cough, shortness of breath, sore throat, and dry mouth</li></ul>
Oral	<ul><li>Easy and convenient</li><li>Patient compliance</li><li>Easily accessible route</li></ul>	<ul><li>Low bioavailability (1%)</li><li>Proteolytic degradation in gastrointestinal tract</li><li>First-pass hepatic metabolism</li><li>Large quantity insulin required</li><li>High resistance by intestinal epithelial barriers</li></ul>

Continued

SECTION 4: Pharmacological Management

Continued

Route	Advantage	Disadvantage
Transdermal	• Large surface area • Microneedle approach increases insulin permeability • Can use iontophoresis and sonophoresis techniques	• Skin is impermeable • Variability in dosing
Nasal	• Large absorptive surface • High vascularity	• Low bioavailability (8–15%) • Degraded by proteolytic enzymes • Nasal irritation • Nasal tolerance • High rates of treatment failure • Mucociliary clearance • Inconsistent absorption
Ocular	• Fast systemic absorption • No first-pass hepatic metabolism	• Low bioavailability • Local irritation
Rectal	• Avoids local enzymatic degradation • Insulin enters systemic circulation via the lymphatic system. • No first-pass hepatic metabolism	• Local adverse reactions • Low and variable levels of absorption • Local irritation
Buccal	• No first-pass hepatic metabolism • Good accessibility • Drug is in direct mucosal contact • Avoids acidic pH of stomach • Large surface for absorption • High vascularity • Quite robust • Improved compliance	• No first-pass hepatic metabolism • Good accessibility • Drug is in direct mucosal contact • Avoids acidic pH of stomach • Large surface for absorption • High vascularity • Quite robust • Improved compliance
Patch Pad33	• Ease of use, accuracy • Predictability • Ability to calculate bolus insulin doses based on user-input	• Temporary unavailability of a controller device • Pump size (form factor) • Adhesive intolerance • Poor adherence

For many patients, administering insulin by subcutaneous injection seems like a daunting therapy option. Consequently, research is being undertaken on alternative methods for administering insulin (Table 6). An ideal route for insulin delivery should have the ability to provide effective and predictable lowering of blood glucose level.

CONCLUSION

Although not curable, T1DM is eminently controllable. Considering the remarkable advances in contemporary therapy, including MDI and CSII, the likelihood of even greater future improvements in quality of life and survivability can be anticipated. Success requires patient engagement and education, an informed primary care provider, and an interdisciplinary team to maximize the benefits of insulin therapy and avoid the risks of hypoglycemia.

REFERENCES

1. Stephens E. Insulin therapy in type 1 diabetes. Med Clin N Am. 2015;99:145-56.
2. The effect of intensive treatment of diabetes on the development and progression of long-term complications in insulin-dependent diabetes mellitus. The Diabetes Control and Complications Trial Research Group. N Engl J Med. 1993;329:977-86.
3. Nathan DM. Intensive diabetes treatment and cardiovascular disease in patients with type 1 diabetes. N Engl J Med. 2005;353:2643-53.
4. Effect of intensive diabetes treatment on the development and progression of long-term complications in adolescents with insulin-dependent diabetes mellitus: Diabetes Control and Complications Trial. Diabetes Control and Complications Trial Research Group. J Pediatr. 1994;125:177-88.
5. Writing Group for the DCCT/EDIC Research Group, Orchard TJ, Nathan DM, Zinman B, Cleary P, Brillon D, et al. Association between 7 years of intensive treatment of type 1 diabetes and long-term mortality. JAMA. 2015;313:45-53.
6. Vajo Z, Fawcett J, Duckworth WC. Recombinant DNA technology in the treatment of diabetes: insulin analogs. Endocr Rev. 2001;22:706-17.
7. Heinemann L, Linkeschova R, Rave K, Hompesch B, Sedlak M, Heise T. Time-action profile of the long-acting insulin analog insulin glargine (HOE901) in comparison with those of NPH insulin and placebo. Diabetes Care. 2000;23:644-9.
8. Eli Lilly and Company. (2011). Humulin® 70/30 70% human insulin isophane suspension and 30% human insulin injection (rDNA origin) 100 units per ML (U-100). [online] Available from: https://dailymed.nlm.nih.gov/dailymed/archives/fdaDrugInfo.cfm?archiveid=43271 [Accessed February, 2017].
9. Novo Nordisk Inc. (2010). Novolin® 70/30, 70% NPH, Human Insulin Isophane Suspension and 30% Regular, Human Insulin Injection (recombinant DNA origin) [online] Available from: https://dailymed.nlm.nih.gov/dailymed/fda/fdaDrugXsl.cfm?setid=8c7038f4-60d4-4604-814d-74921cdc1ad8&type=display [Accessed February, 2017].
10. Tibaldi JM. Evolution of insulin development: focus on key parameters. Adv Ther. 2012;29:590-619.
11. Mudaliar SR, Lindberg FA, Joyce M, Beerdsen P, Strange P, Lin A, et al. Insulin aspart (B28 asp-insulin): a fast-acting analog of human insulin: absorption kinetics and action profile compared with regular human insulin in healthy nondiabetic subjects. Diabetes Care. 1999;22:1501-6.
12. Howey DC, Bowsher RR, Brunelle RL, Woodworth JR. [Lys(B28), Pro(B29)]-human insulin. A rapidly absorbed analogue of human insulin. Diabetes. 1994;43:396-402.
13. Becker RH, Frick AD, Burger F, Potgieter JH, Scholtz H. Insulin glulisine, a new rapid-acting insulin analogue, displays a rapid time-action profile in obese non-diabetic subjects. Exp Clin Endocrinol Diabetes. 2005;113:435-43.
14. Owens DR. Insulin preparations with prolonged effect. Diabetes Technol Ther. 2011;13:S5-14.
15. Poon K, King AB. Glargine and detemir: Safety and efficacy profiles of the long-acting basal insulin analogs. Drug Healthc Patient Saf. 2010;2:213-23.
16. Rolla A. Pharmacokinetic and pharmacodynamics advantages of insulin analogues and premixed insulin analogues over human insulins: impact on efficacy and safety. Am J Med. 2008;121:S9-19.
17. Garber AJ, Ligthelm R, Christiansen JS, Liebl A. Premixed insulin treatment for type 2 diabetes: analogue or human? Diabetes Obes Metab. 2007;9:630-9.
18. Indian National Consensus Group. Premix Insulin: Initiation and Continuation Guidelines for Management of Diabetes in Primary Care. J Assoc Physicians India. 2009;57:42-6.
19. Heise T, Heinemann L, Hovelmann U, Brauns B, Nosek L, Haahr HL, et al. Biphasic insulin aspart 30/70: pharmacokinetics and pharmacodynamics in comparison with once-daily biphasic human insulin and basal-bolus therapy. Diabetes Care. 2009;32:1431-3.

SECTION 4: Pharmacological Management

20. Danne T, Bangstad HJ, Deeb L, Jarosz-Chobot P, Mungaie L, Saboo B, et al. ISPAD Clinical Practice Consensus Guidelines 2014. Insulin treatment in children and adolescents with diabetes. Pediatr Diabetes. 2014:15:115-34.
21. Jonassen I, Havelund S, Hoeg-Jensen T, Steensgaard DB, Wahlund PO, Ribel U. Design of the novel protraction mechanism of insulin degludec, an ultra-long-acting basal insulin. Pharm Res. 2012;29:2104-14.
22. Unnikrishnan AG, Singh AK, Modi KD, Saboo B, Garcha SC, Rao PV. Review of Clinical Profile of IDegAsp. J Assoc Physicians India. 2015;63:15-20.
23. Kalra S, Singh Balhara YP, Baruah MP, Chadha M, Chandalia HB, Chowdhury S, et al. Forum for Injection Techniques, India: The First Indian Recommendations for Best Practice in Insulin Injection Technique. Indian J Endocrinol Metab. 2012;16:876-85.
24. Pickup J. Insulin pumps. Int J Clin Pract Suppl. 2011;170:16-9.
25. Becker R, Frick A, Wessels D, Scholtz H. Evaluation of the pharmacodynamic and pharmacokinetic profiles of insulin glulisine—a novel, rapid-acting, human insulin analogue. Diabetologia. 2003;46 (Abstract 775).
26. Frick A, Becker R, Wessels D, Scholtz, H. Pharmacokinetic and glucodynamic profiles of insulin glulisine: an evaluation following subcutaneous administration at various injection sites. Diabetologia. 2003;46 (Abstract 776).
27. Didangelos T, Iliadis F. Insulin pump therapy in adults. Diabetes Res Clin Pract. 2011;93:S109-13.
28. Bangstad HJ, Danne T, Deeb L, Jarosz-Chobot P, Urakami T, Hanas R, et al. Insulin treatment in children and adolescents with diabetes. Pediatr Diabetes. 2009;10:82-99.
29. Kesavadev J, Jain SM, Muruganathan A, Das AK; Diabetes Consensus Group. Consensus evidence-based guidelines for use of insulin pump therapy in the management of diabetes as per Indian clinical practice. J Assoc Physicians India. 2014;62:34-41.
30. Chiang JL, Kirkman MS, Laffel LM, Peters AL. Type 1 Diabetes Sourcebook Authors. Type 1 diabetes through the life span: a position statement of the American Diabetes Association. Diabetes Care. 2014;37:2034-54.
31. Woo VC. New Insulins and New Aspects in Insulin Delivery. Can J Diabetes. 2015;39:335-43.
32. Kumria R, Goomber G. Emerging trends in insulin delivery. J Diabetology. 2011;2:1.
33. Anhalt H, Bohannon NJ. Insulin patch pumps: their development and future in closed-loop systems. Diabetes Technol Ther. 2010;12:S51-8.

14
CHAPTER

Noninsulin Therapy

Sanjay Kalra, Manash P Baruah

INTRODUCTION

While insulin is the mainstay of treatment of type 1 diabetes mellitus (T1DM), interest in noninsulin therapies for this condition has grown in recent years. Availability of newer drugs, with non-insulin dependent and indirect β-cell tropic mechanisms of action has encouraged research in this field. While no firm recommendations can be made regarding the use of noninsulin therapies in T1DM, data are promising enough to support a call for large randomized controlled trials.[1,2]

This chapter describes the various noninsulin therapies available, and discusses how best they may fit in the T1DM therapeutic landscape.

CLASSIFICATION

A proposed classification of noninsulin therapies is presented in table 1.[3] This divides all glucose-lowering drugs into three classes: (i) insulin secretagogues, (ii) sensitizers, and (iii) nutrient load reducers. While directly acting secretagogues cannot be used in T1DM, all others may be tried in specific situations (Table 2).

INSULIN SENSITIZERS

Metformin

An exhaustive review showed that metformin is associated with reductions in: insulin-dose requirement (5.7–10.1 U/day in six of seven studies); glycosylated hemoglobin (HbA1c) (0.6–0.9% in four of seven studies); weight (1.7–6.0 kg in three of six studies); and total cholesterol (0.3–0.41 mmol/L in three of seven studies). It was also found that the metformin is well-tolerated, and leads to significant reduction in insulin dose (6.6 U/day, p <0.001) but no significant reduction in HbA1c (absolute reduction 0.11%, p = 0.42) levels.[4]

SECTION 4: Pharmacological Management

TABLE 1: Classification of noninsulin glucose lowering drugs

Insulin secretagogues	Insulin sensitizers	Nutrient load reducers
Directly acting	**Directly acting**	**Absorption inhibitors**
• Sulfonylureas • Meglitinides	• Metformin • Pioglitazone	• AGIs • Colesvelam • Orlistat
Indirectly acting, via incretin pathway	**Indirctly acting, via counter-regulatory hormone pathway**	**Excretion enhancers**
• GLP1-1RA • DPP4i	• Pramlintide • Bromocriptine	• SGLT2i

GLP-1RA, glucagon-like peptide 1 receptor agonist; DPP4i, dipeptidyl peptidase 4 inhibitor; SGLT2i, sodium-glucose cotransporter 2 inhibitor; AGIs, α-glucosidase inhibitors.

TABLE 2: Patient-centered choice of noninsulin therapy in type 1 diabetes mellitus

Aim of therapy	Choice of drug
To limit weight gain	• Pramlintide • Metformin • Sodium-glucose cotransporter 2 inhibitor
To reduce cardiovascular risk	• Glucagon-like peptide 1 receptor agonist • Sodium-glucose cotransporter 2 inhibitor • Metformin
To improve insulin sensitivity/reduce insulin requirement	• Metformin • Pioglitazone • Glucagon-like peptide 1 receptor agonist
To reduce glycemic variability	• Acarbose • Dipeptidyl peptidase 4 inhibitor • Glucagon-like peptide 1 receptor agonist
To provide post-lunch coverage with twice daily pre-mixed regimes; or provide post-snack coverage at school	• Acarbose

Thiazolidinediones

In a randomized, double-blind, placebo-controlled crossover clinical trial (24-week each, with a 4-week washout period), rosiglitazone resulted in decreased insulin dose (5.8% decrease vs. 9.4% increase with placebo, p = 0.02), but no significant change in HbA1c (–0.3 vs. –0.1, p = 0.57).[5] In another 8-month long randomized, double-blind clinical trial study of 50 overweight T1DM subjects, rosiglitazone in combination with insulin resulted in improved glycemic control and blood pressure without an increase in insulin requirements, compared with insulin- and placebo-treated subjects, with the greatest effect seen in subjects with significant insulin resistance.[6]

INCRETIN-BASED THERAPY

Incretin-based therapies, including dipeptidyl peptidase 4 (DPP4) inhibitors and glucagon-like peptide 1 receptor agonists (GLP-1RA), are indirectly acting secretagogues which act to preserve β-cell mass and prevent apoptosis, while suppressing glucagon secretion and enhancing α-cell sensitivity. These twin mechanisms have led to their use in T1DM, especially newly diagnosed patients. The fact that human islet regeneration persists a long time after the onset of T1DM,[7] suggests that the type 1 diabetic pancreas may still respond to treatments capable of expanding β-cell mass.

Dipeptidyl Peptidase 4 Inhibitors

In a pilot double blind crossover randomized controlled trial (RCT), conducted in 20 adult T1DM participants, sitagliptin 100 mg once daily significantly reduced postprandial glucose, mean blood glucose, 24 hours area under the curve, and time spent in euglycemic range. It also reduces HbA1c by $0.27 \pm 0.11\%$ ($p = 0.025$) while reducing total and prandial dose.[8] In a double blind randomized parallel 20-week study involving 141 subjects, sitagliptin use led to higher post-meal glucagon-like peptide 1 (GLP-1) ($p <0.001$), and lower glucose-dependent insulinotropic polypeptide (GIP) ($p = 0.03$), with glucagon suppression at 30 minutes, at 16 weeks. While there were no statistically significant changes, sitagliptin users demonstrated a nonsignificant trend toward decrease in HbA1c, and mean glucose if they were C-peptide positive.[9]

Glucagon-like Peptide 1 Receptor Agonists

In a randomized open label study, newly diagnosed T1DM patients were prescribed either exenatide or sitagliptin. In both groups, insulin requirements were reduced without increasing endogenous insulin production or hypoglycemic events.[10]

In a three part double blinded RCT of exenatide, two doses (1.25 and 2.5 μg) were compared with insulin monotherapy in eight participants. Both doses significantly reduced postprandial glycemic excursion ($p <0.0001$), and delayed gastric emptying ($p <0.004$), while reducing insulin dose by 20%. No suppression of glucagon was noted.[11]

Liraglutide has been tried in T1DM patients, both with and without residual β-cell function. In a 4-week long study, insulin dose decreased significantly in both C-peptide positive (0.50 ± 0.06 to 0.31 ± 0.08 U/kg/day; $p <0.001$) and C-peptide negative (0.72 ± 0.08 to 0.59 ± 0.06 U/kg/day; $p <0.01$) patients. Relative reduction in daily insulin dose correlated positively with baseline β-cell function. Two patients were able to discontinue insulin of the 19 patients treated with liraglutide, 18 lost weight (2.3 ± 0.3 kg; ≤ 0.001). Transient gastrointestinal adverse effects were experienced by almost all subjects.[12]

In a 12-week long study, 72 patients (placebo = 18, liraglutide = 54) with T1DM received either placebo and 0.6, 1.2, and 1.8 mg liraglutide daily. In the 1.2 and 1.8 mg groups, the mean weekly reduction in average blood glucose was -0.55 ± 0.11 mmol/L (10 ± 2 mg/dL) and -0.55 ± 0.05 mmol/L (10 ± 1 mg/dL), respectively ($p <0.0001$), while it remained unchanged in the 0.6 mg and placebo groups. In the 1.2 mg group, HbA1c fell significantly ($-0.78 \pm 15\%$, $-8.5 \pm$

1.6 mmol/mol, p <0.01), while it did not in the 1.8 mg group (−0.42 ± 0.15%, −4.6 ± 1.6 mmol/mol, p = 0.39) and 0.6 mg group (−0.26 ± 0.17%, −2.8 ± 1.9 mmol/mol, p = 0.81) versus the placebo group (−0.3 ± 0.15%, −3.3 ± 1.6 mmol/mol). Glycemic variability was reduced by 5 ± 1% (p <0.01) in the 1.2 mg group only. Total daily insulin dose fell significantly only in the 1.2 and 1.8 mg groups (p <0.05). There was a 5 ± 1 kg weight loss in the two higher-dose groups (p <0.05) and by 2.7 ± 0.6 kg (p <0.01) in the 0.6 mg group versus none in the placebo group. In the 1.2 and 1.8 mg groups, postprandial plasma glucagon concentration fell by 72 ± 12% and 47 ± 12%, respectively (p <0.05). Liraglutide led to higher gastrointestinal adverse events (p <0.05) and ≤1% increases (not significant) in percent time spent in hypoglycemia (<55 mg/dL, 3.05 mmol/L).[13]

In a 24-week long study (Lira-1), 100 patients with T1DM were equally allocated to placebo or liraglutide, in combination with insulin. At the end of treatment, change in HbA1c from baseline did not differ between groups, but hypoglycemic events were reduced with liraglutide, with an incident rate ratio of 0·82 [95% confidence interval (CI) 0.74 to 0.90]. There were no changes in glycemic variability both bolus insulin (difference −5·8 IU, 95% CI −10.7 to −0.8, p = 0.0227) and bodyweight (difference −6.8 kg, 95% CI −12.2 to −1.4, p = 0.0145) decreased with liraglutide treatment compared with placebo. Heart rate increased with liraglutide, with a difference between groups of 7·5 bpm (95% CI 2.8–12.2, p = 0.0019). Postprandial plasma glucagon and GLP-1 concentrations did not differ between groups. Gastric emptying was delayed after 3 weeks of treatment with liraglutide (19.9 minute, 95% CI 0.8 to 39.0, p = 0.0412), but no difference was detected after 24 weeks of treatment. Liraglutide was associated with more frequent nausea, dyspepsia, diarrhea, decreased appetite, and vomiting.[14]

Sodium-glucose Cotransporter 2 Inhibitors

The sodium-glucose cotransporter 2 (SGLT2) inhibitor dapagliflozin has been studied formally in a randomized double blind pilot study. Over 2 weeks, 70 adults with T1DM were randomized to varying (1, 2.5, 5, and 10 mg) dosed of dapagliflozin. There was an increase in glycosuria of 88 g 24 hours with 10 mg dapagliflozin, as compared to a decrease of 21.5 g with placebo. Dose-related reduction in 24 hours glucose, glycemic variability, and insulin dose were noted.[15]

Dapagliflozin has also been studied in conjunction with liraglutide in T1DM. Thirty patients on insulin and liraglutide therapy for at least last 6 months were randomized (in 2:1 ratio, drug:placebo) to receive either dapagliflozin 10 mg or placebo daily for 12 weeks. Glycosylated hemoglobin fell by 0.6 ± 0.08% in the dapagliflozin group (p <0.01 vs. placebo) with no changes in placebo group. The average weekly glucose concentration fell in the dapagliflozin group by 15 ± 6 mg/dL (p <0.05 vs. baseline, p = 0.07 vs. placebo) with no changes in placebo group. There was no additional hypoglycemia (<70 mg/dL; p = 0.52 vs. placebo). The basal insulin dose fell by 0.72 ± 0.96 from 33.70 ± 4.53 units while it increased by 1.9 ± 0.5 units (p <0.01 vs. baseline) in placebo (p <0.05 vs. placebo). However, total insulin dose remained unchanged in both groups. The body weight fell by 1.9 ± 0.54 kg (p <0.05 vs. placebo) in the dapagliflozin group while it remained unchanged in placebo group. Two dapagliflozin patients developed diabetic ketoacidosis (DKA) within 24 hours of increasing the dose to 10 mg daily.[16]

In another study, 75 patients with T1DM were randomized to receive once-daily empagliflozin 2.5 mg, empagliflozin 10 mg, empagliflozin 25 mg, or placebo as adjunct to insulin for 28 days. Empagliflozin significantly increased 24-hour urinary glucose excretion versus placebo on days 7 and 28. On day 28, adjusted mean differences with empagliflozin versus placebo in changes from baseline in: HbA1c were −0.35 to −0.49% (−3.8 to −5.4 mmol/mol; all p < 0.05 vs. placebo); total daily insulin dose −0.07 to −0.09 U/kg (all p < 0.05 vs. placebo); and weight were −1.5 to −1.9 kg (all p < 0.001 vs. placebo).[17]

An 18-week, double-blind, phase 2 study randomized 351 patients on insulin to canagliflozin 100 or 300 mg or placebo. More patients had both HbA1c reduction more than or equal to 0.4% and no increase in body weight with canagliflozin 100 and 300 mg versus placebo at week 18 (36.9%, 41.4%, and 14.5%, respectively; p <0.001). Both canagliflozin doses provided reductions in HbA1c, body weight, and insulin dose versus placebo over 18 weeks. Increased incidence of ketone-related adverse events (AEs) (5.1, 9.4, and 0%), including the specific AE of DKA (4.3, 6.0, and 0%), was seen with canagliflozin 100 mg and 300 mg versus placebo.[18]

Alpha Glucosidase Inhibitors

Acarbose is approved for use in T1DM in India.

Alpha-glucosidase inhibitors (acarbose) have been evaluated in several well-designed randomized controlled clinical trials in T1DM. Acarbose in combination with insulin reduces postprandial plasma glucose levels, decreases insulin requirement, but has no significant effect on HbA1c levels.[1] In a double-blind, randomized, placebo-controlled, 6-week run-in study, 121 patients were randomized to acarbose or placebo and to high- or low-fiber diet for 24 weeks. Acarbose compared with placebo decreased 2-hour postprandial plasma glucose levels (12.23 ± 0.83 vs. 14.93 ± 0.87 mmol/L; F = 6.1, p <0.02) (least square means ± standard error of the mean), but did not impact HbA1c or the number of hypoglycemic episodes.[19]

Pramlintide

Three placebo-controlled randomized controlled trials on pramlintide as adjunct to either intensive insulin therapy[20] or to therapy with short- and long-acting insulin, have been published.[21,22] Pramlintide did not improve HbA1c when added to intensive insulin therapy for 29 weeks.[20] There was significantly greater improvement in HbA1c levels with pramlintide at 26 and 52 weeks, when added to conventional insulin therapy, with between-group (pramlintide vs. placebo) differences in HbA1c of 0.2 and 0.3%, respectively.[21,22] Severe hypoglycemia was generally reported more frequently with pramlintide than with placebo in these trials, with severe hypoglycemia occurring more often during the first 4 weeks of treatment as pramlintide doses were being adjusted. Patient satisfaction was significantly greater with pramlintide treatment than placebo at 29 weeks of follow-up on 12 of 14 patient-reported outcome measures.[23]

SECTION 4: Pharmacological Management

PRAGMATIC GUIDANCE

Pragmatic guidance regarding the use of noninsulin therapy in T1DM is listed in table 2 and boxes 1 and 2.

Insulin is the gold standard for treatment of T1DM and there is no substitute for insulin. At best, noninsulin therapy can complement insulin. Noninsulin therapy has a role to play as adjuvant to insulin. They are not the drug of choice in T1DM. However, they do have an important place in management, provided they are used in a rational manner. Noninsulin therapy may be considered in patients with suboptimal response to insulin, insulin resistance, or those with high cardiovascular risk (Box 1). Noninsulin therapy may also be considered to negate the adverse effects associated with insulin therapy, e.g., weight gain and glycemic variability or to utilize the benefits provided with any particular class of drug, e.g., reduction of cardiovascular risk, improvement of insulin sensitivity/reduction of insulin requirement, etc. (Box 1).

BOX 1: Pragmatic indications of non-insulin therapy in type 1 diabetes mellitus

Caveats
- Noninsulin therapy is not a substitute for insulin
- At best, noninsulin therapy can complement insulin

Noninsulin therapy may be considered in patients with
- Suboptimal response to insulin, as identified by
  - High insulin requirement
  - High glycemic variability
  - Postprandial hyperglycemia
  - Preprandial hypoglycemia
  - Rapid weight gain
- Insulin resistance, as identified by
  - Acanthosis nigricans
  - Skin tags
  - Central obesity
  - Hypertension
  - Dyslipidemia
  - Polycystic ovarian syndrome
  - Nonalcoholic fatty liver disease
- High cardiovascular risk, as identified by
  - Past history of cardiovascular disease
  - Family history of cardiovascular disease
  - History of atrial fibrillation
  - History of smoking

BOX 2: Do's and don'ts with noninsulin therapy in type 1 diabetes mellitus

Must	Must not
• Plan therapy based on sound pathophysiologic principles	• Prescribe therapy without an understanding of mechanism of action
• Educate and counsel patient about rationale of prescription	• Neglect proper history taking and physical examination
• Maintain close observation	• Prescribe to unstable patients with life-threatening or organ-threating complications
• Monitor general health, glycemia, and ketonuria	• Prescribe to patients with active infection, ketosis
• Remain alert for potential side effects	• Leave patients unmonitored

CONCLUSION

The choice of therapy should be informed of a detailed knowledge of the concerned drug. It should be concordant with the pathophysiologic mechanisms underlying T1DM. Prescription of any noninsulin therapy should be accompanied by an in-depth biopsychosocial assessment of the patient, explanation and discussion of potential limitations and side effects, and documentation of the reason why they are being considered. Maintain close observation, monitor general health, glycemia, and ketonuria, and remain alert for potential side effects. Active patient participation goes a long way to achieving the desired specific endpoints as well as avoid side effects.

REFERENCES

1. Garg V. Noninsulin pharmacological management of type 1 diabetes mellitus. Indian J Endocr Metab. 2011;15:5-11
2. Munir KM, Davis SN. The treatment of type 1 diabetes mellitus with agents approved for type 2 diabetes mellitus. Expert Opin Pharmacother. 2015;16:2331-41.
3. Kalra S. Classification of non-insulin glucose lowering drugs. J Pak Med Assoc. 2016;66:1497-8.
4. Vella S, Buetow L, Royle P, Livingstone S, Colhoun HM, Petrie JR. The use of metformin in type 1 diabetes: a systematic review of efficacy. Diabetologia. 2010;53:809-20.
5. Stone ML, Walker JL, Chisholm D, Craig ME, Donaghue KC, Crock P, et al. The addition of rosiglitazone to insulin in adolescents with type 1 diabetes and poor glycaemic control: a randomized-controlled trial. Pediatr Diabetes. 2008;9:326-34.
6. Yang Z, Zhou Z, Li X, Huang G, Lin J. Rosiglitazone preserves islet beta-cell function of adult-onset latent autoimmune diabetes in 3 years follow-up study. Diabetes Res Clin Pract. 2009;83:54-60.
7. Meier JJ, Bhushan A, Butler AE, Rizza RA, Butler PC. Sustained beta cell apoptosis in patients with long-standing type 1 diabetes: indirect evidence for islet regeneration? Diabetologia. 2005;48:2221-8.
8. Ellis SL, Moser EG, Snell-Bergeon JK, Rodionova AS, Hazenfield RM, Garg SK. Effect of sitagliptin on glucose control in adult patients with type 1 diabetes: a pilot, double-blind, randomized, crossover trial. Diabetic Medicine. 2011; 28:1176-81.
9. Garg S, Moser E, Bode B, Klaff L, Hiatt W, Beatson C, et al. Effect of sitagliptin on post-prandial glucagon and GLP-1 levels in patients with type 1 diabetes: Investigator-initiated, double-blind, placebo-controlled trial. Endocrine Practice. 2012;19:19-28.
10. Hari Kumar KV, Shaikh A, Prusty P. Addition of exenatide or sitagliptin to insulin in new onset type 1 diabetes: a randomized, open label study. Diabetes Res Clin Pract. 2013;100:e55-8.
11. Raman VS, Mason KJ, Rodriguez LM, Hassan K, Yu X, Bomgaars L, et al. The role of adjunctive exenatide therapy in pediatric type 1 diabetes. Diabetes Care. 2010;33:1294-6.
12. Pieber TR, Deller S, Korsatko S, Jensen L, Christiansen E, Madsen J, et al. Counter-regulatory hormone responses to hypoglycaemia in people with type 1 diabetes after 4 weeks of treatment with liraglutide adjunct to insulin: a randomized, placebo-controlled, double-blind, crossover trial. Diabetes Obes Metab. 2015;17:742-50.
13. Kuhadiya ND, Dhindsa S, Ghanim H, Mehta A, Makdissi A, Batra M, et al. Addition of liraglutide to insulin in patients with type 1 diabetes: a randomized placebo-controlled clinical trial of 12 weeks. Diabetes Care. 2016;39:1027-35.
14. Dejgaard TF, Frandsen CS, Hansen TS, Almdal T, Urhammer S, Pedersen-Bjergaard U, et al. Efficacy and safety of liraglutide for overweight adult patients with type 1 diabetes and insufficient glycaemic control (Lira-1): a randomised, double-blind, placebo-controlled trial. Lancet Diabetes Endocrinol. 2016;4:221-32.
15. Henry RR, Rosenstock J, Edelman S, Mudaliar S, Chalamandaris AG, Kasichayanula S, et al. Exploring the potential of the SGLT2 inhibitor dapagliflozin in type 1 diabetes: a randomized, double-blind, placebo-controlled pilot study. Diabetes Care. 2015;38:412-9.
16. Kuhadiya ND, Mehta A, Ghanim H, Garg M, Hejna J, Makdissi A, et al. FRI-708: Dapagliflozin as additional treatment to liraglutide and insulin in patients with type 1 diabetes. Randomized clinical trial of 12 weeks. [online] Available from http://press.endocrine.org/doi/abs/10.1210/endo-meetings.2016.DGM.23.FRI-708. [Accessed January, 2017].

SECTION 4: Pharmacological Management

17. Pieber TR, Famulla S, Eilbracht J, Cescutti J, Soleymanlou N, Johansen OE, et al. Empagliflozin as adjunct to insulin in patients with type 1 diabetes: a 4-week, randomized, placebo-controlled trial (EASE-1). Diabetes Obes Metab. 2015;17:928-35.
18. Henry RR, Thakkar P, Tong C, Polidori D, Alba M. Efficacy and safety of canagliflozin, a sodium-glucose cotransporter 2 inhibitor, as add-on to insulin in patients with type 1 diabetes. Diabetes Care. 2015;38:2258-65.
19. Riccardi G, Giacco R, Parillo M, Turco S, Rivellese AA, Ventura MR, et al. Efficacy and safety of acarbose in the treatment of type 1 diabetes mellitus: A placebo controlled, double blind, multicentre study. Diabet Med. 1999;16:228-32.
20. Edelman S, Garg S, Frias J, Maggs D, Wang Y, Zhang B, et al. A double-blind, placebo-controlled trial assessing pramlintide treatment in the setting of intensive insulin therapy in type 1 diabetes. Diabetes Care. 2006;29:2189-95.
21. Whitehouse F, Kruger DF, Fineman M, Shen L, Ruggles JA, Maggs DG, et al. A randomized study and open-label extension evaluating the long-term efficacy of pramlintide as an adjunct to insulin therapy in type 1 diabetes. Diabetes Care. 2002;25:724-30.
22. Ratner RE, Dickey R, Fineman M, Maggs DG, Shen L, Strobel SA, et al. Amylin replacement with pramlintide as an adjunct to insulin therapy improves long-term glycaemic and weight control in type 1 diabetes mellitus: A 1-year, randomized controlled trial. Diabet Med. 2004;21:1204-12.
23. Marrero DG, Crean J, Zhang R, Kellmeyer T, Gloster M, Herrmann K, et al. Effect of Adjunctive pramlintide treatment on treatment satisfaction in patients with type 1 diabetes. Diabetes Care. 2007;30:210-6.

CHAPTER 15

Continuous Glucose Monitoring System and Insulin Pump

Sunil M Jain

INTRODUCTION

Insulin pump technology is under development since 1970. In last one decade, a significant improvement has happened. Earlier continuous subcutaneous insulin infusion (CSII) or insulin pump was existing as standalone technology. Later, continuous glucose monitoring system (CGMS) technology added to pumps. This initially led to continuous availability of glucose reading on pump screen. Subsequently, algorithms were developed which allowed pump to get shut down if patient is in hypoglycemia. Further improvement in algorithms made it possible for pump to predict hypoglycemia and stop insulin delivery before patient goes in hypoglycemia. In near future, it will be possible that more and more dose adjustments will be done by pump and there may be a time when our patients will be using fully functional artificial pancreas. Continuous glucose monitoring system and insulin pump have been discussed separately and then sensor and pump unit have been explained in combination.

CONTINUOUS GLUCOSE MONITORING SYSTEM

Various methodologies have been used for assessment of glycemic control. In current era of technology, we are now moving toward continuous monitoring of glucose. Once upon a time, laboratory glucose measurement and urine glucose testing were the only methods to know the glucose level and physician had to take treatment decisions based on this limited information. Advent of home glucose testing technology in the 1970s started a new era and subsequently made urinary glucose testing obsolete. Simultaneously, glycosylated hemoglobin (HbA1c) measurement became possible which gave us overall glycemic assessment of last 3 months. In spite of so many ways to assess glucose control of a patient, need of a technology to know a continuous change in glucose trend was felt because the biggest challenge in diabetes management is to achieve normoglycemia with minimizing hypoglycemia.[1,2] The so far used traditional methods to assess glucose control limited our ability to meet glycemic goals. Need of a better technology was always felt. This need has been fulfilled by CGMS. Urine glucose was giving indirect and incorrect information, laboratory testing was giving very limited information, self-monitoring of plasma glucose (SMPG) provides "snapshot" information, thus missing many peaks and troughs, HbA1c giving an average only that may be a mix of extreme highs and extreme lows while CGMS can provide all information and variations in glucose values, what we now label as glycemic variability. In addition, ADAG (A1c-Derived Average Glucose) study has shown the wide range of average glucose for the same HbA1c. Thus, the current understanding of glycemia based on HbA1c seems to be incomplete and thus the era of "actual control" measurement by CGMS is going to begin soon. Physicians and diabetologists should understand this new technology of glycemic control assessment. Many patients have started using CGMS as a monitoring tool and no wonder if SMPG is replaced by continuous home glucose monitoring (CHMG).[3]

What is Continuous Glucose Monitoring System?

This is a technology which measures glucose levels continuously and hence the only technology which provides information about glycemic variability in an individual. In glucose meter, a strip is used and a drop of blood is placed on this strip. This strip contains enzymes which generate hydrogen peroxide (H_2O_2) and this then leads to generation of a signal which is measured by reader in glucose meter and converted to glucose number which is then displayed on glucose meter screen as glucose value. Higher glucose means more H_2O_2 generation, and thus, higher glucose value and vice versa. Same technology is used in CGMS where a similar enzyme-coated platinum sensor is placed in subcutaneous tissue. Glucose present in subcutaneous tissue comes in contact with sensor. Enzyme present in sensor generates H_2O_2 and this quantity of generated H_2O_2 depends on glucose levels in subcutaneous tissue. Hydrogen peroxide is measured by sensor every 10 seconds and an average value during a period of 5 minutes is transferred to a system which then converts this to glucose value as done by glucose meter.[4]

How Continuous Glucose Monitoring System is Performed?

In continuous glucose monitoring technology, a glucose sensor, which looks like a needle (Fig. 1) is placed into the subcutaneous tissue.

This sensor is then attached to a recorder or a transmitter (Fig. 2). If sensor is attached to a recorder, it will save all data. Sensor will measure glucose and these values will be saved in recorder. Once CGMS is completed, sensor will be removed and this recorder will be connected to computer and all data will be extracted and a report will be generated. This is also known as retrospective CGMS. Here, during CGMS glucose values are stored in recorder, patient is not aware of these values. These values will become visible at the end of CGMS process when sensor will be removed and data from recorder are transferred to a computer (Fig. 3).

If sensor is attached to a transmitter, glucose values measured by sensor will be sent to transmitter which then will send this data to a display screen and thus glucose value will be

CHAPTER 15: Continuous Glucose Monitoring System and Insulin Pump

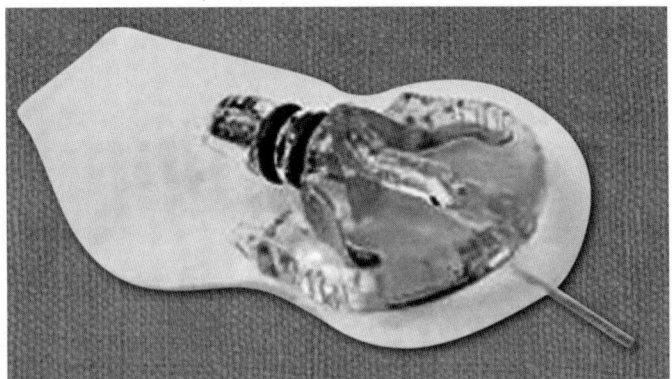

Fig. 1: Glucose sensor

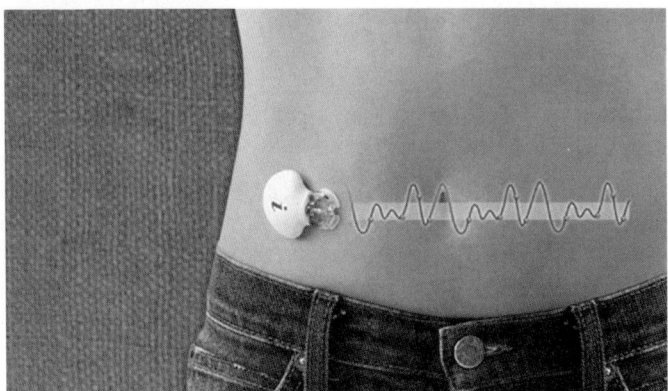

Fig. 2: Sensor attached to a recorder

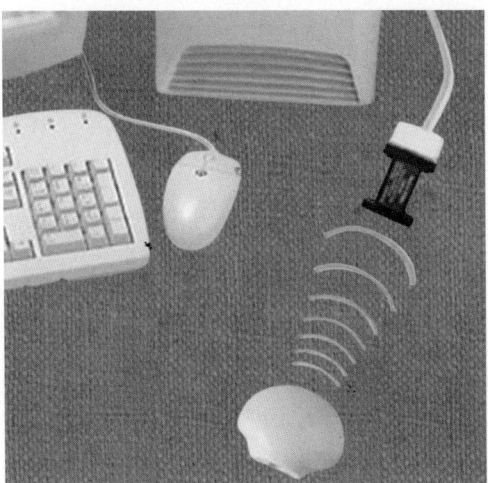

Fig. 3: Data from the recorder transferred to the computer

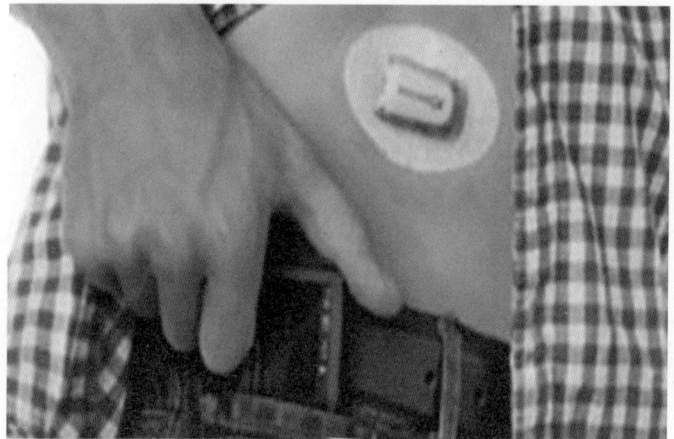

Fig. 4: Continuous glucose monitoring system with glucose values continuous display

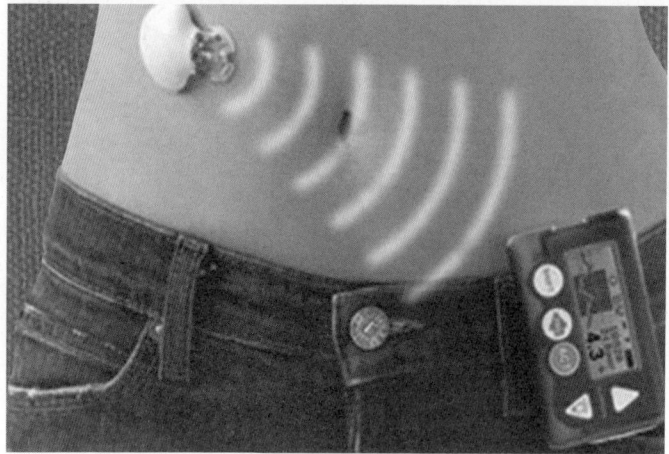

Fig. 5: Continuous glucose monitoring system with glucose value and trend display

continuously visible on a monitor screen as shown in figure 4. This is also known as prospective CGMS. One more CGMS system is shown in figure 5. In prospective CGMS, patient can see their glucose levels as well as rate of change of glucose levels on their monitor.[4]

Where to Insert Sensor?

For sensor insertion, generally abdomen is a preferred place (Fig. 6), though it can be placed at arms also (Fig. 7). In addition, arms can also be used. If a patient is on insulin therapy, it is a must that insulin should be injected in subcutaneous tissue at least 3 inches away from sensor site. This needle-like sensor is inserted with help of a device which makes sensor insertion virtually painless.

CHAPTER 15: Continuous Glucose Monitoring System and Insulin Pump

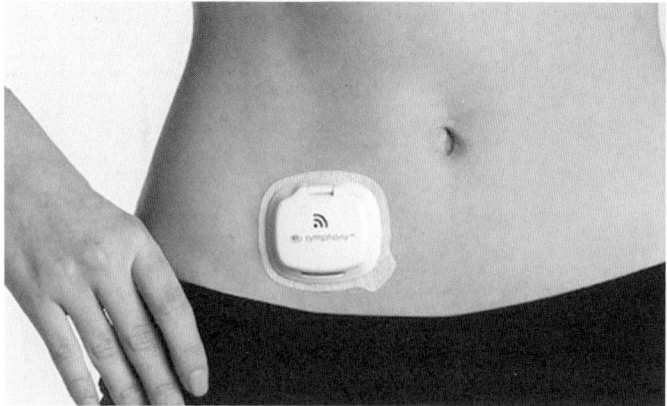

Fig. 6: Placement of sensor on the abdomen

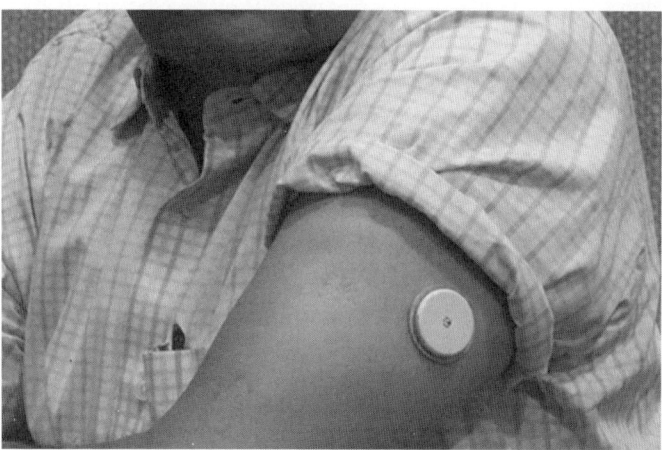

Fig. 7: Placement of sensor on the arms

Which Glucose is Measured by Continuous Glucose Monitoring System?

Glucose measurements in laboratory are done in venous plasma, while glucose meter measures estimated capillary plasma glucose (Fig. 8).

While in CGMS, glucose level in another compartment that is, interstitial fluid is measured (Fig. 9).

For the understanding and interpretation of glucose measured by CGMS, there is need to understand concept of interstitial fluid glucose. Interstitial fluid glucose and capillary glucose have a difference due to physiology of glucose movement from capillaries to interstitial fluid. Thus to understand how interstitial fluid glucose differs from capillary or venous plasma glucose, we need to understand difference of glucose kinetics between interstitial fluid and blood vessels including capillaries. Glucose in blood will reach first to arterioles and

SECTION 4: Pharmacological Management

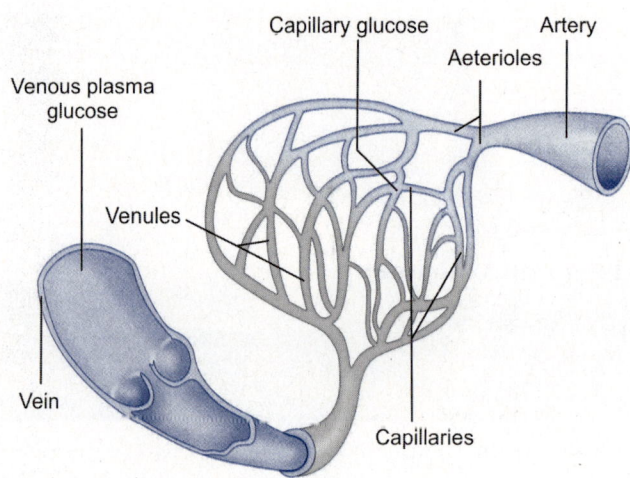

Fig. 8: Blood glucose level measurement: Venous plasma (laboratory) or capillary plasma (glucose meter)

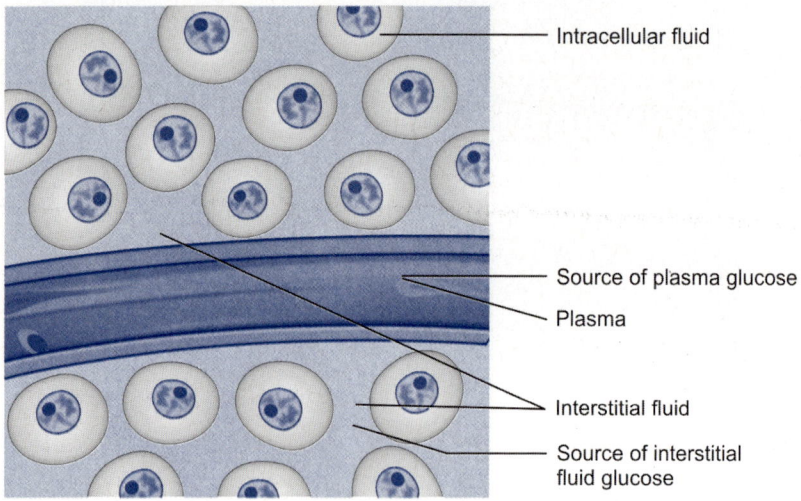

Fig. 9: Continuous glucose monitoring system measures interstitial fluid glucose level

capillaries, from here, it will diffuse to interstitial fluid space, and will be delivered to cells (Fig. 10).[5]

Continuous glucose monitoring sensor is placed in subcutaneous tissue, and thus, it measures glucose in the interstitial fluid, while glucose meters measure glucose from mixed capillaries. Glucose takes time to move from capillaries to interstitial space. If glucose levels are stable, such as in the fasting or premeal state, both compartments are in equilibrium. In this scenario, glucose levels in both interstitial fluid and capillaries will be nearly identical. If there is rapid change in glucose level, this will happen first at capillary level and after few minutes, it will be in equilibrium with interstitial fluid compartment (Fig. 11).[5]

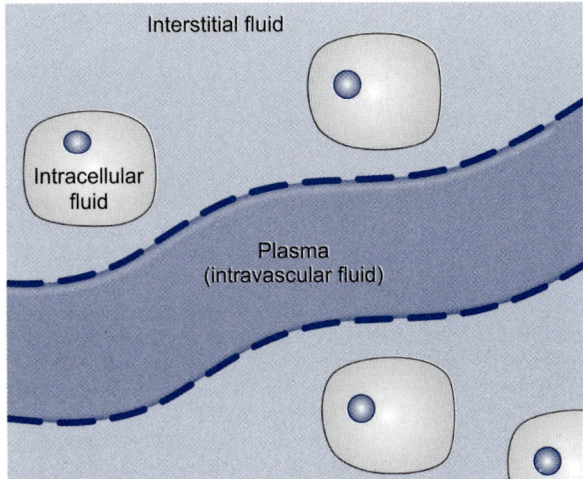

Fig. 10: Concept of interstitial fluid glucose

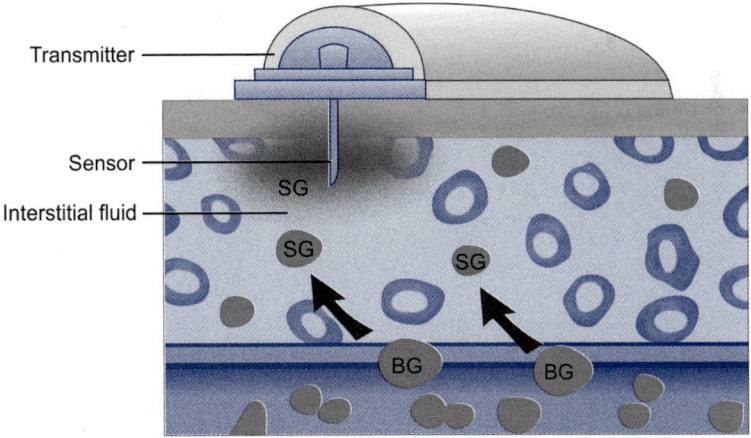

Fig. 11: Capillary glucose reaches to interstitial fluid and measured by sensor

Thus, when glucose levels are rapidly changing, such as after a meal, glucose will rise first in blood vessels and capillaries and then will move to interstitial space, and if a measurement is done at this time, capillary glucose and thus glucose meter value will be higher than interstitial fluid glucose or continuous glucose monitoring sensor measured value (Fig. 12).

Similarly, if glucose is falling rapidly as it happens in hypoglycemia, changes in glucose level will happen first in capillary glucose and thus glucose meter value will be lower than continuous glucose monitoring sensor value (Fig. 13).

Thus, as a concept, during steady state, capillary glucose values are similar to interstitial fluid glucose while during rapid change in glucose level, continuous glucose monitoring sensor value or interstitial fluid glucose lag behind capillary/metered glucose. This delay is physiological and called lag time. Any interpretation and understanding of CGMS values has to be done in the light of lag time concept.

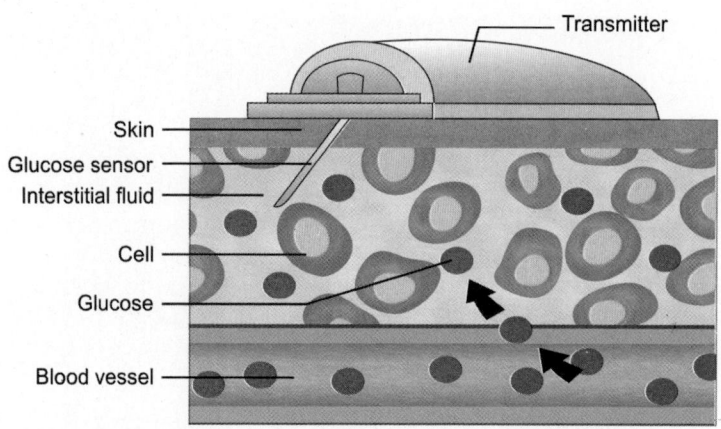

Fig. 12: Rapid rise in glucose, interstitial fluid values relatively low

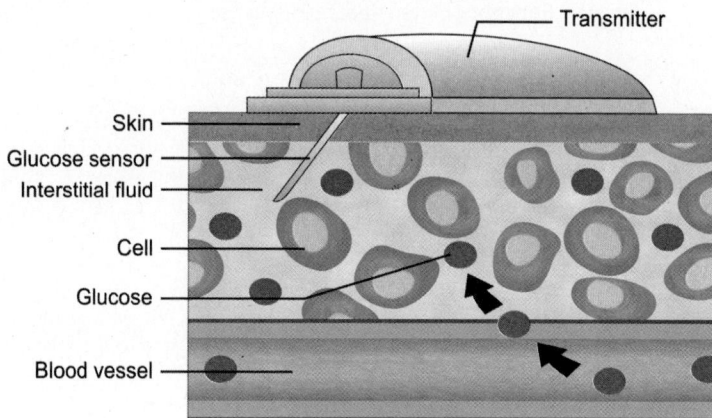

Fig. 13: Rapid fall in glucose, interstitial fluid values relatively high

How Continuous Glucose Monitoring Sensor Works?

Continuous glucose monitoring system sensor consists of two semipermeable membranes containing glucose oxidase enzyme (Fig. 14).

Once inserted in subcutaneous tissue, glucose present in interstitial space passes through the semipermeable membrane of sensor to react with the glucose oxidase enzyme in the presence of oxygen. This generates H_2O_2 which leads to electron release and produce an electronic signal. The "signal" is then recorded and converted into glucose value. If glucose levels in interstitial fluid are higher, then, signal strength will be higher, while when glucose levels are lower, signal strength will be lower. Sensor keeps on measuring glucose continuously in this manner. Current sensor measures glucose every 10 seconds, average of such multiple values is converted every 5 minutes to one figure, and thus, current most CGMS software store and provide glucose value every 5 minutes and 288 glucose values in 24 hours.[4]

CHAPTER 15: Continuous Glucose Monitoring System and Insulin Pump

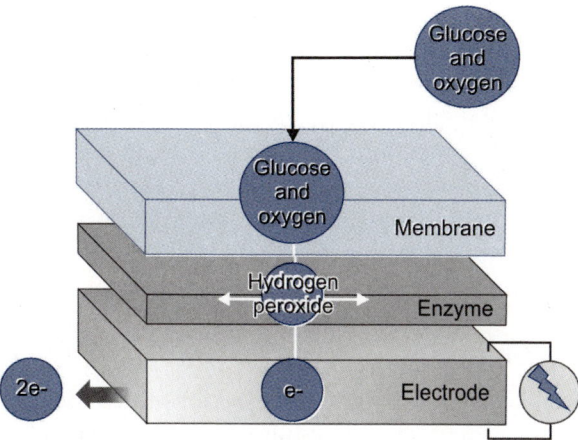

Fig. 14: Glucose measurement by continuous glucose monitoring system sensor

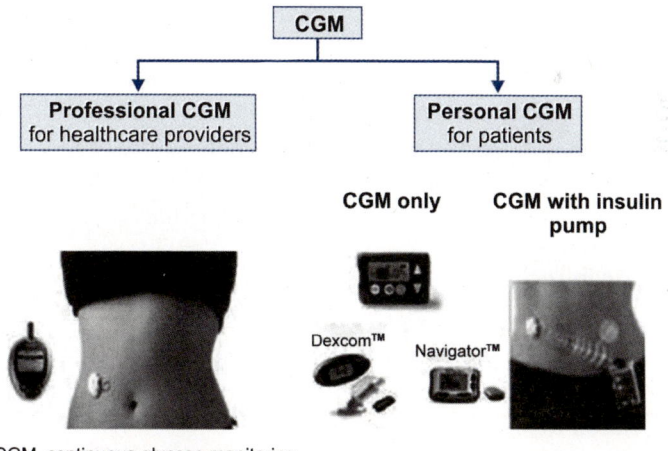

CGM, continuous glucose monitoring.

Fig. 15: Various types of continuous glucose monitoring systems

Types of Continuous Glucose Monitoring System

Continuous glucose monitoring systems can be for physicians use. In these systems, glucose data are blinded to patient, analysis is done after CGMS and then treatment is planned. These are also called as retrospective CGMS. Similarly, CGMS primarily made for patient use are called personal or prospective CGMS. These systems may be a part of sensor augmented insulin pumps or may be CGMS only system (Fig. 15).

Professional Continuous Glucose Monitoring System

Professional CGMS consists of a glucose sensor and a recorder to store data. The glucose sensor is inserted under the skin to check glucose levels in subcutaneous tissue fluid. The

SECTION 4: Pharmacological Management

glucose sensor has an adhesive patch to hold it on skin. The glucose sensor is inserted with the help of a device. One such CGMS system is iPro 2. The most common site for iPro 2 sensor is abdomen. Sensor lasts for 5 days. Recently, FreeStyle Libre Pro Flash sensor is launched in India. This sensor works for 14 days. Site for insertion of this sensor is arm. Once CGMS duration is over, sensor is removed and data stored in recorder are converted to report by software. This report provides every 5 minutes glucose value, daily graphs, glucose value in relation to meals, medication and physical activity, parameters of glycemic variability, etc. In this system, glucose values are not visible to patient. Physician has to modify treatment based on this retrospective information.[6,7]

Personal Continuous Glucose Monitoring System

Personal CGMS consists of the same sensor as used for professional CGMS, a transmitter to transmit glucose data and a small external monitor (which may be built-in to an insulin pump or a standalone device) to view glucose levels, trends, graphs, etc.

Glucose sensor will measure glucose, the glucose value will be gathered by the transmitter attached to sensor, and information is sent wirelessly to the glucose monitor unit. This glucose monitor unit may be mobile phone-like device (Fig. 16) or in case of sensor augmented pumps insulin pump screen will be a monitor. Thus, patient can see glucose value being displayed on monitor screen every 5 minutes. In addition, glucose trend that is glucose is stable, rising, or falling is also visible on the monitor screen. This kind of information can warn patient about hypoglycemia in advance. Thus, this CGMS provides a prospective information on which patient can react and act so as to keep in normoglycemic range.[7]

Available Options in India

Currently available options in India are:
- Professional CGMS
    - iPro 2
    - FreeStyle Libre Pro Flash
- Personal CGMS
    - Guardian RT
    - Dexcom G4.

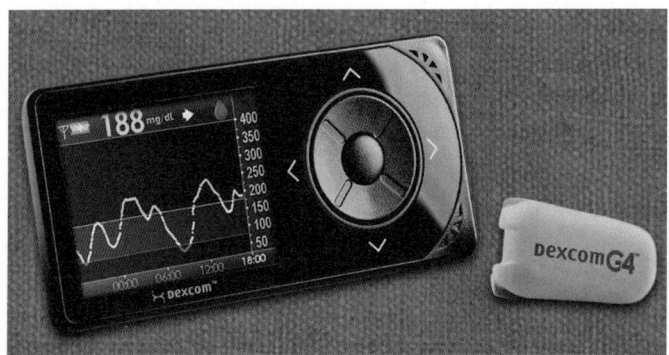

Fig. 16: Personal continuous glucose monitoring system (Dexcom G4)

CHAPTER 15: Continuous Glucose Monitoring System and Insulin Pump

Need of Self-monitoring of Plasma Glucose during Continuous Glucose Monitoring System: Concept of Calibration

With most available CGMS devices, patient has to measure glucose level by glucose meter and enter the data into system. This is called as calibration. The concept of calibration is based on the fact that currently, CGM systems are to be cross checked with glucose meter reading. If sensor interstitial fluid glucose and SMPG value correlate well, only then CGMS will provide glucose readings. This is a must at beginning as well as at nearly 12-hour interval. This process of cross check of SMPG value with sensor value is called calibration. Self-monitoring of plasma glucose is the reference for glucose levels, so the CGM sensor needs to be calibrated using a meter blood glucose value as the reference. In simple words, CGMS sensor measures and generates a raw glucose value, it needs a confirmation from glucose meter reading and if both values are similar or nearly equal, only then CGMS sensor will provide continuous data. As a rule, calibration has to be done during steady state, at a time when interstitial fluid and capillary glucose are expected to be same. The new FreeStyle Libre Pro Flash CGMS system will not require such calibration.

Clinically useful Information from Continuous Glucose Monitoring System

Personal Continuous Glucose Monitoring System

Personal CGMS (Guardian RT, Dexcom G4 systems) provides continuous trends in a graph diagram as well as information about parameters of glycemic variability. Data of this CGMS can be downloaded and a report can be prepared for treatment planning by physician.

Professional Continuous Glucose Monitoring System

Here, CGMS is done; data will not be visible to patient. When patient comes to clinic, data from CGMS will be downloaded and then all glucose values will become visible. In India, as of now, there are two CGMS systems in use for professional—iPro 2 and FreeStyle Libre Pro.

In iPro 2, sensor is fixed mostly on abdomen and data are downloaded after sensor removal. We get 5 days data with information shown in figure 17.

Daily graphs and one summary showing all graphs together. Through this summary, we can see pattern of glucose control in a patient. These graphs start from 12 in the midnight to the same time on next day. First look at overnight glucose trend and then look at pre- and postmeal glucose trends. Table below these graphs (Fig. 17) gives information about highest, lowest, and average glucose of the day as well as standard deviation. Numbers of excursions are shown in a table in the same report and duration of time spent in hypo-, hyper-, and normoglycemia is depicted by pie diagrams. In addition, a data table with time and every 5 minute, glucose value is also available.[8,9]

In FreeStyle Libre Pro, sensor is fixed on arm, it works for 14 days, data can be downloaded with the help of a reader during these 14 days (Fig. 18).

Multiple downloads are possible during these 14 days.

SECTION 4: Pharmacological Management

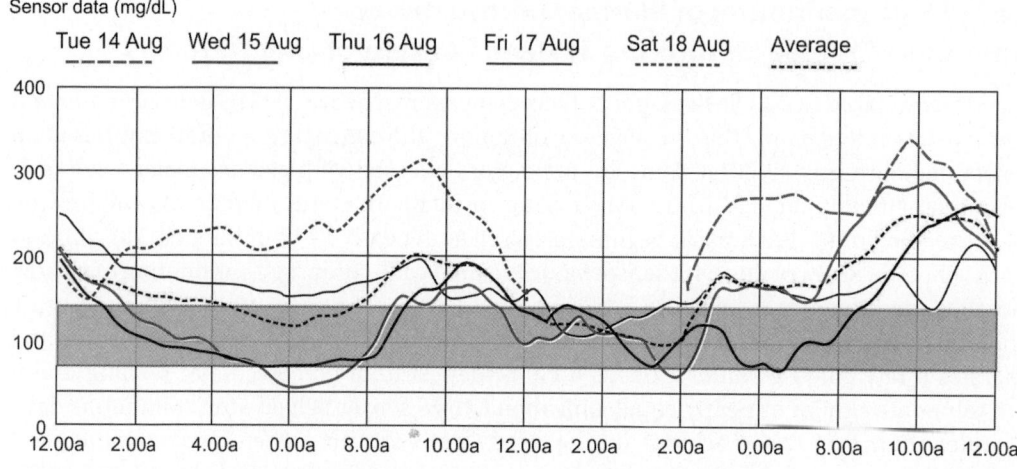

Fig.17: Information from iPro 2 continuous glucose monitoring system

The software of this CGMS system provides data in a format called ambulatory glucose profile (AGP) (Fig. 19). The graph in AGP shows 1 standard deviation variability from mean.

These data can help in a precise and accurate decision making for choosing therapies for diabetes, particularly selecting regimen and adjusting dose for insulin-based treatment.

CHAPTER 15: Continuous Glucose Monitoring System and Insulin Pump

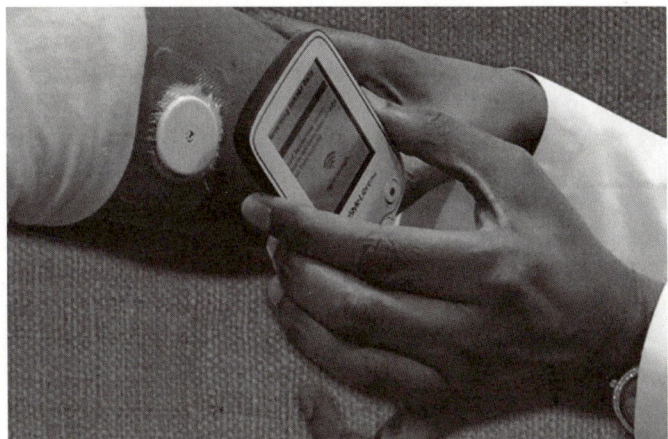

Fig. 18: Data downloading from the FreeStyle Libre Pro Sensor

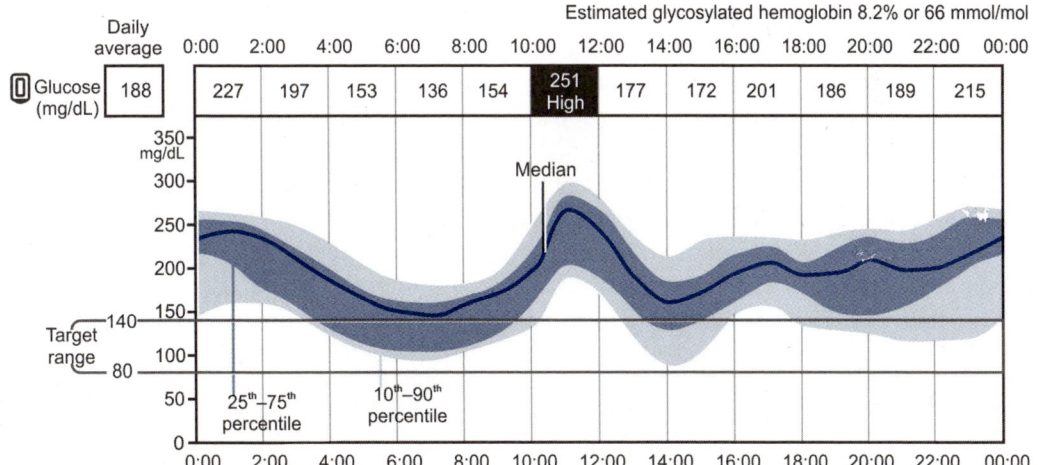

Fig. 19: Data of continuous glucose monitoring system in the ambulatory glucose profile format

Continuous Glucose Monitoring System during Emergencies and Hospitalized Patients[10-12]

Few studies are performed in critically ill hospitalized patients. These studies have shown that CGMS is reliable in critically ill patients but since CGMS measures interstitial fluid glucose which may be affected with hypotension in sick patients and many drugs may also interfere in sensor function, CGMS is not approved for use in critically ill patients. It may be used in noncritically ill hospitalized patients. More studies are needed in this area, and may be in future, CGMS may be cleared for critically ill patients as well.

SECTION 4: Pharmacological Management

INSULIN PUMP[13,14]

Normally, our pancreas secretes small amount of insulin continuously throughout the day and this is called basal insulin secretion. When a meal or snack is eaten, our β-cells then secrete large bursts of insulin called bolus insulin. Aim of insulin replacement in diabetes management, is to replace insulin in a similar way. Before availability of insulin pumps, the only way was insulin injections. In type 1 diabetes mellitus (T1DM), it is often challenging to replace β-cell function, and in many patients, it is difficult to achieve optimal glycemic control without severe hypoglycemia. Insulin pump or CSII provides an option for insulin delivery where basal rates can be customized and each meal can be covered with a bolus insulin thus achieving better glycemic control with minimizing risks of severe hypoglycemia.

Limitations of Insulin Injections

When injections are used, two type of Insulin are needed that is basal and prandial. On injections, it is possible to achieve normal glucose pattern but it demands a much regulated life style, a rigid eating pattern with the same amounts of carb in each meal, fixed exercise plan, etc. This is difficult to achieve and maintain by many patients particularly young patients.
Insulin shots have four major problems:
1. The action of both short- and long-acting insulin is unpredictable. In clinical studies, the amount of insulin that reaches a person's blood varies by 15–50% from 1 day to the next with injections.
2. Multiple injections are often inconvenient and may not be acceptable.
3. Bolus insulin delivery cannot be customized for the type of meal.
4. Long-acting like NPH (neutral protamine Hagedorn) or analogs, like glargine and detemir, can provide basal insulin but this may not necessarily match the variable background needs of an individual like dawn phenomenon in morning, or a different basal need in late evening.

What does a Pump Do?

Insulin (preferably rapid-acting analog) is filled in a syringe, and the syringe is kept inside the pump. The syringe is attached to a tube called infusion set. Infusion set has a cannula at its end which is inserted in subcutaneous tissue with the help of a needle. Then, the needle is removed.
   Pump delivers insulin in two ways—basal and bolus. Basal insulin refers to the steady pumping of small amount of insulin continuously with option of different basal rates for different time of the day. Bolus insulin means insulin to cover carbohydrates in the meal and pump user decides its quantity as per meal size and type.

Who should Use Pump?

Insulin replacement by pump makes life very easy and flexible. The pump gives option to tackle day-to-day lifestyle issues and still manage precise insulin delivery. When a person starts "thinking like a pancreas" and thus sets a right basal or modifies it as per need and takes a

CHAPTER 15: Continuous Glucose Monitoring System and Insulin Pump

TABLE 1: Indications of pump insulin

Clinical indications	Lifestyle indications
• Type 1 diabetes mellitus • Inadequate glycemic control in spite of multiple subcutaneous insulin • Recurrent hyperglycemia • Hypoglycemia unawareness • Dawn phenomenon difficult to manage pregnancy • Gastroparesis with brittleness • Postrenal transplant patients	• Erratic schedule • Varied work shifts • Desire for flexibility • Inconvenience of multiple dose injections

correct bolus to cover meal, then this patient can easily manage day-to-day changes in lifestyle and at the same time remain in safe glucose range. Objective of precise insulin delivery and dose adjustment is possible only when patient is doing regular SMPG. Pump is a good option for many clinical settings (Table 1).

Why Pump is a Better Option for Indian Patients?

- Indian has higher carbohydrate content in their diet and there is a lot of variability in carbohydrate as well as sucrose intake which leads to postprandial hyperglycemia
- Eating at unpredictable timing is very common in Indian society due to social reasons and is unavoidable. These food intakes remain uncovered on injection therapy leading to high HbA1c though many fasting and 2 hour postmeal may not be that high. These situations can be very easily managed by the pump
- Festivals, marriages, fast, etc., are very common in Indian culture, and during these occasions, it is difficult to manage life with injections therapy while the pump makes it a smooth event
- Many patients of T1DM do not disclose about their disease due to teasing, comments, negative remarks by people about pricks, etc. Injection is considered a tough treatment in Indian society. Using a pump makes it simple and such problems are easily tackled
- Issue of marriage can become more comfortable with pump therapy.

Candidate Selection

Insulin pump is an ideal option for insulin replacement but, it is not for everyone. Those patients having following characteristics are good candidates for insulin pump therapy who:
- Are interested in glucose control
- Are willing to monitor glucose regularly
- Are capable intellectually and technically
- Are willing to quantify food intake
- Can afford.

In last 10 years, there is a revolution in insulin pump technology. After availability of CGMS, now insulin pump is no more solo technology. It has been replaced by sensor-augmented insulin pumps like Paradigm 722, Paradigm Veo, Medtronic G 640, etc.

SECTION 4: Pharmacological Management

In these pumps, glucose values are visible on screen at every 5-minute interval. In addition, real-time information about rate of change and direction of change is also visible on screen. Rate and direction of change is represented by arrows coming with glucose value. For example, if screen shows a glucose value of 108 mg and there is one arrow with downward (Fig. 20) direction, it indicates glucose is currently falling at 1 mg/min.

If there are two arrows and a down arrow, it indicates that glucose is falling at a rate of 2 mg/min or more. The opposite is also true that is one up arrow indicates glucose rising by 1 mg/min and two arrows indicate glucose rising by 2 mg/min. If there is no arrow, this is an indication that glucose value is stable. This real-time trend is very helpful to detect hypoglycemia very early and thus prevent a hypoglycemic episode. If a patient see glucose as 78 mg and there is no arrow that means no need to worry, while glucose 78 mg with two arrows down is an indication of hypoglycemia in next few minutes and by needful action, patient can prevent this episode to happen.

In initial sensor-augmented pumps, like Paradigm 722, glucose information with real-time trend was available on pump screen but pump was not allowed to take any decision. The first pump which had an automation feature was Paradigm Veo. This pump goes in a suspend mode when there is hypoglycemia.

The next generation technology, which became available in 2015, made it possible to predict hypoglycemia and to act prior to actual hypoglycemia. The recently launched G640 pump can predict and prevent hypoglycemia. If a patient has a glucose value of 118 mg as measured by CGMS, and the rate of fall is such that there is a possibility of hypoglycemia then G640 pump will stop delivering insulin. It will restart only when CGMS detects rise in glucose at a level which can be considered safe (Fig. 21).

Thus, insulin was discovered in 1921 and saved life of T1DM patients. Around 100 years after this insulin discovery, we will probably have technology which will work like pancreas, and thus, may provide all automatic insulin delivery and dream of cure of T1DM may become a reality.

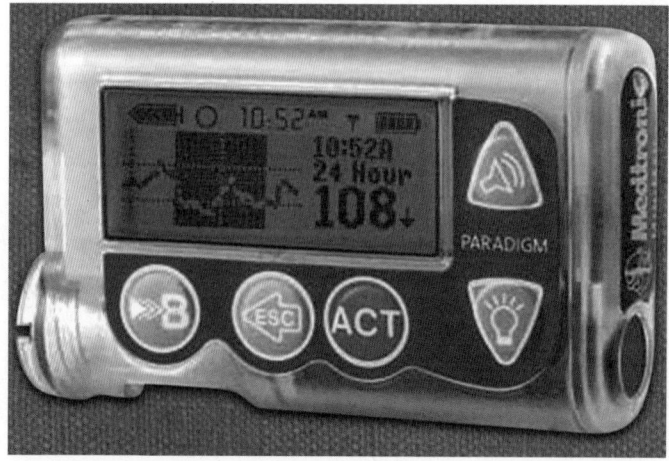

Fig. 20: Sensor pump with continuous glucose monitoring system for direction of change of glucose value

CHAPTER 15: Continuous Glucose Monitoring System and Insulin Pump

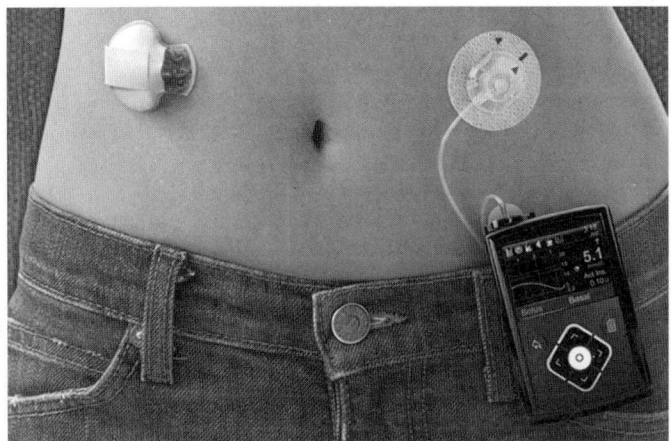

Fig. 21: G640 pump continuous glucose monitoring system with low glucose suspend

REFERENCES

1. Blevins TC, Bode BW, Garg SK, Grunberger G, Hirsch IB, Jovanovic˘ L, et al. Statement by the American Association of Clinical Endocrinologists Consensus Panel on continuous glucose monitoring. Endocr Pract. 2010;16 (5):730-45.
2. Rice MJ, Coursin DB. Continuous Measurement of Glucose: Facts and Challenges. American Society of Anesthesiologists, Inc. Lippincott Williams & Wilkins. Anesthesiology. 2012;116:199-204.
3. Bruce W Bode. The Accuracy and Interferences in SMPG. US Endocrine Disease. 2007;46-8.
4. Günther Schmelzeisen-Redeker et al. Overview of a Novel Sensor for Continuous Glucose Monitoring. J Diabetes Sci Technol. 2013; 7(4):808-14.
5. Cengiz E, Tamborlane WV. A tale of two compartments: interstitial versus blood glucose monitoring. Diabetes Technol Ther. 2009;11 Suppl 1:S11-6.
6. Blevins TC. Professional continuous glucose monitoring in clinical practice 2010. J Diabetes Sci Technol. 2010;4(2):440-56.
7. De Groot LJ, Chrousos G, Dungan K, et al. Monitoring Technologies – Continuous Glucose Monitoring, Mobile Technology, Biomarkers of Glycemic Control. EndoText. South Dartmouth (MA): MDText.com, Inc.; April 30, 2014.
8. Hill NR, Oliver NS, Choudhary P, Levy JC, Hindmarsh P, Matthews DR. Normal reference range for mean tissue glucose and glycemic variability derived from continuous glucose monitoring for subjects without diabetes in different ethnic groups. Diabetes Technol Ther. 2011;13(9):921-8.
9. Siegelaar SE, Holleman F, Hoekstra JB, DeVries JH.. Glucose variability: does it matter? Endocr Rev. 2010;31(2):171-82.
10. Holzinger U, Warszawska J, Kitzberger R, Wewalka M, Miehsler W, Herkner H, et al. Real-time continuous glucose monitoring in critically Ill patients: a prospective randomized trial. Diabetes Care. 2010;33:467-72.
11. Siegelaar SE, Barwari T, Hermanides J, Stooker W, van der Voort PH, DeVries JH. Accuracy and reliability of continuous glucose monitoring in the intensive care unit: a head-to-head comparison of two subcutaneous glucose sensors in cardiac surgery patients. Diabetes Care. 2011;34(3):e31
12. Zhu W, Jiang L, Jiang S, Ma Y, Zhang M. Real-time continuous glucose monitoring versus conventional glucose monitoring in critically ill patients: a systematic review study protocol. BMJ Open. 2015;5(1):e006579.
13. Saboo BD, Talaviya PA. Continuous subcutaneous insulin infusion: practical issues. Indian J Endocr Metab 2012;16, Suppl S2:259-62
14. Scheiner G1, Sobel RJ, Smith DE, Pick AJ, Kruger D, King J, Green K. Insulin pump therapy: guidelines for successful outcomes. Diabetes Educ. 2009;35 Suppl 2:29S-41S; quiz 28S, 42S-43S.

CHAPTER 16

Pancreas and Islet Cell Transplant in Children

Sujoy Ghosh

BACKGROUND

Pancreas transplantation was first carried out in humans in 1966 to treat type 1 diabetes mellitus. Around 10,000 pancreatic transplantations were recorded by the end of 1997. In patients with diabetes, the pancreatic transplantation with renal failure was considered at once or after kidney transplantation.

THE RATIONALE

Intensive insulin therapy, either with continuous insulin infusion using insulin pump or basal bolus therapy is often unsuccessful in achieving treatment goals, especially in brittle type 1 diabetes patients. Alternative treatment options like pancreatic transplantation and islet cell transplantations have to be explored in such situations. The goals of transplantation are primarily to achieve insulin independence, reduce complications, and improve quality of life.

However, all transplants require immunosuppressive therapy to avoid graft rejection. Hence, transplantation is contemplated in patients with significant and grave diabetic complications where the benefits of transplant outweigh the risks of complications.

The American Diabetes Association has placed in the following criteria for eligibility for transplantation:
- Patients with end stage renal disease having decided to go for it, either as sequential kidney transplant followed by pancreatic transplant or a simultaneous kidney-pancreas transplant
- Patients without renal disease only if they have persistent acute severe metabolic complications such as recurrent ketoacidosis, marked hyperglycemia, recurrent hypoglycemia, and debilitating symptomatic and emotional issues with external insulin and constant failure of insulin management
- Islet cell transplant should be restricted to research setting only.

Patients Outcome

Patient outcome is best in patients with type 1 diabetes having low body mass index (BMI), without cardiovascular complications. Younger patients (<45 years) tend to do better. Patients undergoing simultaneous kidney-pancreas transplant fare better than patients undergoing pancreas only transplantation.

The insulin requirement and serum C peptide levels are assessed to determine possible benefit of patient. In general patients requiring insulin more than 1 IU/kg/day may not achieve euglycemia following transplant. Candidates will have to meet the following criteria for pancreas listing:
- C-peptide ≤2 ng/mL and on insulin and/or
- C-peptide >2 ng/mL and BMI ≤28 kg/m^2 and on insulin.

TECHNIQUE

Cadaver donors are the source for most of the pancreatic grafts. Venous drainage of the pancreatic graft is usually established by draining into the systemic circulation. Sometimes pancreas are sourced from living donors but restricted to the donors who are willing to undergo a hemipancreatectomy. In most pancreatic transplants, quadruple immunosuppression with antibody induction therapy utilizes a monoclonal or polyclonal agents. Antimetabolite (mycophenolate mofetil or azathioprine), a calcineurin inhibitor (cyclosporine or tacrolimus), and corticosteroid termed as, the triple therapy, is used as maintenance immunosuppression. Some centers conduct the transplant without antibody induction as it is not required in case of newer immunosuppressants. Patients with diabetes find it easier to manage these immunosuppressive regimens though being complex, than continued diabetes with hyperglycemia and insulin-based therapy.

This utilizes total pancreas attached to a portion of the donor duodenum containing the exit of the pancreatic duct. In the pelvis, the pancreas is placed laterally. Blood supply includes the arterial flow from the iliac artery and venous return via the iliac vein. The duodenal segment and pancreatic duct outlet are sutured on the urinary bladder, receiving the exocrine drainage. Portal drainage of the endocrine pancreas and enteric drainage of the exocrine pancreas can also be utilized. Urinary amylase to monitor for rejection and avoidance of small-bowel complications such as obstruction and infection are the benefits of bladder over enteric drainage. The avoidance of hematuria, urinary tract infection, and reflux pancreatitis are the benefits of enteric over bladder drainage. The freedom of hyperinsulinemia which occurs when systemic drainage bypasses hepatic metabolism of insulin secreted by the allograft is the benefit of portal over systemic venous drainage of the transplanted pancreas.

Patient and Graft Survival

The morbidity, mortality, and results are contingent on the experience of the center for transplantation. Cardiovascular disease accounts for majority of deaths. Reported patient survival ranges from 95 to 98%, 91 to 92%, and 78 to 88% at 1 year, 3 year, and 5 years respectively. The pancreatic graft survival as defined by insulin free normoglycemia,

SECTION 4: Pharmacological Management

i.e., normal fasting glucose and glycosylated hemoglobin for simultaneous kidney pancreas graft is 86% and 54% at 1 year and 10 years, and for pancreas alone graft the rates were 78–88% and 27% at 1 year, and 10 years respectively.

BENEFITS OF TRANSPLANTATION

Restoration of glycemic control and freedom from insulin therapy (as mentioned above) are the major benefits of transplantation.

Hyperinsulinemia tends to occur after transplantation and the main cause is systemic venous drainage of the allograft. It is unlikely that post-transplantation hyperinsulinemia has adverse effect on cardiovascular risk.

Glucose counterregulation after hypoglycemia is significantly improved by pancreatic transplantation as glucagon and epinephrine responses are restored. Identification of symptoms of hypoglycemia is upgraded.

Renal pancreatic transplantation may improve lipid profile and blood pressure without changing weight and might lead to improvement of atherosclerotic risk.

Reversal of renal dysfunction has been observed, including improvement in renal histopathology has been demonstrated in long-term studies. Clinical neuropathy has been shown to stabilize. Progression of retinopathy has been shown to improve in few small studies. The life span in patients with autonomic imbalance has been dramatically improved.

Acute and Chronic Rejection

Graft rejection can take place within days or after years of transplantation. The management of the rejection includes hospitalization and intensive acceleration of immunosuppression. If both pancreas and kidney are transplanted then the detection of rejection can be monitored based on serum creatinine levels. Warnings for pancreas rejection in case of pancreas transplant alone with bladder drainage decrease in urinary amylase, increase in serum amylase, and increase in blood glucose levels. If rejection is suspected it can be confirmed using cystoscopy transduodenal or percutaneous biopsy with ultrasound. The chances of autoimmune attack may be very less because the recipients usually receives immunosuppressant. If autoimmune attack is detected, the reason may be inadequate or improper immunosuppressant therapy.

NONIMMUNOLOGIC COMPLICATIONS

General

Technical failure rate following pancreatic transplantation occurs frequently (up to 10% cases). Technical failure is the irreversible graft loss due to hemorrhage, thrombosis, local infection, graft pancreatitis, or anastomotic leak compelling graft removal. The most common, graft thrombosis, occurs primarily in the first week following transplant and is associated with graft pancreatitis, hypotension, reperfusion injury, and prolonged cold-ischemia times, as well as hypercoagulable states.

Fever, pancreas allograft tenderness, and/or abdominal pain, and elevated serum lipase warrant prompt investigation for peripancreatic infection, transplant pancreatitis, or leaks from duodenal segment. These duodenal leaks are often nonoperative, and managed by prolonged Foley catheter drainage. Conversely, surgical exploration and broad spectrum antibiotics are indicated for leak in the enteric-drained recipient due to intra-abdominal spillage of enteric contents.

Infection

The aggressive immunosuppressive approach used that exposes the patient to an increased threat of bacterial, fungal, and viral infections. The BK virus is the identified cause of allograft loss in renal transplant recipients and a notable cause of renal graft loss in patients with pancreatic transplant.

Metabolic Disturbances

Drainage of the pancreatic duct into the bladder is linked with the loss of huge quantities of bicarbonate-rich pancreatic secretions into urine, resulting in normal anion gap metabolic acidosis, low sodium levels, and volume depletion.

Concerns with acidosis and volume depletion are to a considerable extent reduced with enteric exocrine drainage of the pancreatic graft. Allograft and patient survival appear similar with either enteric or bladder drainage.

Hyperglycemia

This occurs as a result of two separate mechanisms after pancreas transplantation: (i) due to pancreatic dysfunction either due to rejection or technical problems or (ii) due to toxic effects of cyclosporine or tacrolimus.

Post-transplant Erythrocytosis

It is constantly elevated hemoglobin and hematocrit levels after renal transplantation and continue for more than 6 months in the absence of thrombocytosis, leukocytosis, or any other cause of erythrocytosis.

ISLET CELL TRANSPLANTATION

History of Islet Transplant

Pitfall of insulin management and whole pancreas transplantation caused the development of endocrine cell replacement such as the percutaneous islet cell transplantation for managing type 1 diabetes mellitus. The islet cell transplantation is a minimally invasive cellular replacement therapy which includes the normalization of the metabolism of glucose without the danger of hypoglycemia and surgical complications.[1] In late 1960s, the development of novel collagenase-based cellular isolation method took place.[2] In 1970s, these methods were refined and *in-vivo* experiment were performed which mainly focused on isolation and transplantation of islets in animals.[3-5] The clinical experience of islet transplantation in humans started from late 1970s and early 1980s.[6-8] The successful transplantation in humans were achieved during 1990s.[9-12] In 2000, Shaipiro et al. reported the results of seven consecutive patients with brittle type 1 diabetes mellitus who had a fruitful islet cell transplantation simultaneously with glucocorticoid-free immunosuppressant regimen. This transformed from experiment to a true alternative to conventional diabetes therapy. This was known as Edmonton protocol.[13] In 2006, the immune tolerance network used the Edmonton protocol and carried out a multicenter trial of islet cell transplantation. The trial reported adequate glycemic control in 44% of recipients 1 year after transplant.[14] Few more studies are also available which unveil insulin freedom for 1 year in 80% of islet transplant recipients.[15-18] Collaborative Islet Transplant Registry (CITR) reported after attainment of insulin freedom due to islet cell transplant, 70% of recipients retained at 1 year, 55% at 2 years, 45% at 3 years, and 36% at 4 years.[9] Fiorina et al., Thompson et al., showed depletion in complication[19,20] and Toso, et al., reported improvement in quality of life post-transplant.[21]

Types of Islet Transplant

There are two types of islet cell transplant viz. (i) allotransplant and (ii) autotransplant. Allotransplant means the organ from the diseased donor is isolated, purified, and transferred into another person. Autotransplant is conducted after total pancreatectomy in patients with severe or chronic pancreatitis that cannot be managed by other treatments. Pancreatic islet autotransplantation cannot be performed in type 1 diabetes patients. For type 1 diabetes mellitus, pancreatic islet all-transplantation is recommended.

ISLET CELL PREPARATION

Isolation and Storage of Organ at Donor's Site

Cold perfusion of abdominal organs of the deceased donor is performed first. The pancreas, spleen, and duodenum are eliminated. The transaction of portal vein at the duodenal border and bile duct close to the pancreatic border is done. Cohesion of the pancreatic capsule and duodenum is retained. The isolated organ is transported being packed in a triple barrier bag with a cold preservative. While transportation, the temperature should maintained at 4°C. Cold ischemia can be maintained for maximum of 12 hours. University of Wisconsin solution is most frequently used preservative but histidine-tryptophan-ketoglutarate solution have shown the similar results.[22-24]

Preparation of Islet Cell at Transplant Centre

Organ procured from donor's site undergoes series of steps to obtain the end product. Initially through the main pancreatic duct, the infusion of collagenase is achieved. The collagenase is transported with pressure monitoring focused at duct distension with least leakage of the enzyme. Successful isolation depends upon the type of collagenase used.[25] Next step is to processing tissue digestion. The Ricordi Chamber consists of stainless steel balls, 5-6 in number which contribute to the mechanical fracture of the thick inter-lobar fibrous tissue that collagenase would not be able to digest. The digested tissue is collected under strict

CHAPTER 16: Pancreas and Islet Cell Transplant in Children

temperature control. This tissue consists of endocrine tissue and exocrine tissue. Exocrine tissue is used for extraction of islet cells, centrifuged using density gradient method so that different density materials can be separated. One of the material will contain islet cells. Now the analysis for the purity of the final cell suspension is performed. The cells are washed and placed in culture media for 12 hours in an incubator by maintaining the temperature between 22°C and 37°C. Now the islet cells are ready for transplantation.[26]

Procedure for Islet Cell Transplantation

This is performed through portal veins as it has advantages of being minimally invasive and has freedom from systemic hyperinsulinemia. This is usually performed under intravenous moderate sedation with routine hemodynamic, cardiac, and oxygen saturation monitoring. But portal venous site has certain disadvantages like portal hypertension, bleeding, and portal vein thrombosis. This site also has difficulty to access for surveillance biopsy. Investigators have explored alternative sites like kidney, spleen, pancreas, peritoneum, momentum, gastrointestinal wall, and bone marrow.[27] Wang et al. based on the animal study suggested the utilization of hepatic artery as a route infusion of cellular therapies.[28] Human study is warranted for this site. In spite of research on alternative sites, the carriage of islet cells through portal venous system is the most effective, feasible, standardized, and least complicated site.

Patients undergo periprocedural antimicrobial and antiviral therapy. But limited data are available to support this. Usually, the first-generation cephalosporin like cefazolin sodium is used. One hour before transplantation is administered with 1g cefazolin sodium intravenously. The same is continued every 6 hours for 24 hours post-transplantation. Usually patients are prone to pneumocystis pneumonia and cytomegalovirus infection post-transplant, hence the patients also do receive a 24-week combination treatment of trimethoprim/sulfamethoxazole 80/400 mg orally twice per week and a 12-week treatment of valganciclovir 450 mg orally on a daily basis. Bacteremia and sepsis are rare in patients with islet cell transplant but can expect sporadic cases if cryopreserved islet cells are contaminated.[29]

TRANSPLANTATION OUTCOMES

Complications

Numerous clinically relevant risks are associated with islet cell transplantation.[30] Most common complication is bleeding occurring either at intraperitoneal or liver subcapsular and incidence reported is 13%. But the bleeding can be significantly reduced with effective hepatic parenchymal tract embolization.[31] The prevalence of partial vein thrombosis is 5% in islet cell transplantation and complete portal venous thrombosis is very rare.[32] During the procedure, tracking of portal venous pressure and systemic anticoagulation are required as transplanted islets can activate coagulation. The coagulation is activated by secretion of tissue factor which causes depletion in portal flow, stasis, and development of clot through embolic effects.[33]

Apart from this liver enzyme elevation, abdominal pain, focal hepatic steatosis, and severe hypoglycemia can also with incidence rate of 50%, 50%, 20%, and 3%, respectively.[34] Post-transplant, acute increase in portal venous pressure occurs immediately which is transient in nature. Portal pressure increases with sequential transplantation but will not be typical unless portal vein thrombosis occurs.[35]

Transplantation Efficacy

The C-peptide level defines the function of islet, which should be greater than 0.3 ng/mL.[9] Islet cell is categorized as nonfunctional, partially functional, or fully functional if there is no detectable C-peptide levels, insulin is required or not required respectively.[36] Immediately after transplantation, islet cells generally begins functioning. One of the largest registry by CITR summarized the results of islet transplants performed in North American centers, European centers, and Australian medical centers between 1999 and 2008.[9]

Islet function is defined by a fasting C-peptide level analyzed by local assay or a stimulated C-peptide level greater than 0.3 ng/mL.[9] Islets may be classified as fully functional (i.e., in an insulin-independent patient), partially functional (i.e., insulin is required but C-peptide is detectable), or nonfunctional (i.e., there is no detectable C-peptide).[36] After transplantation pancreatic islet cells begin to function immediately. The National Institute of Diabetes and Digestive and Kidney Diseases funded the CITR, analyzed the data from all islet cell studies from 2009 to the present. This registry is the biggest data on islet cell transplantation outcomes. The 6th annual report of the CITR encapsulated the findings and outcomes of islet allograft transplants performed at 32 North American medical centers (inclusive of all human-to-human islet transplantation programs in North America), 3 European centers, and 2 Australian centers between 1999 and 2008. The report incorporated 828 islet infusions in 412 allograft recipients, who received one, two, three, and four infusions among 26%, 49%, 23%, and eight 2% patients, respectively. Among these, about 84% and the remaining 16% of patients underwent islet cell transplantation without and after kidney transplantation respectively. Repeat infusion was performed in 11% of patients by day 30, in 33% by day 75, in 54% by month 6, and in 65% by end of 1 year to achieve insulin independence. Insulin independence rates among islet cell recipients after achievement of insulin independence were 70%, 55%, 45% and 36%, at the end of 1 year, 2 years, 3 years, and 4 years, respectively.[9] American Diabetes Association recommends the use of islet cell transplantation in benefiting by reversing and delaying the long-term complications of diabetes mellitus.[37] Few studies showed partial graft function communicated by transplanted islet cells, in steadiness or improvement in diabetic retinopathy.[20,38-40] Lee et al. expressed the stabilization and betterment in diabetic retinopathy in all the patients after islet cell transplantation.[40] Similarly, studies by Thompson et al. and Warnock et al. outlined statistically significant fall in diabetic retinopathy progression after islet cell transplantation as compared with intensive therapy (12.2% vs 0%; $p < 0.01$).[20,39] Many studies have described diminution in diabetic nephropathy progression and glomerular filtration rate (GFR) after islet cell transplantation as compared with intensive medical therapy.[38,39,41,42] Fiorina et al. reported an improvement in renal graft survival rates after successful islet transplantation after kidney transplantation with 1 year, 4 years, and 7 years survival rates of 100%, 83%, and 83% versus unsuccessful islet transplantation after kidney transplantation with 1 year, 4 years, and 7 years survival rates of 83%, 72%, and 51%, respectively ($p < 0.02$).[41] A study conducted by Fung et al. in 2007 had shown no statistically significant difference in the reduction of GFR in patients undergoing islet cell transplantation versus intensive therapy.[42] Reduced GFR rate post-transplantation was reported in Warnock et al. study, but statistical significance was not reached (p <0.1 vs intensive therapy).[39]

INDICATIONS FOR REPEAT TRANSPLANTATION

The crucial signal for repeat of islet cell transplantation are in those post-transplant patients who could not achieve insulin independence or maintain insulin independence, or need insulin for 14 or more consecutive days.[9] Witkowski et al. delineated that up to 80% of patients must undergo two islet transplantation to attain insulin independence.[43]

CONCLUSION

Pancreatic islet cell transplantation is the most essential, integral, and biological management of type 1 diabetes. Though, there are many clinically successful pancreatic islet cell transplantation is performed and also many published data on successful pancreatic islet cell transplantation but still more development and accessibility to the patients are much needed.

REFERENCES

1. Hatipoglu B, Benedetti E, Oberhölzer J. Islet transplantation: current status and future directions. Curr Diab Rep. 2005;5:311-6.
2. Lacy PE, Kostianovsky M. Method for the isolation of intact islets of Langerhans from the rat pancreas. Diabetes. 1967;16:35-9.
3. Ballinger WF, Lacy PE. Transplantation of intact pancreatic islets in rats. Surgery. 1972;72:175-86.
4. Kemp CB, Knight MJ, Scharp DW, Lacy PE, Ballinger WF. Transplantation of isolated pancreatic islets into the portal vein of diabetic rats. Nature. 1973;244:447.
5. Scharp DW, Murphy JJ, Newton WT, Ballinger WF, Lacy PE. Transplantation of islets of Langerhans in diabetic rhesus monkeys. Surgery. 1975;77:100-5.
6. Najarian JS, Sutherland DE, Matas AJ, Steffes MW, Simmons RL, Goetz FC. Human islet transplantation: a preliminary report. Transplant Proc. 1977;9:233-6.
7. Sutherland DE. Pancreas and islet transplantation. II. Clinical trials. Diabetologia. 1981;20:435-50.
8. Largiader F, Kolb E, Binswanger U. A long-term functioning human pancreatic islet allotransplant. Transplantation. 1980;29:76-7.
9. CITR. (2009). Collaborative Islet Transplant Registry. Sixth Annual Report. Available from: https://web.emmes.com/study/isl/reports/CITR%206th%20Annual%20Data%20Report%20120109.pdf. [Accessed February, 2017].
10. Oberholzer J, Triponez F, Mage R, Andereggen E, Bühler L, Crétin N, et al. Human islet transplantation: lessons from 13 autologous and 13 allogeneic transplantations. Transplantation. 2000;69:1115-23.
11. Scharp DW, Lacy PE, Santiago JV, McCullough CS, Weide LG, Falqui L, et al. Insulin independence after islet transplantation into type I diabetic patient. Diabetes. 1990;39:515-8.
12. Alejandro R, Lehmann R, Ricordi C, Kenyon NS, Angelico MC, Burke G, et al. Long-term function (6 years) of islet allografts in type 1 diabetes. Diabetes. 1997;46:1983-9.
13. Shapiro AM, Lakey JR, Ryan EA, Korbutt GS, Toth E, Warnock GL, et al. Islet transplantation in seven patients with type 1 diabetes mellitus using a glucocorticoid-free immunosuppressive regimen. N Engl J Med. 2000;343:230-8.
14. Shapiro AM, Ricordi C, Hering BJ, Auchincloss H, Lindblad R, Robertson RP, et al. International trial of the Edmonton protocol for islet transplantation. N Engl J Med. 2006;355:1318-30.
15. Froud T, Ricordi C, Baidal DA, Hafiz MM, Ponte G, Cure P, et al. Islet transplantation in type 1 diabetes mellitus using cultured islets and steroid-free immunosuppression: Miami experience. Am J Transplant. 2005;5:2037-46.

SECTION 4: Pharmacological Management

16. Toso C, Baertschiger R, Morel P, Bosco D, Armanet M, Wojtusciszyn A, et al. Sequential kidney/islet transplantation: efficacy and safety assessment of a steroid-free immunosuppression protocol. Am J Transplant. 2006;6:1049-58.
17. O'Connell PJ, Hawthorne WJ, Holmes-Walker DJ, Nankivell BJ, Gunton JE, Patel AT, et al. Clinical islet transplantation in type 1 diabetes mellitus: results of Australia's first trial. Med J Aust. 2006;184:221-5.
18. Cure P, Pileggi A, Froud T, Messinger S, Faradji RN, Baidal DA, et al. Improved metabolic control and quality of life in seven patients with type 1 diabetes following islet after kidney transplantation. Transplantation. 2008;85:801-12.
19. Fiorina P, Folli F, Bertuzzi F, Maffi P, Finzi G, Venturini M, et al. Long-term beneficial effect of islet transplantation on diabetic macro-/microangiopathy in type 1 diabetic kidney-transplanted patients. Diabetes Care. 2003;26:1129-36.
20. Thompson DM, Begg IS, Harris C, Ao Z, Fung MA, Meloche RM, et al. Reduced progression of diabetic retinopathy after islet cell transplantation compared with intensive medical therapy. Transplantation. 2008;85:1400-5.
21. Toso C, Shapiro AM, Bowker S, Dinyari P, Paty B, Ryan EA, et al. Quality of life after islet transplant: impact of the number of islet infusions and metabolic outcome. Transplantation. 2007;84:664-6.
22. Habwe VQ. Posttransplantation quality of life: more than graft function. Am J Kidney Dis. 2006;47:S98-110.
23. Willoughby LM, Fukami S, Bunnapradist S, Gavard JA, Lentine KI, Hardinger KL, et al. Health insurance considerations for adolescent transplant recipients as they transition to adulthood. Pediatr Transplant. 2007;11:127-31.
24. Salehi P, Hansen MA, Avila JG, Barbaro B, Gangemi A, Romagnoli T, et al. Human islet isolation outcomes from pancreata preserved with histidine-tryptophan ketoglutarate versus University of Wisconsin solution. Transplantation. 2006;82:983-5.
25. Wang Y, Paushter D, Wang S, Barbaro B, Harvat T, Danielson KK, et al. Highly purified versus filtered crude collagenase: comparable human islet isolation outcomes. Cell Transplant. 2011;20:1817-25.
26. Ricordi C, Lacy PE, Scharp DW. Automated islet isolation from human pancreas. Diabetes. 1989;38:140-2.
27. Rajab A. Islet transplantation: alternative sites. Curr Diab Rep. 2010;10:332-7.
28. Wang W, Liu S, Zheng W, Gao F, Hawthorne WJ, Yi S. Hepatic artery vs. portal vein infusion of microbeads: a large animal pre-clinical model evaluating the intrahepatic capacity for cell infusion and imaging. Xenotransplantation. 2010;17:207-14.
29. Taylor GD, Kirkland T, Lakey J, Rajotte R, Warnock GL. Bacteremia due to transplantation of contaminated cryopreserved pancreatic islets. Cell Transplant. 1994;3:103-6.
30. Ryan EA, Paty BW, Senior PA, Shapiro AM. Risks and side effects of islet transplantation. Curr Diab Rep. 2004;4:304-9.
31. Villiger P, Ryan EA, Owen R, O'Kelly K, Oberholzer J, Al Saif F, et al. Prevention of bleeding after islet transplantation: lessons learned from a multivariate analysis of 132 cases at a single institution. Am J Transplant. 2005;5:2992-8.
32. Ryan EA, Paty BW, Senior PA, Bigam D, Alfadhli E, Kneteman NM, et al. Five-year follow-up after clinical islet transplantation. Diabetes. 2005;54:2060-9.
33. Moberg L, Johansson H, Lukinius A, Berne C, Foss A, Källen R, et al. Production of tissue factor by pancreatic islet cells as a trigger of detrimental thrombotic reactions in clinical islet transplantation. Lancet. 2002;360:2039-45.
34. CITR. (2006). Collaborative Islet Transplant Registry. Third Annual Report. [online] Available from: https://web.emmes.com/study/isl/reports/110912_citr_bibliography.pdf. [Accessed February, 2017].
35. Casey JJ, Lakey JR, Ryan EA, Paty BW, Owen R, O'Kelly K, et al. Portal venous pressure changes after sequential clinical islet transplantation. Transplantation. 2002;74:913-5.
36. Berney T, Toso C. Monitoring of the islet graft. Diabetes Metab. 2006;32:503-12.
37. Robertson RP, Davis C, Larsen J, Stratta R, Sutherland DE; American Diabetes Association. Pancreas and islet transplantation in type 1 diabetes. Diabetes Care. 2006;29:935.
38. Thompson DM, Meloche M, Ao Z, Paty B, Keown P, Shapiro RJ, et al. Reduced progression of diabetic microvascular complications with islet cell transplantation compared with intensive medical therapy. Transplantation. 2011;91:373-8.
39. Warnock GL, Thompson DM, Meloche RM, Shapiro RJ, Ao Z, Keown P, et al. A multi-year analysis of islet transplantation compared with intensive medical therapy on progression of complications in type 1 diabetes. Transplantation. 2008;86:1762-6.
40. Lee TC, Barshes NR, O'Mahony CA, Nguyen L, Brunicardi FC, Ricordi C, et al. The effect of pancreatic islet transplantation on progression of diabetic retinopathy and neuropathy. Transplant Proc. 2005;37:2263-5.
41. Fiorina P, Folli F, Zerbini G, Maffi P, Gremizzi C, Di Carlo V, et al. Islet transplantation is associated with improvement of renal function among uremic patients with type I diabetes mellitus and kidney transplants. J Am Soc Nephrol. 2003;14:2150-8.
42. Fung MA, Warnock GL, Ao Z, Keown P, Meloche M, Shapiro RJ, et al. The effect of medical therapy and islet cell transplantation on diabetic nephropathy: an interim report. Transplantation. 2007;84:17-22.
43. Witkowski P, Zakai SB, Rana A, Sledzinski Z, Hardy MA. Pancreatic islet transplantation, what has been achieved since Edmonton breakthrough. Ann Transplant. 2006;11:5-13.

SECTION 5

Acute Complications

Editor
Nalini Shah

Diabetic Ketoacidosis in Children

Alok Kanungo

INTRODUCTION

Diabetic ketoacidosis (DKA) is a complex metabolic state consisting of hyperglycemia, ketosis with acidosis. It is the leading cause of morbidity and mortality in children with type 1 diabetes mellitus (T1DM), with a case fatality rate ranging from 0.15 to 0.31%.[1,2] Incidence of T1DM is 2 per 1,000. The exact incidence of DKA is unknown but is estimated to be 4–8 per 1,000 diabetic patients. Diabetic ketoacidosis, occurring at the time of diagnosis of diabetes mellitus, is more common in younger children.[3] Globally, the frequency of DKA at diagnosis ranged from 12.8 to 80%, with highest frequencies in the United Arab Emirates, Saudi Arabia, and Romania, and the lowest in Sweden, the Slovak Republic, and Canada.[4] Data on incidences in Asia, and especially India, is very limited. An association with human leukocyte antigen (HLA) groups DR3 and DR4 (which occur more commonly in white populations) has been established, and hence, T1DM and DKA are more common in White children. The exact racial frequency is unknown. With current medical therapy, DKA has a mortality rate of 2–5%. The prognosis is excellent if aggressive fluid and insulin therapy commence in the first few hours of diagnosis.

ETIOLOGY

Diabetic ketoacidosis is the presenting complaint in approximately one-fourth of newly diagnosed T1DM patients. Infection is the most frequent cause of DKA, particularly in patients with known diabetes.[5] Poor compliance with existing insulin regimens, underlying endocrine changes of adolescence (thelarche, adrenarche, menarche), caregiver's lack of competence, and insulin pump failure may be the other causes. Risk factors for DKA have been listed in box 1.

SECTION 5: Acute Complications

BOX 1: Risk factors for diabetic ketoacidosis	
In newly diagnosed cases	**In known diabetic patients**
• Younger age (<2 years) • Delayed diagnosis • Lower socioeconomic status • Countries with low prevalence of type 1 diabetes mellitus	• Insulin omission • Poor metabolic control • Previous episodes of diabetic ketoacidosis • Psychiatric (including eating) disorders • Challenging social and family circumstances • Peripubertal and adolescent girls • Limited access to medical services • Failures in insulin pump therapy • Gastroenteritis with persistent vomiting and inability to maintain hydration

PATHOPHYSIOLOGY

Diabetic ketoacidosis results from deficiency of insulin and increased levels of the counter-regulatory hormones (catecholamines, glucagon, cortisol, and growth hormone). The combination of absolute or relative insulin deficiency and high counter-regulatory hormone concentrations results in an accelerated catabolic state with increased glucose production by the liver and kidney (via glycogenolysis and gluconeogenesis), and simultaneously impaired peripheral glucose utilization, which combine to result in hyperglycemia and hyperosmolality; insulin deficiency and high counter-regulatory hormones also increase lipolysis and ketogenesis and cause ketonemia and metabolic acidosis. Ketone bodies provide alternative source of energy in the absence of intracellular glucose. The ketoacids [acetoacetate, β-hydroxybutyrate (β-OHB), acetone] are products of proteolysis and lipolysis.[6]

Hyperglycemia causes an osmotic diuresis and resultant hypovolemia leads to tissue hypoperfusion and lactic acidosis. Ketosis and lactic acidosis produce a metabolic acidosis. This further enhances the production of counter-regulatory hormones and leads to a vicious cycle. Electrolyte imbalances are the consequences of hyperglycemia, hyperosmolality, and acidosis. Serum hyperkalemia occurs as potassium ions shift from the intracellular to extracellular space because of acidosis from insulin deficiency and decreased renal tubular secretion. Similar decreases in serum phosphate and magnesium concentrations are the result of ion shifts. Hyponatremia results from a dilutional effect as free water shifts extracellularly because of high serum osmolarity. The pathophysiology of DKA in children[7] is summarized in figure 1.

As serum osmolarity increases from hyperglycemia, intracellular osmolality in the brain also increases. Overly rapid correction of serum hyperglycemia and osmolarity may create a large gradient between intracerebral and serum osmolarity. Free water then shifts into the brain and may cause cerebral edema with herniation.[8] Cerebral and other autoregulatory mechanisms may not be well-developed in younger children. Hence, greater severity at presentation in younger children together with less maturity of autoregulatory systems combine to predispose children to cerebral edema. Therefore, fluid resuscitation and correction of hyperglycemia should be gradual and closely monitored.

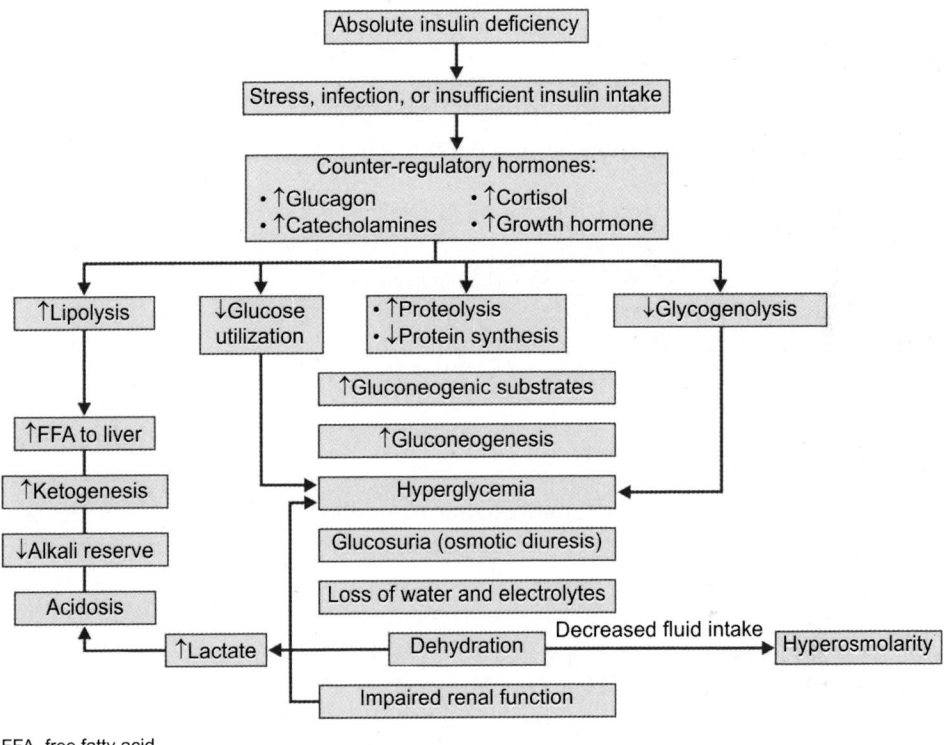

Fig. 1: Pathophysiology of diabetic ketoacidosis

CLINICAL FEATURES

Classic symptoms of DKA are often insidious and are as follows:
- Fatigue and malaise
- Nausea/vomiting, abdominal pain
- Polydipsia, polyuria, and polyphagia
- Weight loss
- Fever.

Physical examination may reveal the following:
- Altered mental status without evidence of head trauma
- Tachycardia, tachypnea, or hyperventilation (Kussmaul's respirations)
- Normal or low blood pressure
- Increased capillary refill time, poor perfusion
- Lethargy and weakness
- Acetone odor of the breath reflecting metabolic acidosis.

Classic symptoms of DKA are often absent in toddlers. If a patient has known diabetes, obtain a history for compliance with insulin regimens. The younger the child, the more difficult it is to obtain the classical history of polyuria, polydipsia, and weight loss.

DIAGNOSIS

The biochemical criteria for the diagnosis of DKA are:
- Hyperglycemia [blood glucose >11 mmol/L (~200 mg/dL)]
- Venous pH less than 7.3 or bicarbonate less than 15 mmol/L
- Ketonemia and ketonuria.

Although not universally available, blood β-OHB concentration should be measured whenever possible; a level more than or equal to 3 mmol/L is indicative of DKA.[9]
The severity of DKA is categorized by the degree of acidosis:[10]
- Mild: Venous pH <7.3 or bicarbonate <15 mmol/L
- Moderate: pH <7.2, bicarbonate <10 mmol/L
- Severe: pH <7.1, bicarbonate <5 mmol/L.

DIFFERENTIAL DIAGNOSIS

Differential diagnosis includes fever, pancreatitis, alcoholic ketoacidosis, metabolic acidosis due to other causes, bowel obstruction, dehydration, gastroenteritis, pneumonia, pyloric stenosis, and salicylate toxicity.

INVESTIGATIONS

Following laboratory tests are helpful in diagnosing and/or monitoring the treatment:
- Serum glucose: (By a glucometer) provides the opportunity for rapid diagnosis and treatment. However, a urine analysis (dip for sugar and ketones) is also acceptable.
- Serum potassium: Most important electrolyte disturbance in DKA (Table 1)
- Arterial blood gas level: Venous blood gas also is an acceptable alternative in limited resource setting
- Glycosylated hemoglobin: High glycosylated hemoglobin indicates poor compliance with insulin therapy
- Complete blood count: Increased white blood cell may be a response to stress and not necessarily due to infection
- Other studies: Serum sodium, chloride, bicarbonate, blood urea nitrogen, creatinine, magnesium, calcium, and phosphate levels, urine glucose, ketones, and osmolality, serum osmolality, blood, urine, and throat cultures, along with any other study appropriate for suspected infections. An electrocardiography is helpful when results of serum potassium concentration are not rapidly available
- Imaging studies: For suspected infection, obstructive abdominal processes, or cerebral edema.

TABLE 1: Potassium replacement in children with diabetic ketoacidosis

Serum potassium (mEq/L)	Intravenous fluid potassium (mEq/L)
<3	40–60
3–4	30–40
4–5	20–30
>5	0–20

MANAGEMENT OF DIABETIC KETOACIDOSIS

Goals of therapy are to correct dehydration, acidosis and reverse ketosis, slowly correct hyperosmolality and restore blood glucose to near normal, monitor for complications of DKA and its treatment, and identify and treat any precipitating event.[11] Fluid replacement should begin before starting insulin therapy. Fluid, glucose, and insulin administration have to be modified in response to the dynamic and often volatile metabolic changes that occur during treatment.[12] Meticulous monitoring of the clinical and biochemical response to treatment is necessary. Progression of DKA management has to be documented and a flow sheet is maintained to monitor the response (Fig. 2). Management in the emergency department has been highlighted in box 2.

Management during 1st Hour

The goal of the 1st hour of treatment is volume resuscitation and confirmation of DKA by laboratory studies. Isotonic sodium chloride solution bolus should be given at 20 mL/kg intravenously over an hour or less. Dextrose infusion can be considered if serum glucose levels fall rapidly to 250–300 mg/dL during rehydration (Fig. 3).

Management during 2nd Hour till 6th Hour

The goals of the 2nd and succeeding hours are slow correction of hyperglycemia (with glucose level falling at a rate <100 mg/dL/h), metabolic acidosis, and ketosis, in addition to continued volume replenishment. This should be achieved in a manner that prevents too rapid a decrease in serum osmolarity. It is prudent to carefully observe the patient in order to avoid hypoglycemia which may occur suddenly, as insulin resistance resolves. Glucose levels should be maintained above 150–250 mg/dL.
- Fluids: Isotonic sodium chloride solution (0.9% NaCl) or 0.45% isotonic sodium chloride solution (0.45% NaCl) should be administered along with supplemental potassium at twice the maintenance rate. Potassium can be given as potassium chloride, potassium phosphate, or potassium acetate. If serum potassium levels are very low and life-threatening, consider

BOX 2: Management of diabetic ketoacidosis in the emergency department
Emergency department care
• Should follow the general guidelines for pediatric advanced life support
• Access two large intravenous (IV) catheter lines for fluids, insulin infusion, and drips
• Arterial catheterization is performed if profoundly altered mental status, signs of severe shock, or signs of severe acidosis
• Provide oxygen and advanced airway management
• Provide isotonic IV fluids (e.g., isotonic sodium chloride or lactated Ringer's solution)
• If there is a history of recent large consumption of glucose-containing fluids, consider emptying the stomach
• Patients with diabetic ketoacidosis should be on nil per os, receive supplemental oxygen and, if bacterial infection is suspected, empiric antibiotic therapy should be started

Hour	Time	Chemistry status						Treatment status				
		Serum pH	Glucose (fingerstick)	Glucose (chem panel)	Anion gap	CO_2	K^+	PO_4^{3-}	Insulin given (units)	Route (IV/IM/SC)	Cumulative fluid input	Present fluid type	Cumulative urine output
0													
1													
2													
3													
4													
5													
6													
7													
8													
9													
10													
11													
12													
13													
14													
15													
16													
17													
18													
19													
20													

Patient: _____ Date beginning: _____ Time beginning: _____

CO_2, carbon dioxide; K^+, potassium; PO_4^{3-}, phosphate; IV, intravenous; IM, intramuscular; SC, subcutaneous.

Fig. 2: Sample flow sheet of diabetic ketoacidosis management

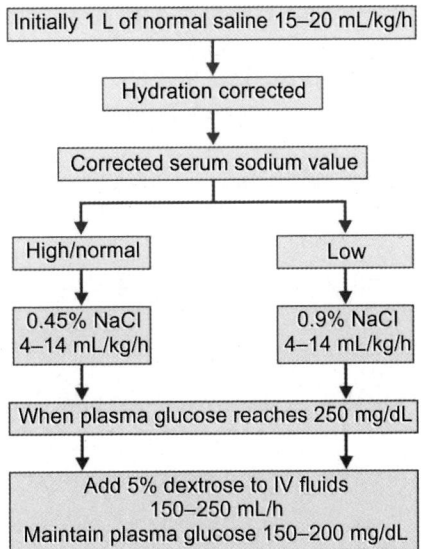

Fig. 3: Fluid replacement in children with diabetic ketoacidosis

giving orally (or by nasogastric tube) in a liquid formulation. This corrects hypokalemia much quicker than intravenous replenishment, since the rate of infusion needs to be kept low due to cardiac considerations
- Insulin: Withhold insulin until severe hypokalemia is corrected. Then administer an intravenous bolus dose at the rate of 0.1 U/kg, followed by a constant infusion at the rate of 0.1 U/kg. The intravenous tubing needs to be primed before the bolus dose is administered since insulin binds to the tubing. The insulin bolus dose may be foregone if the serum glucose level is less than 500 mg/dL or if there is a history of hypersensitivity to exogenous insulin. To prepare the drip, add units of regular insulin equal to the patient's weight in kilograms to 100 mL saline. Saturate the IV tubing with 20 mL of the insulin solution and set the infusion rate to 10 mL/h. This will provide 0.1 U/kg/h.
- Glucose: Add 5 or 10% dextrose (D5 or D10) to the intravenous fluids if patient remains in ketoacidosis and serum glucose level reaches 250–300 mg/dL. Do not discontinue the insulin drip as it is critical in eliminating ketoacidosis. Maintain serum glucose concentration at 150–250 mg/dL during insulin infusion. Titrate insulin and glucose infusions keeping in mind that 1 unit of regular insulin metabolizes 3 g of glucose.

Management after 6 Hours

The final goal is to attain a serum glucose level as close to normal as possible, attain neutral blood pH (pH: 7.4, serum bicarbonate: 15–18 mEq/dL) and eliminate ketones. This phase includes transitioning from parenteral to subcutaneous insulin and from a fasting state to oral feed, initially with fluids and later solids.

- Fluids: Give 0.45% sodium chloride solution with dextrose and potassium up to twice maintenance rate. Consider oral fluids if nausea is absent
- Insulin: Set the intravenous infusion at 0.05–0.10 U/kg/h
- Glucose: Consider 5–10% dextrose in intravenous fluids to maintain serum glucose level at least 150 mg/dL.

Transfer to a pediatric intensive care unit is prudent for the patient with persistent altered mental status, resistant acidosis, and hemodynamic instability, and for the first-time newly diagnosed patient.

An algorithmic approach and protocol for management of DKA has been depicted in figure 4 and table 2, respectively.

Caveats in the Management of Diabetic Ketoacidosis

- Anion gap = Na − (Cl + HCO_3). Normal range is 12 ± 2 mmol/L. In DKA, the anion gap is typically 20–30 mmol/L; an anion gap more than 35 mmol/L suggests concomitant lactic acidosis
- Corrected sodium = Measured Na + 2 [(plasma glucose−5.6)/5.6] mmol/L or measured Na + 2[(plasma glucose−100)/100] mg/dL.
- Effective osmolality (mOsm/kg) = 2 × (plasma Na) + plasma glucose (mmol/L)
- The degree of sodium loss may be overestimated because of the presence of hyperglycemia. For each increase in glucose of 100 mg/dL (5.5 mmol/L), serum sodium may be decreased by 2 mEq/L. An increase in corrected serum sodium is a goal of therapy
- Serum potassium may be normal, but total body potassium moves to the extracellular compartment and may be lost in urine or vomitus. Hyperkalemia in DKA is, therefore, uncommon unless renal shutdown has occurred. In contrast, hypokalemia may develop rapidly after treatment is initiated because the provision of insulin in the presence of hyperglycemia and the correction of acidosis promote the return of potassium to the intracellular compartment
- A patient with a low serum potassium level should be assumed to have a potentially life-threatening total body potassium level. Patients with evidence of hypovolemia or history of polydipsia who have normal or high serum potassium level should be assumed to have moderate total potassium depletion. Therapy should begin with volume resuscitation. As a result of the potential for hypokalemia-induced malignant dysrhythmias, do not give insulin to patients known to have profound potassium depletion until potassium replenishment is underway
- Ketone bodies may cause spurious elevation in creatinine values in some assays. Urine and blood ketone tests measure different metabolites: urine ketone tests measure acetoacetate and blood ketone tests measure β-OHB. Since β-OHB is the predominant ketone body in DKA, urine measurement may give false-negative results. The concentration of β-OHB is 4- to 10-fold higher than that of acetoacetic acid at initial presentation. With correction of acidosis, β-OHB is oxidized back to acetoacetate and then measured. Hence, physicians should not be misled by the persistence of a strong ketone reaction as long as the patient manifests evidence of clinical and biochemical improvement in acidosis

CHAPTER 17: Diabetic Ketoacidosis in Children

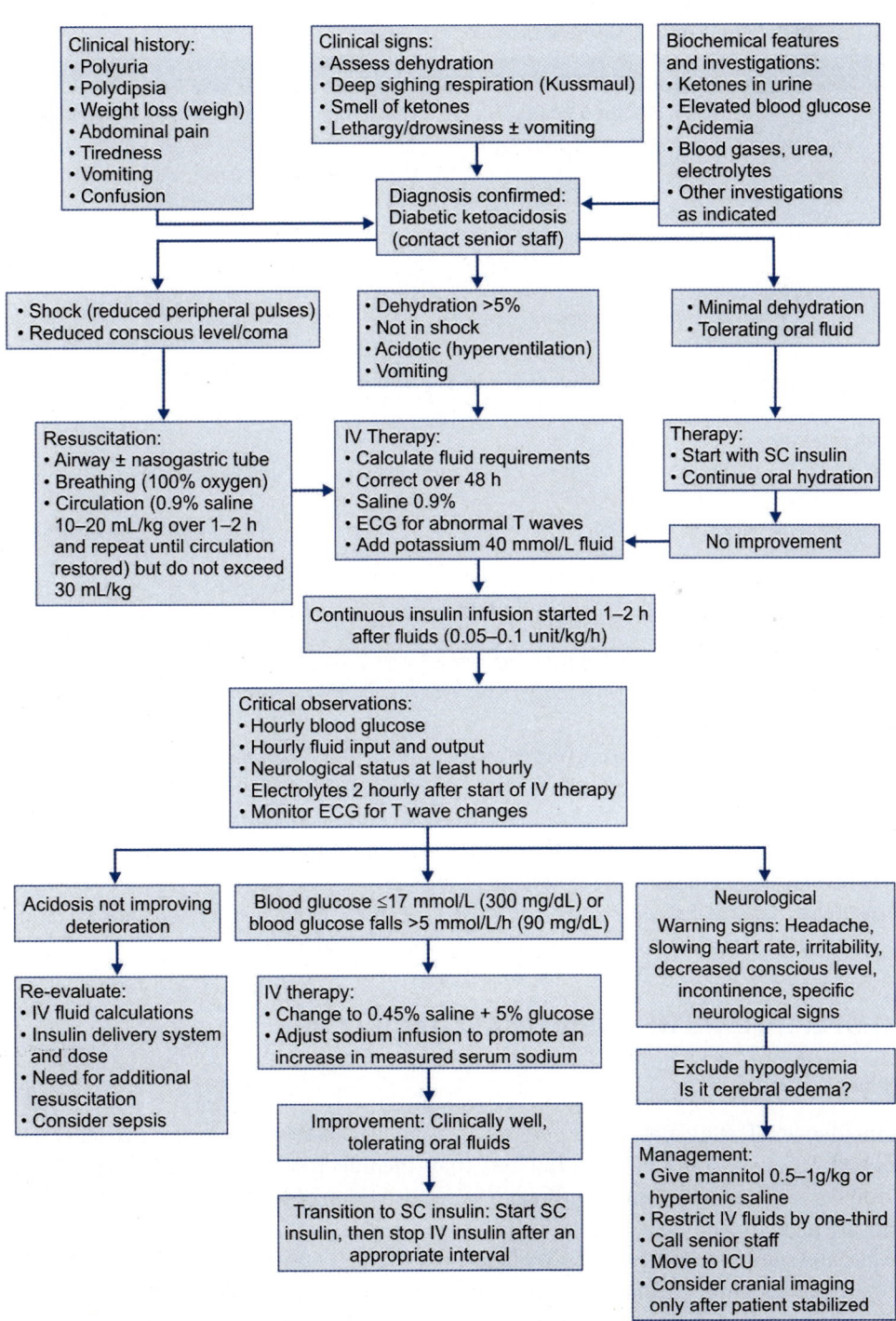

SC, subcutaneous; ICU, intensive care unit; IV, intravenous; ECG, electrocardiogram.

Fig. 4: Algorithm for management of diabetic ketoacidosis

TABLE 2: Diabetic ketoacidosis treatment protocol[3]

Time	Therapy	Comments
1st h	10–20 mL/kg IV bolus 0.9% NaCl or LR Insulin drip at 0.05–0.10 units/kg/hr	Quick volume expansion; may be repeated. NPO. Monitor I/O, neurologic status Use flow sheet. Have mannitol at bedside; 1 g/kg IV push for cerebral edema
2nd h until DKA resolution	0.45% NaCl, plus continue insulin drip 20 mEq/L KPhos and 20 mEq/L KAc	IV rate = $\dfrac{85\ \text{mL/kg} + \text{maintenance bolus}}{23\ \text{h}}$
	5% glucose if blood sugar >250 mg/dL (14 mmol/L)	If K <3 mEq/L, give 0.5–1.0 mEq/kg as oral K solution or increase IV K to 80 mEq/L
Variable	Oral intake with subcutaneous insulin	No emesis; CO_2 ≥16 mEq/L; normal electrolytes

Note that the initial IV bolus is considered part of the total fluid allowed in the first 24 hours and is subtracted before calculating the IV rate.

Maintenance (24 h) = 100 mL/kg (for the first 10 kg) + 50 mL/kg (for the second 10 kg) + 25 mL/kg (for all remaining kg)

Sample calculation for a child weighing 30 kg:

1st hour = 300 mL IV bolus 0.9% NaCl or LR

2nd and subsequent hour = $\dfrac{(85\ \text{mL} \times 30) + 1750\ \text{mL} - 300\ \text{mL}}{23\ \text{h}} = 175\ \text{mL/h}$

(0.45% NaCl with 20 mEq/L Kphos and 20 mEq/L KAc).

DKA, diabetic ketoacidosis; I/O, input and output (urine, emesis); K, potassium; KAc, potassium acetate; KPhos, potassium phosphate; LR, lactated Ringer solution; NaCl, sodium chloride; NPO, nothing by mouth; CO_2, carbon dioxide.

- Ketoacidosis takes longer to correct than hyperglycemia. Therefore, insulin therapy should not be discontinued if ketoacidosis has not cleared, even if glucose concentrations are approaching 300 mg/dL (17 mmol/L). Glucose should be provided in the intravenous solutions because the provision of substrate in the form of intravenous glucose and insulin will reverse ketogenesis
- The higher basal metabolic rate and large surface area relative to total body mass in children require greater precision in delivering fluids and electrolytes.

COMPLICATIONS OF DIABETIC KETOACIDOSIS

Cerebral Edema

The incidence of clinically overt cerebral edema is 0.5–0.9% and the mortality rate is 21–24%.[13,14] Causes are multifactorial but may include too rapid infusion of fluids and electrolytes, overhydration, and overly aggressive correction of acidosis or hyperglycemia. Risk factors are highlighted in box 3.

Signs and symptoms of cerebral edema include headache and slowing of heart rate, change in neurological status (restlessness, irritability, increased drowsiness, and incontinence), specific neurological signs (e.g., cranial nerve, palsies, papilledema), rising blood pressure, and decreased oxygen saturation.[15] Clinically significant cerebral edema usually develops within the first 12 hours after treatment has started, but can occur before treatment has begun

CHAPTER 17: Diabetic Ketoacidosis in Children

or, rarely, may develop as late as 24–48 hours after the start of treatment. A method of clinical diagnosis based on bedside evaluation of neurological state has been developed to diagnose cerebral edema. One diagnostic criterion, two major criteria, or one major and two minor criteria have a sensitivity of 92% and a false-positive rate of only 4% (Box 4).

Treatment of cerebral edema includes reduction in the rate of fluid administration by one-third and intravenous mannitol, 0.5–1 g/kg over 10–15 minutes. Repeat mannitol if there is no initial response in 30 minutes to 2 hours. Hypertonic saline (3%) 2.5–5 mL/kg over 10–15 minutes may be used as an alternative, especially if there is no initial response to mannitol. Elevate the head of the bed to 30°. Intubation may be necessary for the patient with impending respiratory failure. Cranial imaging may be considered as with any critically ill patient with encephalopathy or acute focal neurologic deficit.[16]

BOX 3: Risk factors for development of cerebral edema at diagnosis or treatment of diabetic ketoacidosis

- Greater hypocapnia at presentation after adjusting for degree of acidosis
- Increased serum urea nitrogen at presentation
- More severe acidosis at presentation
- Bicarbonate treatment for correction of acidosis
- An attenuated rise in measured serum sodium concentrations during therapy
- Greater volumes of fluid given in the first 4 hours
- Administration of insulin in the first hour of fluid treatment
- Younger age
- New onset diabetes
- Longer duration of symptoms

BOX 4: Diagnosis of cerebral edema in diabetic ketoacidosis

Diagnostic criteria
- Abnormal motor or verbal response to pain
- Decorticate or decerebrate posture
- Cranial nerve palsy (especially III, IV, and VI)
- Abnormal neurogenic respiratory pattern (e.g., grunting, tachypnea, Cheyne-Stokes respiration, apneusis)

Major criteria
- Altered mentation/fluctuating level of consciousness
- Sustained heart rate deceleration (decrease more than 20 beats/min) not attributable to improved intravascular volume or sleep state
- Age-inappropriate incontinence

Minor criteria
- Vomiting
- Headache
- Lethargy or not easily arousable
- Diastolic blood pressure >90 mmHg
- Age <5 years

Hypoglycemia

Causes of hypoglycemia include increased sensitivity to exogenous insulin and insufficient serum glucose for insulin to metabolize. Treatment includes adding 5-10% dextrose to intravenous fluids when serum glucose level is 250-300 mg/dL.

Hypokalemia

Serum potassium begins to reflect actual total body potassium depletion as volume depletion and acidosis resolve. Add potassium to intravenous fluids when urine output is present and results of serum potassium level are available.

Cardiac Dysrhythmia

Causes include hyperkalemia, hypokalemia, and hypocalcemia. Treatment involves correcting the specific cause.

Pulmonary Edema

Causes include low plasma oncotic pressure and increased pulmonary capillary permeability. Treatment includes oxygen and diuresis.

PREVENTION

Patients with known diabetes have to maintain compliance with an insulin therapy regimen and are to be monitored periodically by the treating physician.[17] This is especially important in the presence of nausea, vomiting, and abdominal pain. Admit children with DKA for further evaluation, observation, management, diabetes education, and assessment of compliance by responsible caretakers. Awareness by patient education camps on sick day management and identification of risk factors may help in preventing such episodes.

REFERENCES

1. Umpierrez G, Korytkowski M. Diabetic emergencies - ketoacidosis, hyperglycaemic hyperosmolar state and hypoglycaemia. Nat Rev Endocrinol. 2016;12(4):222-32.
2. Curtis JR, To T, Muirhead S, Cummings E, Daneman D. Recent trends in hospitalization for diabetic ketoacidosis in ontario children. Diabetes Care. 2002;25(9):1591-6.
3. Bui H, To T, Stein R, Fung K, Daneman D. Is diabetic ketoacidosis at disease onset a result of missed diagnosis? J Pediatr. 2010;156(3):472-7.
4. Usher-Smith JA, Thompson M, Ercole A, Walter FM. Variation between countries in the frequency of diabetic ketoacidosis at first presentation of type 1 diabetes in children: a systematic review. Diabetologia. 2012;55(11):2878-94.
5. Szypowska A, Skorka A. The risk factors of ketoacidosis in children with newly diagnosed type 1 diabetes mellitus. Pediatr Diabetes. 2011;12(4 Pt 1):302-6.
6. Wolfsdorf JI. The International Society of Pediatric and Adolescent Diabetes guidelines for management of diabetic ketoacidosis: Do the guidelines need to be modified? Pediatr Diabetes. 2014;15(4):277-86.

7. Wolfsdorf J, Glaser N, Sperling MA, American Diabetes Association. Diabetic ketoacidosis in infants, children, and adolescents: A consensus statement from the American Diabetes Association. Diabetes Care. 2006;29(5):1150-9.
8. Tasker RC, Acerini CL. Cerebral edema in children with diabetic ketoacidosis: vasogenic rather than cellular? Pediatr Diabetes. 2014;15(4):261-70.
9. Sheikh-Ali M, Karon BS, Basu A, Kudva YC, Muller LA, Xu J, et al. Can serum beta-hydroxybutyrate be used to diagnose diabetic ketoacidosis? Diabetes Care. 2008;31(4):643-7.
10. Maniatis AK, Goehrig SH, Gao D, Rewers A, Walravens P, Klingensmith GJ. Increased incidence and severity of diabetic ketoacidosis among uninsured children with newly diagnosed type 1 diabetes mellitus. Pediatr Diabetes. 2005;6(2):79-83.
11. Rosenbloom AL. The management of diabetic ketoacidosis in children. Diabetes Ther. 2010;1(2):103-20.
12. Kapellen T, Vogel C, Telleis D, Siekmeyer M, Kiess W. Treatment of diabetic ketoacidosis (DKA) with 2 different regimens regarding fluid substitution and insulin dosage (0.025 vs. 0.1 units/kg/h). Exp Clin Endocrinol Diabetes. 2012;120(5):273-6.
13. Glaser NS, Wootton-Gorges SL, Buonocore MH, Marcin JP, Rewers A, Strain J, et al. Frequency of sub-clinical cerebral edema in children with diabetic ketoacidosis. Pediatr Diabetes. 2006;7(2):75-80.
14. Edge JA, Hawkins MM, Winter DL, Dunger DB. The risk and outcome of cerebral oedema developing during diabetic ketoacidosis. Arch Dis Child. 2001;85(1):16-22.
15. Siwakoti K, Giri S, Kadaria D. Cerebral edema among adults with diabetic ketoacidosis and hyperglycemic hyperosmolar syndrome: incidence, characteristics, and outcomes. J Diabetes. 2017;9(2):208-9.
16. Barrot A, Huisman TA, Poretti A. Neuroimaging findings in acute pediatric diabetic ketoacidosis. Neuroradiol J. 2016;29(5):317-22.
17. Choudhary A. Sick Day Management in Children and Adolescents with Type 1 Diabetes. J Ark Med Soc. 2016;112(14):284-6.

CHAPTER 18

Management of Diabetes in Hospitalized Children

PV Rao, Daruru Ranganath

INTRODUCTION

Diabetes mellitus in children is a polygenic disease with age of onset between 6 months and young adulthood. Clinical presentation in almost all, about 99% in India, is acute and rapid with signs of ketoacidosis, and rarely, hyperosmolar without ketoacidosis. In all these cases, a preceding history of polyuria, polydipsia, and polyphagia of about 2 weeks is usually present. Very rarely, children can also be diagnosed with diabetes, when they are evaluated routinely either by fasting or post prandial blood glucose levels or glycated hemoglobin.

Markers of the immune destruction of the β-cell include islet cell autoantibodies, autoantibodies to insulin, glutamic acid decarboxylase-65), and tyrosine phosphatases islet antigen (IA)-2 and IA-2β. One or more of these autoantibodies are usually present in about 90% of individuals when fasting hyperglycemia is initially detected. As autoimmunity is invariably present on testing, testing for diabetes antibodies is neither cost-effective nor practical for diagnosing diabetes. History of parental diabetes is present in 2–4% of children at the time of detection of diabetes.

Rarely, a child has transient hyperglycemia with glycosuria while under substantial physical stress. This usually resolves permanently during recovery from the stressors. Stress-produced hyperglycemia can reflect a limited insulin reserve temporarily revealed by counter-regulatory hormones. Transient diabetes mellitus is rare and is encountered only in newborns. It usually manifests as dehydration, loss of weight, or acidosis in infants who are small for gestational age.

PROTOCOL FOR DIABETES MANAGEMENT IN CHILDREN

This is mainly a management protocol for diabetic ketoacidosis (DKA). Following presentation of a child with diabetes in an acute situation, management of diabetes is individualized while considering the basic principles of child care to achieve the targets of growth, and both physical and mental milestones of development.

CHAPTER 18: Management of Diabetes in Hospitalized Children

Criteria for Diagnosing Diabetic Ketoacidosis[1]

Criteria for diagnosing DKA is mentioned in table 1.

In a child with acidosis, casual blood glucose may be normal if there is no diabetes. Associated diabetes or sepsis invariably manifests high blood glucose with acidosis.

Urine test for glucose and ketone bodies is positive. Venous blood pH is below 7.2 in severe DKA.

Electrolytes in DKA-serum sodium may be normal, serum chloride may be normal or low, and serum potassium is low.

Serum creatinine is normal or increased, and serum phosphorous is elevated in associated renal failure.

For confirmation of a diagnosis, management protocol considers presence or absence of vomiting and abdominal pain, polyuria, polydipsia, polyphagia, fever, altered sensorium, cough, and chest pain.

Differential diagnosis of type 1 diabetes mellitus (T1DM) and tests to be considered are mentioned in table 2.

TABLE 1: Criteria for diagnosing diabetic ketoacidosis

Hyperglycemia	Blood glucose >200 mg/dL
Acidosis	Venous pH <7.3 and/or bicarbonate <15 mEq/L
Ketosis	Glycosuria and ketonuria; ketonemia (β-hydroxybutyrate); ketones in serum >5 mg/dL

Note: Euglycemic ketoacidosis may develop in young or partially treated children, pregnant women, and children treated 'off-label' with sodium glucose cotransporter-2 inhibitors.

TABLE 2: Differential diagnosis of type 1 diabetes mellitus and tests to consider

	Differential diagnosis	Tests
Vomiting	• Gastroenteritis • Toxic ingestion • Metabolic disorders	• Serum glucose • Serum electrolytes • Electrolyte disturbances and acidosis without hyperglycemia suggest other disorders requiring more directed testing
Abdominal pain	• Gastroenteritis • Appendicitis • Intra-abdominal abscess	• Careful clinical and systemic examination will help in excluding surgical causes • Measurement of serum glucose and urine analysis helps to differentiate diabetes
Hyperpnea	• Pneumonia • Asthma • Anxiety	• Kussmaul's respiration • Serum glucose and electrolytes helps to differentiate diabetes from metabolic acidosis
Hyperglycemia	• Medication, stress	• May be mistaken for diabetes, although careful history does not demonstrate characteristic features of diabetes

Markers of the Immune Destruction of β-cell

Other autoimmunities associated with T1DM should be sought, including celiac disease [by tissue transglutaminase immunoglobulin A (IgA) and total IgA] and thyroiditis (by antithyroid peroxidase and antithyroglobulin antibodies). About 15–30% of subjects with T1DM have elevated thyroid stimulating hormone and antithyroid antibody, and close to 5–10% have evidence for celiac disease.

MANAGEMENT[2]

Assuming 5–10% of dehydration, diabetes management in hospitalized children is started with intravenous fluid replacement. Fluid of choice is normal saline for first 4–6 hours followed by any fluid with 0.45% sodium chloride, half-normal saline.

Insulin infusion is begun without a bolus at a rate of 0.1 units/kg/hr within 2 hours after starting fluid replacement therapy and continued for up to 48 hours. Insulin drip is for resolution of ketosis, but not for treating hyperglycemia. Subcutaneous bolus insulins are not given in hospitalized children.

Potassium is added to intravenous fluids when serum potassium is less than 5.5 mEq/L and child has reestablished urination. Potassium replacement is continued throughout intravenous fluid therapy.

Real-time bedside measurement of β-hydroxybutyrate may help to optimize treatment of DKA and shorten the duration of hospitalization.

There is no major clinical benefit from bicarbonate therapy. It is indicated only in children with severe acidemia (arterial pH <6.9) or life-threatening hyperkalemia.

The most-feared complication during diabetes management in an acute setup is cerebral edema, despite the widespread introduction of gradual rehydration protocols. If glucose elevation and dehydration are severe and persist for several hours, the risk of cerebral edema increases. This is evident in 0.3–1% of all episodes of ketoacidosis. However, its etiology remains unknown. Baseline acidosis and abnormalities of sodium, potassium, and blood urea nitrogen concentrations as well as early bolus administration of insulin and high volumes of fluid were identified as risk factors. It is necessary to treat cerebral edema in pediatric intensive care units, with mannitol and supportive care as required, while watching for hypokalemia and hypoglycemia, which can occur rapidly.

Insulin drip should be continued for at least half an hour to 1 hour after giving a subcutaneous bolus insulin, because absorption of insulin from subcutaneous sites is delayed. Subcutaneous insulin does not act as quickly as intravenous insulin.

After the child is shifted to subcutaneous insulin, insulin doses are titrated to achieve ideal glycemic control. Diabetes education is given to parents, sick-day guidelines explained and prevention and management of hypoglycemia are also explained. The treating doctors ensure that the family is adequately trained for monitoring the child's blood glucose and urine ketones, preparing and injecting the correct insulin dose subcutaneously at a proper time, recognizing and treating low blood glucose reactions, and having a basic meal plan.

Management during Infections

Infections are more common in diabetic children; they always worsen glucose control and may precipitate DKA. Children with any infection are dehydrated due to polyuria from osmotic diuresis and may have ketosis through emesis. Glucose levels are elevated due to increased catabolism and secretion of counter-regulatory hormones. Glucose may be low due to emesis and lack of adequate caloric intake. While hypoglycemia is common in children younger than 3 years of age, older children have a tendency towards hyperglycemia. Frequent blood glucose monitoring and adjustment of insulin doses are thus essential in the management of sick children. The main objectives of management of children are to maintain hydration, control glucose levels, and avoid ketoacidosis, in that order.

Hospitalization of a child is necessary if home treatment does not control ketonuria, hyperglycemia, or hypoglycemia, or if the child shows signs of dehydration. A child whose blood glucose declines to less than 50–60 mg/dL and who cannot maintain oral intake may need intravenous glucose, especially if further insulin is needed to control ketonemia. A child with large ketonuria and emesis should be seen in the emergency department for a general examination, to evaluate hydration and to determine whether ketoacidosis is present by checking serum electrolytes, glucose, pH, and total carbon dioxide.

Management during Surgery

Stress hormones are usually above normal, during surgery and due to underlying conditions, such as infections. Anesthesia itself may cause insulin resistance. Associated counter-regulatory hormones and insulin antagonists are in excess, raising blood glucose, thereby fluid losses through osmotic diuresis, and potentiating ketogenesis. If caloric intake is not adequate as it is usually restricted, glucose levels may fall. Thus, the clinical manifestations of hyperosmolarity, acidosis, and ketosis are variably present during an infection or surgery.

More frequent monitoring of fluid, electrolyte and glucose levels, and rapid insulin titrations are required during surgery or any hospitalization. Avoiding DKA is best achieved by maintaining euglycemia with intravenous insulin and fluids, based on body weight and blood glucose level. After surgery, the intravenous insulin is continued till oral intake is adequate. When full oral intake is achieved, subcutaneous insulin is begun. While the child begins to take oral fluids, the intravenous fluids are gradually decreased and oral intake is encouraged.

Any surgery is scheduled early in the day to enable resuming oral feeds and subcutaneous insulin injections in the evening by allowing maximal recovery time. When preoperatively oral feeds are withheld for a few hours and full oral feeds are resumed shortly after surgery, intravenous insulins are not required. Short-acting insulins are given subcutaneously 6 hourly, and glucose corrections are monitored frequently. With long-acting basal insulins, full dose is given in the evening before surgery. For intermediate-acting insulins, half of the morning dose is given before surgery. The child is kept hospitalized till oral feeds are adequately resumed and blood glucose levels are consistently near-normal.

REFERENCES

1. Lawrence SE, Cummings EA, Gaboury I, Daneman D. Population-based study of incidence and risk factors for cerebral edema in pediatric diabetic ketoacidosis. J Pediatr. 2005;146(5):688-92.
2. Brink S, Joel D, Laffel L, Lee WW, Olsen B, Phelan H, et al. ISPAD Clinical Practice Consensus Guidelines 2014. Sick day management in children and adolescents with diabetes. Pediatr Diabetes. 2014;15(Suppl 20):193-202.
3. Svoren BM, Jospe N. Diabetes mellitus in children. In: Kliegman RM, Stanton BMD, St Geme J, Schor NF (Eds). Nelson Textbook of Pediatrics, 20th edition. Philadelphia, PA: Saunders; 2016. pp. 2773-5.

CHAPTER 19

Surgery in a Child with Diabetes

Sneha M Kothari, Manoj D Chadha

INTRODUCTION

The incidence of both type 1 diabetes mellitus (T1DM) and type 2 diabetes mellitus (T2DM) in children is increasing in India.[1] Type 1 diabetes mellitus is caused by autoimmune destruction of β-cells. Type 2 diabetes mellitus is usually due to resistance to the action of insulin followed later on by decline in its secretion. Type 2 diabetes mellitus is seen in overweight/obese children and usually have a history of diabetes in first and second degree relative. Rarely, diabetes in children may be due to maturity onset diabetes of the young (MODY), fibrocalcific disease of pancreas, genetic syndrome like Down's syndrome, Prader-Willi syndrome, etc.[2]

For optimal perioperative management of children with diabetes, one must not only consider the pathophysiology of diabetes, but also previous treatment regimen, glycemic control, type of surgery, and postoperative care.[3]

End-organ damage from diabetes is an important predictor of perioperative outcome than the presence of diabetes itself. The major risk factors in diabetic patients undergoing surgery include cardiovascular dysfunction, renal insufficiency, autonomic neuropathies (cardiovascular and gastrointestinal effects), all of which may influence the effects of anesthetics.[4] In addition, persistent hyperglycemia leads to immune dysfunction.[5]

TYPE 1 VERSUS TYPE 2 DIABETES MELLITUS

Although both type 1 and type 2 people with diabetes have hyperglycemia, the underlying mechanism is not same. Patients with T1DM completely lack insulin production, whereas people with type 2 diabetes have insulin resistance accompanied with progressive defect in insulin secretion.[6] To inhibit lipolysis, proteolysis, and ketogenesis, minimal amount of insulin is needed. Due to absolute deficiency of insulin, type 1 diabetics are more susceptible to ketoacidosis.[7]

Metabolic Response of a Diabetic Patient to Surgery and Anesthesia

The immediate perioperative problems faced by the diabetic patients are:[5,7,8]
- Induction of "stress response" with catabolic hormone secretion
- Altered consciousness which necessitates frequent glucose monitoring to detect hypoglycemia
- Circulatory disturbances which affect subcutaneous insulin absorption
- Interrupted food intake.

Insulin is an anabolic hormone which promotes the reuptake of glucose by the muscle and adipose tissue, as well as suppresses the metabolic pathways that promote glucose production by the liver (glycogenolysis and gluconeogenesis). Surgery is frequently accompanied by a period of starvation, which leads to catabolic state. In addition, surgery induces stress response which mostly invokes secretion of catecholamines and cortisol. Increased sympathetic activity decreases insulin secretion whereas it increases growth hormone and glucagon production. In diabetic patients, insulin production is already compromised. All the above stated metabolic changes lead to a marked catabolic state with increased gluconeogenesis, glycogenesis, proteolysis, lipolysis, and ketogenesis. This ultimately results into hyperglycemia and ketosis as illustrated in figure 1.

Anesthetic Agents, techniques, and Their Effect on Glucose Metabolism[4,8]

There are numerous anesthetic agents which can have variable effect on glucose metabolism.

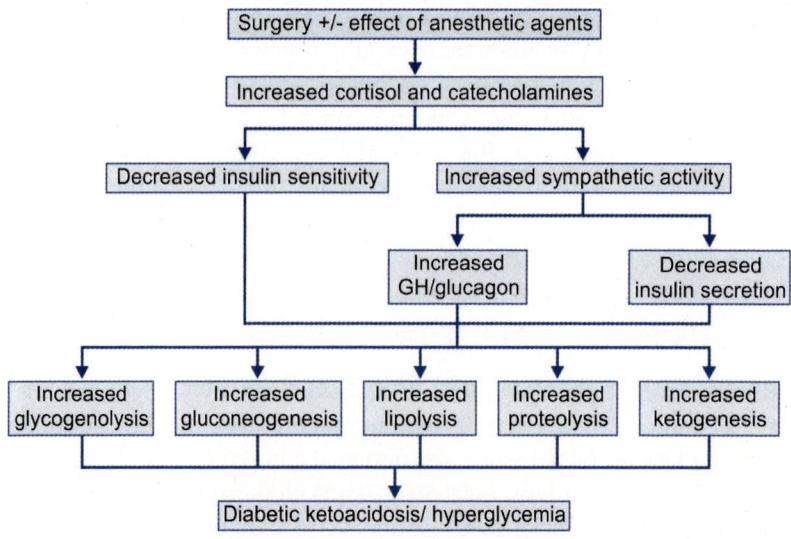

Fig. 1: Pathophysiology of stress response to surgery leading to hyperglycemia/ketoacidosis

Intravenous Agents[4,8]

Baring few, most of the intravenous induction agents have negligible effect on glucose homeostasis.
- Etomidate suppresses cortisol production by inhibiting 11β-hydroxylase, thereby suppressing hyperglycemic response to surgery
- High dose benzodiazepine suppresses adrenocorticotropic hormone production and stimulates growth hormone production
- High dose opiates suppress hypothalamic pituitary axis as well as sympathetic nervous system, thus abolishing hyperglycemic response to surgery.

Volatile Agents[4,8]

In vitro studies have shown that volatile agents, such as halothane, enflurane, and isoflurane, inhibit the insulin secretion in response to glucose in a reversible and dose-dependent manner thus leading to hyperglycemia.

Preanesthetic Medications[4,8]

Some neuromuscular blocking agents like succinylcholine should be avoided in diabetic patients with hyperkalemia as they transiently increase serum potassium concentrations by 0.5–1 mEq/L.

Sometimes, glucocorticoids are given as premedication to prevent nausea and vomiting. Glucocorticoids have anti-insulin effects which thereby lead to hyperglycemia.

Anesthetic Technique[4,8]

There is no evidence stating morbidity and mortality of various anesthetic techniques in diabetic patients. Acute insulin response to glucose is reduced with spinal anesthesia (dermatome level T2–T6) whereas such an effect is not seen with low spinal anesthesia (dermatome level T9–T12). Epidural anesthesia blocks sympathetic efferent signal and inhibits catecholamine release, thus blunts surgical stress response.

In patients with autonomic neuropathy, neuraxial blockade may lead to cardiovascular instability. Also, peripheral neuropathy may worsen as nerves are exposed to higher concentration of anesthetic agents due to impaired blood flow.

It is imperative that the anesthetic technique should allow for rapid recovery after surgery to prevent concealment of hyperglycemic or hypoglycemic coma.

RATIONALE FOR MAINTENANCE OF EUGLYCEMIA

Perioperative Hyperglycemia

As discussed, surgery leads to metabolic stress response which alters glucose homeostasis. Many studies have shown that poor perioperative glycemic control increases the risk of adverse outcomes. Hyperglycemia leads to poor wound healing.[5-8]

The physiological process of wound healing is divided into four phases: (i) hemostasis, (ii) inflammation, (iii) proliferation, and (iv) maturation or remodeling. A number of cellular and humoral factors play role in this process.[9,10]

In patients with diabetes, there is thickening of the basement membrane of the capillaries and arterioles. In addition, long standing hyperglycemia leads to formation of advanced glycation end products (AGEs) which induce the production of inflammatory molecules (tumor necrosis factor-α and interleukin-1) and interfere with collagen synthesis. Impaired collagen synthesis affects the tensile strength of the wound. Altered immune function leads to decreased chemotaxis, phagocytosis, bacterial killing, and reduced heat shock protein expression which leads to poor wound healing in patients with diabetes.[6,7,9,10]

The growth factor production and angiogenesis is impaired in people with diabetes. The wound healing requires critical balance between collagenous and noncollagenous extracellular matrix tissue inhibitors of matrix metalloproteinases. Altered balance of these components also contributes to poor wound healing.[9,10]

Hyperglycemia is a risk factor for postoperative sepsis, endothelial dysfunction, and cerebral ischemia. Studies in adults have shown that good glycemic control perioperatively improves overall outcome.[9,10]

Perioperative Hypoglycemia

Like hyperglycemia, unrecognized hypoglycemia is also associated with increased morbidity, mortality, and hospital stay. Hypoglycemia, if undetected can lead to increased somnolence, seizures, or irreversible neurological insult. It is difficult to recognize symptoms of hypoglycemia if patient is under the effect of general anesthesia or sedatives; hence it is imperative to monitor blood glucose (BG).[11-13]

Glycemic Variability

Glycemic variability means intraday excursions in BG readings which includes hyperglycemia and hypoglycemia. Apart from absolute BG values and glycosylated hemoglobin, glycemic variability has been linked to macrovascular diseases. Acute changes in BG levels lead to oxidative stress and formation of AGEs. The rapid decline in glycosylated hemoglobin (HbA1c) may have contributed to increased mortality. Thus perioperatively, it is imperative to maintain stable BG and avoid excursions.[6,14]

PERIOPERATIVE ASSESSMENT AND MANAGEMENT GOALS FOR THE DIABETIC PATIENT[4,5,15]

Children with diabetes rarely exhibit any vascular, neurological, or renal complications that are usually present in adult people with diabetes; thus the goal is to strike good glucose homeostasis. The key objectives for perioperative management of glucose levels are:
- Avoidance of hyperglycemia, hypoglycemia, and glycemic variability
- Reduction of morbidity and mortality

TABLE 1: Recommended inpatient target glucose values for children

Inpatient	Plasma blood glucose range (mg/dL)	
Critically ill	140–180	
Noncritically ill	Before meals	After meals
Toddlers and preschoolers (0–6 years)	<180	150–200
School aged (6–12 years)	<180	150–200
Adolescents and young adults (13–19 years)	<140	150–200

- Prevention of diabetic ketoacidosis
- Maintenance of fluid and electrolyte balance
- Achieve BG within the recommended target as shown in table 1.

Glycemic Targets for Surgery

Studies in adults have shown that hyperglycemia is associated with increased risk of infections postoperatively.[3,16]

Van Den Berghe study showed that achieving tight glycemic control (~80-110 mg/dL) using continuous intravenous insulin infusion significantly decreased mortality and morbidity in critically ill patients, however there were more episodes of hypoglycemia.[17] Randomized controlled trials have shown that hypoglycemia is associated with increased morbidity and mortality in adults.[11-13]

There are no conclusive randomized controlled trials recommending inpatient glycemic goals in pediatric critical illness. The expert groups differ in the recommendations in children with type 1 diabetes and are mainly studied in surgical settings. They differ in glycemic targets. No guidelines exist for steroid induced hyperglycemia. For patients undergoing minor surgery, there is no consensus so as to perioperative glycemic targets and different methods to attain them.[15]

International Society for Pediatric and Adolescent Diabetes 2009 guidelines recommend maintaining BG between 90-180 mg/dL.[16] American Diabetes Association 2005[18] recommendations modified by Tridgell et al.[15] are as given in table 1.

The total daily dose of insulin for a prepubertal child is around 0.7-1.0 U/kg per day, whereas a pubertal child may need 1.0-2.0 U/kg per day. If the child has recently been detected with diabetes, insulin requirement is close to 0.5 U/kg per day.[15]

Perioperative management of diabetes will be influenced by:[3,5,15,16,19]
- Duration of procedure/period of fasting (minor vs major surgery)
- Current diabetes regimen (premix, basal bolus, pump or oral hypoglycemia agents)
- Time of surgery (morning vs afternoon)
- Urgency of surgery (elective vs emergency).

SURGICAL SETTINGS

To simplify management, surgical setting is divided in two categories:[3,5,6,7,17,19]
1. Minor surgery or procedure
2. Major surgery.

Minor Surgery or Procedure

- Requires a short general anesthesia or heavy sedation
- Usually does not have a major impact on glycemic control
- Usually discharged on the day of procedure, e.g., endoscopies, jejunal biopsy, adenotonsillectomy, and grommet insertion.

Major Surgery

- Prolonged general anesthesia
- Associated with greater risks of metabolic decompensation
- Unlikely to be discharged from hospital on the day of procedure.

Most of the surgical procedures may be elective; however they may occur on emergency basis.

Elective Surgery

For elective surgery or procedure, good metabolic control should be obtained before surgery. This means
- No ketonuria
- Normal serum electrolytes
- Close to normal HbA1c:
    - 7–9%: Less than 5 years old
    - 6–8.5%: 5–13 years old
    - 6–8%: Over 13 years of age.

Preoperative consultation should be sought at least 10 days prior to the date of surgery for adequate metabolic control. Patients with poor glycemic control may be admitted prior to surgery for assessment and stabilization of hyperglycemia.

Emergency Surgery

Diabetic ketoacidosis may present as an "acute abdomen" and acute illness may precipitate diabetic ketoacidosis. These patients are usually dehydrated and electrolyte imbalance, which should be corrected before subjecting patient for surgery.

Based on this, perioperative management usually deals with the following circumstances:
- Elective surgery of a minor nature
- Elective major surgery
- Emergency surgery.

CHAPTER 19: Surgery in a Child with Diabetes

PERIOPERATIVE MANAGEMENT

- Scheduling of surgery[3,5,16,19]
    - Aim to schedule in the morning and preferably first on surgical lists
    - For major surgery, admit patient to the hospital day prior to surgery. For minor surgery admit early on the day of surgery
- Evening prior to surgery[3,5,16,19]
    - Patient is advised to do frequent BG monitoring specially before meals and snacks and at bedtime
    - If BG is more than 250–300 mg/dL, measure blood β-hydroxybutyrate and/or urinary ketone concentration
    - Patient should take the usual evening or bedtime insulin(s) and bedtime snack
    - In case patient develops ketosis or severe hyperglycemia, this should be corrected preferably by overnight intravenous insulin infusion, and if needed, surgery may be delayed.

Elective Surgery of Minor Nature[3,5,16,19]

- No solid food for at least 6 hours prior to general anesthesia (GA)
- Clear fluids (including breast milk) are allowed up to 4 hours before anesthesia
- Aim for BG between 90–180 mg/dL during and after surgery.

Management will vary, depending on the patient's usual insulin regimen:
- Twice daily insulin regimen
- Multiple daily injections
- Insulin pump therapy.

Minor Procedures

Patients Treated With Twice Daily (BID) Insulin Regimens

- Morning operations scheduled:[3,5,16,19]
    - Patients should receive 50% of the usual morning dose of intermediate-acting insulin (NPH and lente)
    - The short- or rapid-acting insulin should be omitted unless needed to correct hyperglycemia
    - If surgery is likely to be completed by 10 AM, can delay the morning dose of insulin and have late breakfast
    - Commence intravenous fluids (use glucose 5–10%, as necessary, to prevent hypoglycemia) as shown in table 2
    - After surgery, patient may be started on oral intake or intravenous glucose may be continued depending on the child's condition
    - Once patient is started on orals, usual dose of short or rapid acting insulin and if needed, correction should be given to reduce hyperglycemia
    - The dinner or evening dose of insulin is given as usual.

TABLE 2: Infusion guide for surgical procedures[16]

Maintenance fluid guide
• Glucose
○ Usually started on 5% glucose; 10% if there is concern about hypoglycemia
○ If blood glucose (BG) is more than 250 mg/dL, use normal saline without glucose and increase insulin supply but add 5% dextrose when BG falls less than 250 mg/dL
• Sodium
○ Use saline 0.45–0.9% (77–154 mmol Na/L).
• Potassium
○ Add potassium chloride 20 mmol to each liter of intravenous fluid
○ Maintenance fluid requirement should be calculated as per the chart below:

	Body weight	Fluid requirement/24 h
For each kg between	3–9 kg	100 mL/kg
For each kg between	10–20 kg	Add an additional 50 mL/kg
For each kg over (max 2,000 mL female, 2,500 mL male)	20 kg	Add an additional 20 mL/kg

Insulin infusion
- Soluble insulin 50 units is added to 50 mL normal saline 0.9%, making a solution of 1 U insulin/mL. It is attached to syringe pump
- Insulin infusion is started at following rate:

Blood glucose (mg/dL)	Infusion rate (U/kg/hour)
100–140	0.025
140–210	0.05
210–270	0.075
>270	0.1

- Drip rate is adjusted based on hourly BG levels monitored trying to maintain between 90–180 mg/dL
- The insulin infusion should not be stopped if BG less than 90 mg/dL as this will cause rebound hyperglycemia. Instead, the drip rate should be reduced.

- Afternoon operations scheduled:[3,5,16,19]
    ○ Child is allowed to eat light breakfast in the morning and clear liquids are allowed for up to 4 hours before anesthesia
    ○ About 50% of the usual dose of intermediate acting insulin (NPH and lente) and the usual dose of short- or rapid-acting insulin should be given
    ○ Alternatively, 30–40% of the usual morning insulin dose of short- or rapid-acting insulin (but no intermediate- or long-acting insulin) can be given and intravenous insulin infusion beginning at least 2 hours before surgery should be used as shown in table 2
    ○ Start intravenous fluids and if need be, intravenous insulin 2 hours before surgery
    ○ Rest of the protocol is like morning scheduled surgery.

Patients on Basal-bolus Insulin Regimens
- Morning operations scheduled:[3,5,16,19]
  - If patient takes basal insulin in the morning, this should be administered to prevent ketosis. If the child takes his basal insulin in the afternoon, this should not be administered before surgery
  - Short- or rapid-acting insulin should be withheld in the morning unless necessary to correct hyperglycemia
  - Intravenous fluids containing glucose 5% should be commenced to prevent hypoglycemia as shown in table 2
  - Alternatively, intravenous regular insulin infusion can be started at breakfast time. Morning doses of subcutaneous insulin are omitted
  - Blood glucose is measured before, during, and immediately after GA, at least hourly. The glucose infusion and insulin are adjusted to maintain perioperative BG in the range of 90–180 mg/dL
  - In the postoperative period, supplemental midmorning short-/rapid-acting insulin may be given if required (10–25% of total daily dose) and, when tolerated, a light meal
  - The aim is to resume normal meals later in the day. The pre-meal insulin doses are resumed as soon as the child is able to tolerate oral feeds
- Afternoon operations scheduled:[3,5,16,19]
  - The patient is usually allowed to eat breakfast and drink clear fluids until 4 hours preoperatively
  - At breakfast, patient can take the usual dose of rapid-acting or 50–60% dose of the short-acting insulin. Basal intermediate- or long-acting insulin is taken as usual (if usually given at this time)
  - Intravenous fluids containing 5% glucose are commenced at a maintenance rate of approximately 2 hours after breakfast as shown in table 2
  - Measure capillary BG hourly and glucose concentration of intravenous fluids is adjusted to prevent hypoglycemia
  - If needed, supplemental intravenous insulin is given to keep perioperative BG concentration in the target range
  - After surgery, intravenous insulin or additional short or rapid acting may be required
  - Once patient can tolerate oral intake, meals should be resumed along with routine insulin dose.

Summary of perioperative protocols for the patients on morning list and afternoon list are given in figures 2 and 3, respectively and insulin dose modifications are given in table 3.

Patients on Insulin Pumps (Continuous Subcutaneous Insulin Infusion)[3,5,16,19]
- Before sending the child to operation theater, it is important to secure the subcutaneous infusion site to prevent dislodgement and interruption of insulin supply during the procedure
- If procedure takes 1–2 hours, the pump can be continued to infuse basal insulin while giving 5% glucose at the maintenance rate
- Morning bolus dose is withheld unless necessary to correct hyperglycemia

SECTION 5: Acute Complications

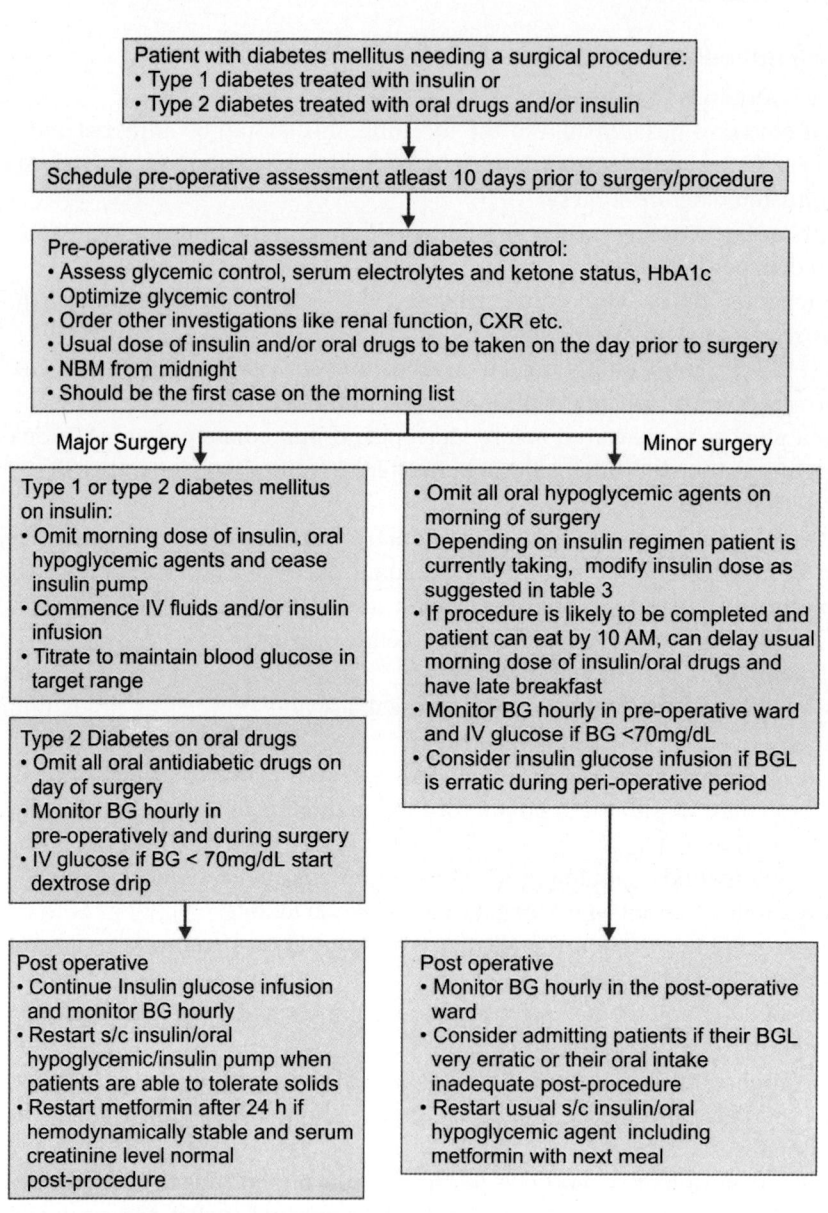

HBA1c, glycosylated hemoglobin; CXR, chest X-ray; NBM, nil by mouth; s/c, subcutaneous.

Fig. 2: Summary of perioperative protocol for the patients on the morning list[3,5,16,19]

- Monitor BG levels hourly preoperatively and at least half hourly during GA
- For hyperglycemia, correction doses of insulin can be given with the pump preoperatively and postoperatively. Alternatively, intravenous insulin can be given to keep perioperative BG within target
- Once the patient is ready to eat, meal bolus is given to eat

CHAPTER 19: Surgery in a Child with Diabetes

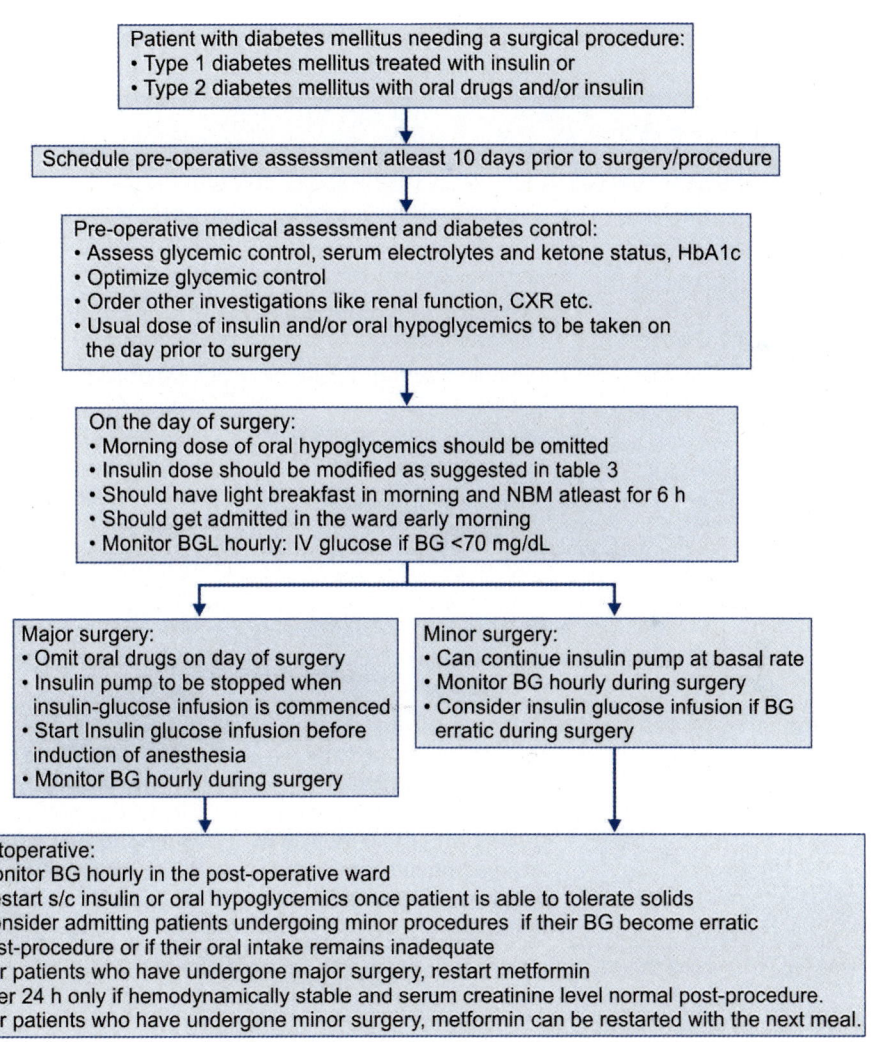

HBA1c, glycosylated hemoglobin; CXR, chest X-ray, NBM, nil by mouth, s/c, subcutaneous.

Fig. 3: Summary of perioperative protocol for the patients on the afternoon list[3,5,16,19]

- Alternatively, continuous subcutaneous insulin infusion can be discontinued and a continuous intravenous insulin and glucose infusion can be started, as shown in table 2 until feeding is established satisfactorily.

Elective Major Surgery[3,5,16,19]

- Procedures are best scheduled in the morning, preferably should be first on the list
- No solid food should be given at least 6 hours prior to surgery
- Clear fluids (including breast milk) may be allowed up to 4 hours before surgery (check with anesthetist)

SECTION 5: Acute Complications

TABLE 3: Insulin dose modification based on type of regimen and timing of surgery for minor surgery[3,5,16,19]

Insulins	Day prior to admission	Day of surgery	
		Morning Surgery	**Afternoon Surgery**
Basal insulin—evening (glargine and detemir)	**No dose change***	• Check blood glucose on admission • **Evening dose is given as usual**	• Check blood glucose on admission • Evening dose is given as usual
Basal insulin—morning	No dose change	• Morning dose is given as usual to prevent ketosis	• Evening dose is given as usual
Split mix	No dose change	• Omit rapid acting/regular insulin • Give 50% of intermediate or long acting insulin • Leave evening dose unchanged	• Give usual dose of rapid acting/regular insulin • Give 50% of usual intermediate or long acting insulin in morning with light breakfast • Leave evening dose unchanged
Premixed insulin	No dose change	• Give half the dose in morning • Leave evening dose unchanged	• Give half the dose in morning • Leave evening dose unchanged
Insulin pump	No dose change	• If surgery will last for less than 2 h, basal rate to be continued. Morning bolus dose is omitted. However, if surgery will last for more than 2 h, discontinue pump, start intravenous fluids and insulin infusion	• Morning bolus dose to be given, basal rate is continued. However, if surgery will last for more than 2 h, discontinue pump and start intravenous fluids and insulin infusion

*Some units may recommnd reducing the evening dose of long acting insulin by one third.

- The usual morning insulin dose is omitted
- At least 2 hours before surgery intravenous insulin infusion [dilute 50 units regular (soluble) insulin in 50 mL normal saline, 1 unit = 1 mL] and glucose 5% (10% if there is concern about hypoglycemia) is started
- If BG is more than 250 mg/dL, normal saline without glucose is used and the rate of insulin infusion is increased, but it should be changed to 5% dextrose when BG falls below 250 mg/dL
- Blood glucose is monitored hourly before surgery and every 30–60 minutes during the operation and until the child awakens from anesthesia
- Blood glucose is monitored hourly for 4 hours after surgery or for as long as the patient is receiving intravenous insulin
- The aim is to maintain BG between 90–180 mg/dL. With intravenous insulin, insulin to glucose ratio for prepubertal children is typically 1 U/5 g of intravenous glucose and for adolescents 1 U/3 g of IV glucose. The dose is adjusted based on BG response

- Once the patient is awake, the intravenous insulin is adjusted to maintain BG in the range of 80–160 mg/dL
- When oral intake is not possible, the intravenous infusion should be continued for as long as necessary.

TYPE 2 DIABETES MELLITUS[3,5,16,19]

- For children with T2DM treated with insulin, follow the same protocol as enlisted earlier
- Patients on oral treatment:
  - Metformin:
    - Discontinue 24 hours before the procedure for elective surgery
    - If less than 24 hours have lapsed since the last dose and patient is scheduled for emergency surgery, it is essential to maintain hydration with intravenous fluids before, during and after surgery
  - Sulfonylureas or thiazolidinediones:
    - Stop on the day of surgery
    - Monitor BG hourly and if greater than 180 mg/dL treat with intravenous insulin, as for elective surgery, to normalize levels, or give subcutaneous insulin if it is a minor procedure.

EXTRA INSULIN RECOMMENDATIONS

Short or fast-acting insulin should be avoided in the morning of surgery. However, if BG is more than 250 mg/dL, rapid or short-acting insulin dose should be administered using a "correction factor". The correction factor is calculated using the "1,500 rule". This rule consists of dividing 1,500 into the usual total dose of insulin used by the child. For example, if the child typically uses 50 U of insulin, the correction factor will be $1,500 \div 50 = 30$; this means that 1 U of insulin in this patient should reduce the plasma glucose concentration by 30 mg/dL. For rapid acting insulin, this rule is "1,800". However, for simplicity the rule of 1,500 is used for both rapid acting and regular insulin. Type 2 diabetic patients not previously treated with insulin should receive rapid acting insulin at dose of 0.1 U/kg when BG levels are above 250 mg/dL.

Emergency Surgery

- Patient is kept nil by mouth; rarely the stomach may need to be emptied by a nasogastric tube
- Intravenous access should be secured
- Weight, serum electrolytes, BG, blood gases, and blood β-hydroxybutyrate or urinary ketone concentration should be measured before anesthesia
- If ketoacidosis is present, treat as per the protocol for diabetic ketoacidosis (DKA) and delay surgery till the time circulatory volume and electrolyte deficits are corrected. If there is no DKA, start intravenous glucose and insulin infusion as for elective surgery.

CONCLUSION

Surgery in children and adolescents with diabetes should preferably be performed in a centre with appropriate personnel and facilities to care for children with diabetes. Joint effort by anesthetic, endocrinologist, and surgeon before admission to hospital for elective surgery and as soon as possible after admission for emergency surgery is needed for favorable outcome. In addition to the current insulin regimen; age, weight, puberty, type and length of surgical procedure should be considered to devise management. Both, hypoglycemia and hyperglycemia should be avoided for optimal outcome.

REFERENCES

1. Anjana RM, Pradeepa R, Deepa M, Datta M, Sudha V, Unnikrishnan R, et al. Prevalence of diabetes and prediabetes (impaired fasting glucose and/or impaired glucose tolerance) in urban and rural India: phase 1 results of the Indian Council of Medical Research-India DIABetes (ICMR-INDIAB) study. Diabetologia. 2011;54:3022-7.
2. Mohan V, Amutha A, Ranjani H, Anjana RM, Unnikrishnan R. Clinical approach to diabetes in the young in India. In: Munjal YP, editors. API Textbook of Medicine. 9th ed. New Delhi: Jaypee Brothers Medical Publishers; 2013. pp. 156-61.
3. Rhodes ET, Ferrari LR, Wolfsdorf JI. Perioperative management of pediatric surgical patients with diabetes mellitus. Anesth Analg. 2005;101:986-99.
4. Giquel J, Rodriguez-Blanco YF, Matadial C, Candiotti K. Diabetes mellitus in anaesthesia. Br J Diabet Vasc Dis. 2012;12:60-4.
5. Del Castillo AS, Holder T, Sardi N. Perioperative management of the diabetic child. Rev Colomb Anestesiol. 2011;39:56-69.
6. Vann MA. Perioperative management of ambulatory surgical patients with diabetes mellitus. Curr Opin Anaesthesiol. 2009;22:718-24.
7. McAnulty GR, Robertshaw HJ, Hall GM. Anaesthetic management of patients with diabetes mellitus. Br J Anaesth. 2000;85:80-90.
8. Sudhakaran S, Surani SR. Guidelines for perioperative management of the diabetic patient. Surg Res Pract. 2015;284063.
9. Tsourdi E, Barthel A, Rietzsch H, Reichel A, Bornstein SR. Current aspects in the pathophysiology and treatment of chronic wounds in diabetes mellitus. Biomed Res Int. 2013;385641.
10. Brem H, Tomic-Canic M. Cellular and molecular basis of wound healing in diabetes. J Clin Invest. 2007;117:1219-22.
11. Angelini G, Ketzler JT, Coursin DB. Perioperative care of the diabetic patient. ASA Refresher Courses in Anesthesiology. 2001;29:1-9.
12. NICE-SUGAR Study Investigators, Finfer S, Chittock DR, Su SY, Blair D, Foster D, et al. Intensive versus conventional glucose control in critically ill patients. N Engl J Med. 2009;360:1283-97.
13. Turchin A, Matheny ME, Shubina M, Scanlon JV, Greenwood B, Pendergrass ML. Hypoglycemia and clinical outcomes in patients with diabetes hospitalized in the general ward. Diabetes Care. 2009;32:1153-7.
14. Satya Krishna SV, Kota SK, Modi KD. Glycemic variability: Clinical implications. Indian J Endocrinol Metab. 2013;17:611-9.
15. Tridgell DM, Tridgell AH, Hirsch IB. Inpatient management of adults and children with type 1 diabetes. Endocrinol Metab Clin North Am. 2010;39:595-608.
16. Betts P, Brink S, Silink M, Swift PG, Wolfsdor J, Hanas R. Management of children and adolescents with requiring surgery. Pediatr Diabetes. 2009;10:169-74.
17. van den Berghe G, Wouters P, Weekers F, Verwaest C, Bruyninckx F, Schetz M, et al. Intensive insulin therapy in critically ill patients. N Engl J Med. 2001;345:1359-67.
18. Silverstein J, Klingensmith G, Copeland K, Plotnick L, Kaufman F, Laffel L, et al. Care of children and adolescents with type 1 diabetes. Diabetes Care. 2005:28:186-212.
19. Wong V, Ross G, Wong J, Chipps D. Peri-operative diabetes management guidelines. Australian Diabetes Society. 2012:1-30.

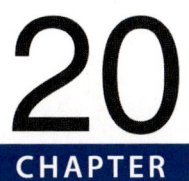

Hypoglycemia

Kranti S Khadilkar, Shivane Vyankatesh, Lila Anurag, Bandgar Tushar, Nalini Shah

INTRODUCTION

Iatrogenic hypoglycemia is the most common and feared complication of intensive glycemic control. It forms the biggest barrier in the quest for maintenance of euglycemia and prevention of complications especially in type 1 diabetes mellitus (T1DM) as depicted by the Diabetes Control and Complications Trial (DCCT).[1] The American Diabetes Association (ADA) Workgroup defines iatrogenic hypoglycemia in people with type 1 diabetes as a plasma glucose level less than 70 mg/dL (3.9 mmol/L).[2] The workgroup has also suggested a classification of hypoglycemia that includes:

- Severe hypoglycemia: An event requiring assistance of another person to raise glucose levels and promote neurologic recovery
- Documented symptomatic hypoglycemia: Symptoms plus documented low glucose
- Asymptomatic hypoglycemia: Low glucose without symptoms
- Probable symptomatic hypoglycemia: Symptoms without a glucose estimate
- Relative hypoglycemia: Symptoms with glucose levels that are not low but are approaching that level.

EPIDEMIOLOGY OF HYPOGLYCEMIA

Incidence of iatrogenic hypoglycemia is quite common in people with type 1 diabetes and long-standing insulin-treated type 2 diabetes. Juvenile diabetes research foundation study utilizing continuous glucose monitoring system (CGMS) in T1DM, found that hypoglycemia [glucose levels ≤70 mg/dL (3.9 mmol/L)] occurred 6.3% of the time, i.e., 1.5 hours per day.[3] Majority of these episodes are asymptomatic but crucial as they impair the counter-regulatory defenses against subsequent hypoglycemia. People with T1DM suffer an average of two episodes of symptomatic hypoglycemia per week and an average of approximately one episode of severe, temporarily disabling, hypoglycemia annually.[4] Hypoglycemia can rarely cause sudden death due to cardiac arrhythmias.[5] Recent reports indicate that 6–10% of deaths of people with T1DM are caused by hypoglycemia.[6]

PHYSIOLOGY OF COUNTER-REGULATION OF GLUCOSE

Glucose being a critical fuel, a multitude of physiologic defenses is present in the normal human body to counteract against falling plasma glucose concentrations.[7] The major counter-regulatory processes are:
- Inhibition of insulin secretion from beta cells of the pancreas
- Stimulation of glucagon secretion from α-cells of the pancreas
- Stimulation of adrenaline secretion from adrenal medulla.

These counter-regulatory steps favor increased glucose production through inhibition of insulin and mobilization of gluconeogenic precursors and decreased glucose utilization. Apart from the hormonal defense mechanism, neuroregulatory mechanisms through behavioral responses of carbohydrate ingestion prompted by neuroglycopenic and sympathetic symptoms also form an important counter-regulatory step.[7]

PATHOLOGY OF COUNTER-REGULATION IN T1DM

The counter-regulatory mechanisms normally occurring in nondiabetics are grossly hampered in T1DM especially with long duration of the disease. An imbalance between caloric supply and glucose utilization in response to therapeutic insulin and exercise forms the basic pathophysiology of hypoglycemia in T1DM.[4] The total dependence on exogenous insulin, alongwith the imperfection in insulin therapies, results in multiple recurrent episodes of iatrogenic hyperinsulinemia which if not effectively countered, result in hypoglycemia. Counter-regulatory mechanisms that autocorrect iatrogenic hypoglycemia often become progressively impaired in these patients resulting in significant morbidity and even mortality.[4] Thus, pathophysiology of hypoglycemia in T1DM is the result of the interplay of relative or absolute therapeutic insulin excess and compromised counter-regulatory hormonal and behavioral responses.[4]

HYPOGLYCEMIA UNAWARENESS

Beta cell failure in established T1DM results in absent first and second tier counter-regulatory responses to hypoglycemia, i.e., inhibition of insulin secretion and hypoglycemia-induced increase in glucagon secretion from α-cells. The lack of glucagon stimulation could be due to loss of paracrine effect of beta cells.[8] The third-tier response, i.e., sympathoadrenal response is commonly attenuated in T1DM. Initially, it is temporarily attenuated due to recent antecedent hypoglycemia, by prior exercise, or by sleep; however, progressively there is irreversibly attenuation of sympathoadrenal response especially the sympathetic neural component causing the clinical condition of hypoglycemia unawareness.[8] As the name suggests, it is lack of awareness of hypoglycemia in the form of loss of protective behavioral response of carbohydrate ingestion. Hypoglycemia unawareness is associated with a sixfold increased risk of iatrogenic hypoglycemia.[9]

HYPOGLYCEMIA-ASSOCIATED AUTONOMIC FAILURE

Hypoglycemia-associated autonomic failure (HAAF) in diabetes denotes that recent antecedent hypoglycemia, or prior exercise or sleep causes defective glucose counter-regulation by attenuating increase in adrenaline in the setting of absent first- and second-tier responses during subsequent hypoglycemia. Coupled with hypoglycemia unawareness, HAAF causes a vicious cycle of recurrent progressive and severe iatrogenic hypoglycemia.[10] Even 2–3 weeks of meticulous avoidance of hypoglycemia reverses hypoglycemia unawareness and improves the defective glucose counter-regulation in most affected patients.[11,12] Pathogenesis is studied but actual reasons for HAAF are still to be known. Multiple theories have tried to explain it which include neurogenic effects of cortisol, altered hypothalamic mechanisms, and activation of an inhibitory neural network relayed through the thalamus.[13]

CLINICAL IMPLICATIONS OF HYPOGLYCEMIA[14,15]

Short-term

Short-term implications include:
- Acute symptoms (autonomic, neuroglycopenic, and general malaise)
- Cognitive impairment and mood change
- Social, sport and travel, scholastic activities affected
- Increased risks of accidents, falls, fractures; dislocations.

Long-term

Long-term implications include:
- Fear of hypoglycemia resulting in reduced quality of life
- Weight gain due to frequent snacking habituated due to fear of hypoglycemia
- Restrictions on employment, profession and social activities
- Glycemic variability resulting in possible worsening of diabetic and/or vascular complications
- Cognitive decline and acceleration of dementia due to recurrent severe hypoglycemia
- Cardiac arrhythmia, myocardial ischemia, and myocardial infarction.

IMPACT OF HYPOGLYCEMIA ON CHILDREN

Children as well as adolescents are risk groups for iatrogenic hypoglycemia due to the challenges presented by insulin dosing, variable eating patterns, erratic activity, and the limited ability of small children to detect hypoglycemia. Puberty is associated with insulin

SECTION 5: Acute Complications

resistance, while at the same time, the stress of normal adolescent developmental stages may lead to inattention to diabetes, rebellious nature, and increased risk for hypoglycemia. Minimizing the impact of hypoglycemia on children with diabetes requires the holistic management of patient as well as the caregivers. The younger patients are most vulnerable to the adverse consequences of hypoglycemia due to the ongoing maturation of the central nervous system.[15]

RISK FACTORS FOR HYPOGLYCEMIA IN TYPE 1 DIABETES

Absolute or relative insulin excess is the most important risk factor for iatrogenic hypoglycemia.[4] Absolute therapeutic hyperinsulinemia occurs in following scenarios:
- Incorrect insulin therapy in terms of incorrect type, timing, or dosage
- Reduced glucose influx occurring in scenarios like missing meals or when glucose absorption is delayed, as in gastroparesis or decreased absorption as in celiac disease
- Increased glucose utilization as in before or just after exercise
- Decreased insulin clearance seen in renal failure
- Differential insulin sensitivity resulting in changing insulin dosage regimens.

Risk Factors for Hypoglycemia-associated Autonomic Failure

Though the exact pathogenesis of HAAF is unknown, the degree of absolute endogenous insulin deficiency denoting the degree of beta cell failure.
- Historical evidence of severe hypoglycemia or hypoglycemia unawareness, especially recent antecedent hypoglycemia causes attenuated sympathoadrenal responses to subsequent hypoglycemia[10]
- Similar to antecedent hypoglycemia, sleep and antecedent exercise also form important causative risk factors for subsequent development of HAAF[13]
- Intensive insulin therapy and strict maintenance of euglycemia. Studies like DCCT with a control group treated to a higher glycosylated hemoglobin (HbA1c) consistently report a higher rate of hypoglycemia in patients treated to a lower HbA1c target, i.e., the intensive therapy group.[1]

Minimizing the Risk of Hypoglycemia in Type 1 Diabetes Mellitus[16,17]

Effective approaches to decrease the risk of iatrogenic hypoglycemia, involves holistic, and individualized diabetes management.
The approaches broadly are as follows:
- Patient education and empowerment
- Dietary and exercise; lifestyle modifications
- Careful, regular, and accurate glucose monitoring
- Regular surveillance by the treating physician.

PATIENT EDUCATION AND EMPOWERMENT

Studies like Dose Adjustment For Normal Eating (DAFNE) have clearly shown the positive impact of diabetes education on the patient outcomes as well as shown to minimize hypoglycemia.[18] Patient education and empowerment involves basic diabetes education imparted to the patient and the immediate caregivers mostly related to recognition of hypoglycemia symptoms (especially crucial in small children) and effective rapid oral self treatment with glucose or parenteral treatment with glucagon.

Patients and caregivers should also be made aware about the basic pharmacokinetics of various types of insulin, importance of regular glucose monitoring, dietary, and exercise adjustments for effective prevention of iatrogenic hypoglycemia. Patient education and empowerment is the most important approach toward prevention of iatrogenic hypoglycemia.

DIETARY INTERVENTION

Patients with diabetes should have basic knowledge of dietary carbohydrates and their effects on blood glucose especially on the background of therapeutic insulin regimens. A balanced, regular, and predictable meal plan should be followed daily especially for those who are on fixed dose combinations of long-acting and regular insulin. Dissociated meal and insulin injection patterns and irregular unpredictable meals and snacking lead to wide fluctuations in plasma glucose levels and high risk of iatrogenic hypoglycemia. Patients on any hypoglycemia-inducing medication should always carry simple carbohydrates with them at all times to treat hypoglycemia. Dietary interventions to prevent hypoglycemia need to be individualized and should be part of a comprehensive holistic strategy involving balanced diet, patient education, optimized insulin regimens, and exercise counseling.

EXERCISE MANAGEMENT

Exercise is an important risk factor for hypoglycemia in people with type 1 diabetes, especially those who are in competitive sports and physical activities. Exercise causes increase in glucose utilization, improvement of insulin sensitivity, and hence is an important cause of relative therapeutic hyperinsulinemia with high risk of iatrogenic hypoglycemia. The risk factors for exercise induced hypoglycemia include prolonged exercise duration, unaccustomed intensity, and inadequate energy supply in the background of insulin therapy.

Hypoglycemia can be prevented or minimized by careful glucose monitoring before and after exercise and taking appropriate preventive actions like altering insulin regimen and shifting to analogs, carbohydrate snacking before and after exercise depending on the trends of blood glucose and carrying readily absorbable carbohydrates. These preventive measures are required not only for exercise but also for unaccustomed strenuous daily activities like working in the yard.

GLUCOSE MONITORING

Glucose monitoring forms an essential cornerstone of diabetes management especially in insulin-treated patients. Regular accurate glucose monitoring helps patient to guide his diet, dose of insulin, exercise schedule, and also to take necessary steps toward prevention of iatrogenic hypoglycemia. Self-monitoring of blood glucose (SMBG) using glucometers; point of care devices is commonly used but it has its own disadvantages and inaccuracies.

Recent technological developments like real-time CGMS by virtue of its ability to display the direction and rate of change, provide helpful information leading to proactive measures to avoid hypoglycemia as against therapeutic interventions after actual glucometer reading of hypoglycemia. The CGMS alarms set at a predetermined threshold help prevent iatrogenic hypoglycemias as well denote the vulnerable periods, i.e., nocturnal hypoglycemia or hypoglycemia unawareness. Ultimate amalgamation of technological advance resulting in complete extinction of iatrogenic hypoglycemia would be an artificial pancreas, coupling a CGM to an insulin pump through sophisticated predictive algorithms. The first step in this direction is the low-glucose suspend pump which shuts off insulin delivery for up to 2 hours once the interstitial glucose concentration reaches a preset threshold thus reducing the duration of nocturnal hypoglycemia.

MEDICATION ADJUSTMENT

Regular review of glucose monitoring logs assists in knowing the vulnerable timings for iatrogenic hypoglycemia. Depending on the specific scenarios leading to iatrogenic hypoglycemia adjustments in timings, dosage and type of insulin would be required. Such adjustments may include substitution of rapid-acting insulin analogs (lispro, aspart, glulisine) for regular insulin, or basal insulin like degludec, glargine or detemir for NPH, to decrease the risk of hypoglycemia. Continuous subcutaneous insulin infusion (insulin pump) offers great flexibility for adjusting the doses and administration pattern of insulin to counteract iatrogenic hypoglycemia. Frequent recurrent hypoglycemia sets in a vicious cycle lead to HAAF. To avoid this vicious cycle and HAAF, adjustments in the treatment regimen that scrupulously avoid hypoglycemia are necessary.

REGULAR SURVEILLANCE: TREATING PHYSICIAN'S DUTY

Treating physicians and diabetes educators should regularly monitor the patient in terms of his awareness for hypoglycemia, training of the immediate caregiver, glucose monitoring records for evidence of hypoglycemia, and the steps taken toward self-treatment of hypoglycemia. Use of hypoglycemia checklists and patient questionnaires has shown to be of benefit. Questions regarding lack of autonomic symptoms or hypoglycemia unawareness should be inculcated in every visit to know the presence and degree of HAAF and other underlying risk factors for iatrogenic hypoglycemia. Physicians should also reiterate importance of patient education and awareness for iatrogenic hypoglycemia in every visit.

TREATMENT OF HYPOGLYCEMIA IN TYPE 1 DIABETES MELLITUS

Oral Treatment

Majority of episodes of asymptomatic or mildly symptomatic hypoglycemia are effectively managed by patients themselves with carbohydrate containing juice, soft drinks, candy, other snacks, or glucose tablets. Generally 20 g of simple carbohydrates, repeated in 15-20 minutes if necessary, is sufficient for self-management. The glycemic response with this management is transient; hence, a subsequent more substantial meal especially of a mixture of simple and complex carbohydrates is essential to prevent recurrence of hypoglycemia.

Parenteral Treatment

In severe symptomatic hypoglycemia where oral management is not possible, parenteral management may be required. Parental management is mostly in the form of glucagon injections (maximum 1 mg or 30 µg/kg) given either subcutaneously or intramuscularly by a trained caregiver of the patient who recognizes the symptoms of severe disabling hypoglycemia. Glucagon causes transient but substantial hyperglycemia, nausea, and vomiting. Smaller doses (e.g., 150 µg) may be repeated if necessary. However, glucagon is ineffective in glycogen depleted states like malnutrition or alcoholic binge. If no response to repeated injections of glucagon, intravenous glucose (25 g initial bolus) is the standard parenteral therapy. Due to transient nature of response a maintenance glucose infusion is usually needed followed by ingestion of a meal when patient recovers consciousness.

FUTURE RESEARCH

Though research has come a long way in terms of iatrogenic hypoglycemia, some unmet needs of knowledge and technology remain. Focused research in these priority areas will ultimately reduce the impact of iatrogenic hypoglycemia on patients with diabetes.
- New educational tools for prevention of hypoglycemia and surveillance methods for consistently reporting hypoglycemia
- Understanding the pathogenesis of HAAF and devising preventive strategies for the same
- Glucose monitoring systems must become more accurate, more reliable, easier to use, and less expensive
- New therapies that do not cause hypoglycemia like glucose-regulated insulin-delivery systems including a dual hormone artificial pancreas need to enhance.

CONCLUSION

This chapter summarizes the awareness about the problem of iatrogenic hypoglycemia and recognition of risk factors for hypoglycemia especially HAAF. Empowering, educating, and counseling the patient and the caregiver to seek a balance between aggressive intensive strategies for euglycemia and occurrence of hypoglycemias has been elaborated. Personalizing glycemic management and utilization of technology to enhance glucose regulated insulin-delivery systems are also discussed.

REFERENCES

1. The Diabetes Control and Complications Trial Research Group. The effect of intensive treatment of diabetes on the development and progression of long-term complications in insulin-dependent diabetes mellitus. N Engl J Med. 1993;329(14):977-86.
2. American Diabetes Association Workgroup on Hypoglycemia. Defining and reporting hypoglycemia in diabetes. Diabetes Care. 2005;28(5):1245-9.
3. Juvenile Diabetes Research Foundation Continuous Glucose Monitoring Study Group. The effect of continuous glucose monitoring in well-controlled type 1 diabetes. Diabetes Care. 2009;32(8):1378-83.
4. Cryer PE. Hypoglycemia in Type 1 Diabetes Mellitus. Endocrinol Metabol Clin North Am. 2010;39(3):641-54.
5. Diabetes Control and Complications Trial/Epidemiology of Diabetes Interventions and Complications Study Research Group. Long-term effect of diabetes and its treatment on cognitive function. N Engl J Med. 2007;356(18):1842-52.
6. Skrivarhaug T, Bangstad HJ, Stene LC, Sandvik L, Hanssen KF, Joner G. Long-term mortality in a nationwide cohort of childhood-onset type 1 diabetic patients in Norway. Diabetologia 2006;49(2):298-305.
7. DeRosa MA, Cryer PE. Hypoglycemia and the sympathoadrenal system: neurogenic symptoms are largely the result of sympathetic neural, rather than adrenomedullary, activation. Am J Physiol Endocrinol Metab. 2004;287(1):E32-41.
8. Cooperberg BA, Cryer PE. Beta-cell-mediated signaling predominates over direct alpha-cell signaling in the regulation of glucagon secretion in humans. Diabetes Care. 2009;32(12):2275-80.
9. Geddes J, Schopman JE, Zammitt NN, Frier BM. Prevalence of impaired awareness of hypoglycaemia in adults with Type 1 diabetes. Diabet Med. 2008;25(4):501-4.
10. Cryer PE. Mechanisms of sympathoadrenal failure and hypoglycemia in diabetes. J Clin Invest. 2006;116(6):1470-3.
11. Cranston I, Lomas J, Maran A, Macdonald I, Amiel SA. Restoration of hypoglycaemia awareness in patients with long-duration insulin-dependent diabetes. Lancet. 1994;344(8918):283-7.
12. Dagogo-Jack S, Rattarasarn C, Cryer PE. Reversal of hypoglycemia unawareness, but not defective glucose counterregulation, in IDDM. Diabetes. 1994;43(12):1426-34.
13. Arbelaez AM, Powers WJ, Videen TO, Price J, Cryer PE. Attenuation of counterregulatory responses to recurrent hypoglycemia by active thalamic inhibition: a mechanism for hypoglycemia-associated autonomic failure. Diabetes. 2008;5(2):470-5.
14. Wright RJ, Frier BM. Vascular disease and diabetes: is hypoglycaemia an aggravating factor? Diabetes Metab Res. 2008;24(5):353-63
15. Perros P, Bjorgaas M. Neurological sequelae of Hypoglycaemia. In: Frier BM, Heller SR, McCrimmon RJ (Eds). Hypoglycaemia in Clinical Diabetes, 3rd edition. Wiley Blackwell; 2014. pp. 305-22.
16. Choudhary P, Rickels MR, Senior PA, Vantyghem MC, Maffi P, Kay TW, et al. Evidence-informed clinical practice recommendations for treatment of type 1 diabetes complicated by problematic hypoglycemia. Diabetes Care. 2015;38(6):1016-29.
17. Seaquist ER, Anderson J, Childs B, Cryer P, Dagogo-Jack S, Fish L, et al. Hypoglycemia and diabetes: a report of a workgroup of the American Diabetes Association and the Endocrine Society. Diabetes Care. 2013;36(5):1384-95.
18. Hopkins D, Lawrence I, Mansell P, Thompson G, Amiel S, Campbell M, et al. Improved biomedical and psychological outcomes 1 year after structured education in flexible insulin therapy for people with type 1 diabetes: the U.K. DAFNE experience. Diabetes Care. 2012;35:1638-42.

SECTION 6

Chronic Complications

Editor

Vaman Khadilkar

CHAPTER 21

Lipid Disorders in Type 1 Diabetes Mellitus

Bipin K Sethi, V Sri Nagesh

INTRODUCTION

Cardiovascular disease (CVD) is the single most important cause for death in people with type 2 diabetes (T2DM) and the story is not dissimilar even in people with type 1 diabetes mellitus mellitus (T1DM).[1] However, unlike in T2DM, not much attention is focused on CVD risk and lipid disorders in T1DM. Some of the factors implicated in this are: lack of data and large-scale studies that have examined the pattern of lipid abnormalities in T1DM and lack of consensus about cut-offs, and targets for lipid levels.

Most of the data about management of lipid disorders and CVD risk reduction in T1DM has been extrapolated from T2DM data. Cardiovascular disease is the major cause of death in persons with T1DM.[2] Dyslipidemia has been shown to be a significant coronary heart disease risk factor in T1DM. Thus, it seems important to pay attention to lipid abnormalities in patients with T1DM, in order to reduce CVD in this population.[3]

PATHOPHYSIOLOGY

Insulin plays a central role in lipid metabolism. In adipose tissue, insulin inhibits the hormone-sensitive lipase. This antipolytic action promotes storage of triglycerides in the adipocytes and reduces release of free fatty acids into circulation.

Insulin inhibits very low-density lipoproteins (VLDLs) production from the liver. In normal subjects, it has been shown that insulin induces a 67% decrease of VLDL-triglyceride production and a 52% decrease of VLDL-apoB production.[4] Insulin also reduces VLDL production by diminishing circulating free fatty acids and also by a direct inhibitory effect on the hepatocytes. Insulin promotes the clearance of low-density lipoproteins (LDL), by increasing LDL B/E receptor expression and activity. Insulin acts also on high-density lipoprotein (HDL) metabolism by activating lecithin-cholesterol acyl transferase and hepatic lipase activities.

SECTION 6: Chronic Complications

In insulin deficient states, the reverse of this is observed, which contributes to the atherogenic profile of lipids in all types of diabetes and consequent CVD risk. Nowhere is this better demonstrated in T1DM than in diabetic ketoacidosis (DKA), which is marked by an absolute insulin deficient state with hyperglycemia. In untreated DKA, triglyceride-rich lipoproteins (chylomicrons, VLDLs) are increased due to decreased lipoprotein lipase activity. Low-density lipoprotein-cholesterol is decreased because of a fall in plasma LDL-cholesterol level via the reduction of triglyceride-rich lipoprotein catabolism, due to decreased lipoprotein lipase activity. High-density lipoprotein-cholesterol is also decreased, due to hypertriglyceridemia that causes the transfer of triglycerides from triglyceride-rich lipoproteins to HDLs through cholesteryl ester transfer protein (CETP) leading to the formation of triglyceride-rich HDL particles.[5] These triglyceride rich-HDL particles are catabolized by hepatic lipase, leading to HDL reduction.

TREATED TYPE 1 DIABETES

Extent of lipid dysfunction in T1DM is essentially a function of glycemic control. In a study by Marcovecchio et al.,[6] glycosylated hemoglobin (HbA1c) was found to be independently correlated with LDL, triglycerides, and non-HDL, and in another large study by Schwab et al.,[7] raised HbA1c was found to have a positive correlation with total and LDL cholesterols and a negative correlation with HDL cholesterol. In the Diabetes Control and Complications Trial, HbA1c correlated positively with total cholesterol, LDL-cholesterol, and triglycerides at baseline.[8] In the SEARCH study by Guy et al.,[9] in 512 young patients with T1DM and in 188 healthy age-matched controls, patients with suboptimal control (HbA1c >7.5%) had much more lipid quantitative disorders than patients with optimal control (HbA1c <7.5%).

In the SEARCH study,[9] youth who exhibited suboptimal glycemic control (n = 348) had elevated total cholesterol, LDL, and non-HDL. In addition, elevated apolipoprotein B (apoB) levels and more small, dense LDL particles were more common among patients with T1DM.

Even well-treated T1DM patients show defects in the regulation of the plasma lipid metabolism that are not routinely evaluated, such as increase in the small dense LDL subfraction, which is more atherogenic, and dysfunctional HDL. In addition, alterations in the transfer of lipids are often found in those patients, involving transfer proteins such as CETP and phospholipid transfer protein.

TREATED TYPE 1 DIABETES WITH OPTIMAL GLYCEMIC CONTROL

In these patients, triglycerides are reduced due to action of endothelial lipoprotein lipase. Plasma LDL-cholesterol is also decreased and maybe due to intense insulin therapy as a consequence of decreased VLDL production by peripheral hyperinsulinemia. Plasma HDL-cholesterol level is normal or slightly increased in well-controlled T1DM patients with different studies reporting an increase in either HDL subfraction 2 or subfraction 3. The increase in plasma HDL-cholesterol may well be the consequence of the elevated lipoprotein lipase/hepatic lipase ratio that is likely due to peripheral hyperinsulinemia as a consequence of the subcutaneous route of insulin administration.[10]

CHAPTER 21: Lipid Disorders in Type 1 Diabetes Mellitus

QUALITATIVE LIPID ABNORMALITIES

Perhaps, more important and pertinent to the genesis of CVD in T1DM are the qualitative, rather than the quantitative changes in the lipid profile. These qualitative lipid abnormalities are not fully reversed by glycemic control and are likely to be atherogenic.

LOW-DENSITY LIPOPROTEINS

In patients with T1DM, LDL is often rich in triglycerides and increased number of small dense LDL particles is observed, which are associated with an increase in CVD risk. In a study by Albers et al.,[11] in 2,657 patients with T1DM, it has been shown that dense LDL increased with HbA1c with buoyant LDL shifting toward dense LDL for HbA1c values above 8%. Small dense LDL particles have reduced affinity for the LDL B/E receptor and are preferentially taken up by macrophages, through the scavenger receptor, leading to the formation of foam cells. These LDL particles have higher affinity for intimal proteoglycans and this may favor the penetration of LDL particles into the arterial wall. Small dense LDL particles are also more susceptible to oxidation. Oxidized LDLs produce chemotactic effects on monocytes by increasing the synthesis of adhesion molecules, such as intercellular adhesion molecule 1 by endothelial cells.

HIGH-DENSITY LIPOPROTEINS

Just like LDL, HDL particles from patients with T1DM are often rich in triglycerides. This modification has been attributed to increased cholesteryl ester transfer between lipoproteins and quite often, glycemic control does not alter these abnormalities. Activity of paraoxonase, an antioxidative enzyme associated with HDLs, is significantly reduced in patients with T1DM, which has a bearing on the antioxidative action of HDL.[12]

VERY LOW-DENSITY LIPOPROTEINS

Very low-density lipoprotein in patients with T1DM is frequently rich in esterified cholesterol at the expense of triglycerides leading to an increased VLDL cholesterol/triglyceride ratio, part of which may be ascribed to an increased cholesteryl ester transfer between lipoproteins.[13]

SCREENING FOR DYSLIPIDEMIA

Screening recommendations for dyslipidemia in children and adolescents with T1DM are required due to the following reasons:
- Characteristic lipid abnormalities (vide supra) have been identified in children with T1DM
- There is a strong signal for tracking of lipid levels from childhood to adulthood
- Adult atherosclerosis might begin in the childhood and T1DM could be a risk factor.

Most of the assumptions about CVD risk, screening, and management in T1DM are nebulous due to absence of wide spread long-term data, but based on the above considerations,

American Diabetes Association has recommended screening and management of lipid abnormalities in T1DM as follows.[14]

Screening

If T1DM is diagnosed after 12 years of age, screening for lipid abnormalities should be done at diagnosis but after glycemic control is achieved, and should be repeated every 5 years if the initial screen is normal (more often if screening is abnormal). If T1DM is diagnosed before 12 years of age, in the absence of a parental history of dyslipidemia or early coronary heart disease, there is no clear indication for a screening lipid examination and it should be done only at 12 years of age. Lipid goals are in concord with the lipid goals as mentioned in Adult Treatment Panel III and American Heart Association guidelines (Box 1).

For children, "borderline" levels of total cholesterol and LDL are defined as 170–199 mg/dL and 110–129 mg/dL, respectively and "elevated" levels are above 200 mg/dL for total cholesterol and above 130 mg/dL for LDL cholesterol. While the guidelines suggest that cut-offs should be lower in children with previous family history of CVD; they have not achieved any consensus on targets in the CVD family history group.

Management

Management is multipronged and is as follows:
- Glycemic control: The initial step in management is optimizing glycemic control. In uncontrolled T1DM, total cholesterol and triglycerides are higher in the presence of poor glycemic control and treatment decisions about lipid management should be taken only after stabilization of blood glucose levels
- Dietary therapy: Components include decreasing fat in diet, limiting saturated fat to below 7% of calories, minimizing intake of trans fat, increasing soluble fiber, and limiting dietary cholesterol to below 200 mg/day. Fasting lipid profiles are repeated at 3 months and then at 6 months. If at target, the lipid profile should be repeated yearly. If after 6 months of glycemic control and dietary therapy, there is no significant improvement in lipids, further intervention is based on LDL levels:
    - LDL 100–129 mg/dL: Maximize nonpharmacologic treatment
    - LDL 130–159 mg/dL: "Consider" medication, based on CVD risk profile, blood pressure, family history, and in older adolescents and adults with T1DM-smoking status
    - LDL more than or equal to 160 mg/dL: Start medication.
- Pharmacotherapy: Initially, experience with statins in children was limited, and bile acid sequestrants were first-line therapy in children. However, acceptability was poor and

---

BOX 1: Lipid targets in children

Goals

- LDL <100 mg/dL
- HDL >35 mg/dL
- Triglycerides <150 mg/dL

LDL reduction was also meagre. As experience with statins has accumulated,[15] they have replaced bile acid sequestrants as the first line. Pharmacotherapy is indicated only in T1DM patients whose age is more than 10 years. Treatment should be initiated with the lowest possible dose, and gradually increased, based on requirement and side effects. Liver function tests (LFTs) should be monitored at periodic intervals and medication should be discontinued if LFTs are greater than three times the upper limit of normal. Medication should be discontinued temporarily in case of any features suggestive of myopathy and etiology evaluated thoroughly. Routine monitoring of creatinine phosphokinase levels is not recommended. Statins should be used cautiously in adolescent females who are sexually active, due to risks associated with statins in pregnancy.
  o If triglycerides are more than 150 mg/dL, glycemic control and dietary modification should be enhanced. Treatment with fibric acid derivatives to forestall pancreatitis is initiated only when triglycerides are more than 1,000 mg/dL.
- Supportive care: In addition to these interventions, optimizing blood pressure control, proper exercise recommendations, weight reduction, and antismoking advice should be reinforced at every visit.

CONCLUSION

Dyslipidemia in T1DM is one of the most significant risks for CVD. While some attention has been focused on this subject in the past few years and a few studies and consensus statements have been released, further work needs to be done on: (i) the association of dyslipidemia with other diabetes complications, particularly the development of microalbuminuria; (ii) gender and race factors; (iii) studies that involve longitudinal tracking of lipid abnormalities from childhood, through adolescence to adulthood in T1DM, and (iv) effect of elevated triglycerides and non-HDL cholesterol on CVD risk in T1DM.

REFERENCES

1. Moss SE, Klein R, Klein BE. Cause-specific mortality in a population-based study of diabetes. Am J Public Health. 1991;81: 1158-62.
2. Libby P, Nathan DM, Abraham K, Brunzell JD, Fradkin JE, Haffner SM, et al; National Heart, Lung, and Blood Institute; National Institute of Diabetes and Digestive and Kidney Diseases Working Group on Cardiovascular Complications of Type 1 Diabetes Mellitus. Report of the National Heart, Lung, and Blood Institute-National Institute of Diabetes and Digestive and Kidney Diseases Working Group on Cardiovascular Complications of Type 1 Diabetes Mellitus. Circulation. 2005;111(25):3489-93.
3. Soedamah-Muthu SS, Chaturvedi N, Toeller M, Ferriss B, Reboldi P, Michel G, et al; EURODIAB Prospective Complications Study Group. Risk factors for coronary heart disease in type 1 diabetic patients in Europe: the EURODIAB Prospective Complications Study. Diabetes Care. 2004;27(2):530-7.
4. Malmström R, Packard CJ, Caslake M, Bedford D, Stewart P, Yki-Jarvinen H, et al. Effects of insulin and acipimox on VLDL1 and VLDL2 apolipoprotein B production in normal subjects. Diabetes. 1998;47:779-87.
5. Weidman SW, Ragland JB, Fisher JN Jr, Kitabchi AE, Sabesin SMJ. Effects of insulin on plasma lipoproteins in diabetic ketoacidosis: evidence for a change in high-density lipoprotein composition during treatment. J Lipid Res. 1982;23:171-82.
6. Marcovecchio ML, Dalton RN, Prevost AT, Acerini CL, Barrett TG, Cooper JD, et al. Prevalence of abnormal lipid profiles and the relationship with the development of microalbuminuria in adolescents with type 1 diabetes. Diabetes Care. 2009;32(4): 658-63.

SECTION 6: Chronic Complications

7. Schwab KO, Doerfer J, Naeke A, Rohrer T, Wiemann D, Marg W, et al; German/Austrian Pediatric DPV Initiative. Influence of food intake, age, gender, HbA1c, and BMI levels on plasma cholesterol in 29,979 children and adolescents with type 1 diabetes--reference data from the German diabetes documentation and quality management system (DPV). Pediatr Diabetes. 2009;10:184-92.
8. The DCCT Research Group. Lipid and lipoprotein levels in patients with IDDM diabetes control and complication. Trial experience. Diabetes Care. 1992;15:886-94.
9. Guy J, Ogden L, Wadwa RP, Hamman RF, Mayer-Davis EJ, Liese AD, et al. Lipid and lipoprotein profiles in youth with and without type 1 diabetes: the SEARCH for Diabetes in Youth case-control study. Diabetes Care. 2009;32(3):416-20.
10. Dullaart RP. Plasma lipoprotein abnormalities in type 1 (insulin-dependent) diabetes mellitus. Neth J Med. 1995;46:44-54.
11. Albers JJ, Marcovina SM, Imperatore G, Snively BM, Stafford J, Fujimoto WY, et al. Prevalence and determinants of elevated apolipoprotein B and dense low-density lipoprotein in youths with type 1 and type 2 diabetes. J Clin Endocrinol Metab. 2008;93(3):735-42.
12. Ferretti G, Bacchetti T, Busni D, Rabini RA, Curatola G. Protective effect of paraoxonase activity in high-density lipoproteins against erythrocyte membranes peroxidation: a comparison between healthy subjects and type 1 diabetic patients. J Clin Endocrinol Metab. 2004;89:2957-62.
13. Vergès B. Lipid disorders in type 1 diabetes. Diabetes Metab. 2009;35(5):353-60.
14. American Diabetes Association. Management of dyslipidemia in children and adolescents with diabetes. Diabetes Care. 2003;26(7):2194-7.
15. De Jongh S, Ose L, Szamosi T, Gagné C, Lambert M, Scott R, et al; Simvastatin in Children Study Group. Efficacy and safety of statin therapy in children with familial hypercholesterolemia: a randomized, double-blind, placebo-controlled trial with simvastatin. Circulation. 2002;106:2231-37.

Hypertension

Sanjay Kalra, Mudita Dhingra, Rakesh Sahay

INTRODUCTION

Diabetes in children is a multifaceted disease, which needs a comprehensive and team effort, rather than glucocentric approach for evaluation and management. Childhood diabetes should be viewed through a biopsychosocial model, and all relevant biomedical aspects, including prevention, limitation, and management of vascular complications, should be addressed. This chapter focuses on hypertension in children with diabetes, its evaluation, nonpharmacological therapy, and pharmacological management.

GUIDANCE

Guidance is provided by the National Institutes of Health and the National Heart, Lung, and Blood Institute, which have produced the Fourth Report on the diagnosis, evaluation and management of high blood pressure (BP) in children and adolescents.[1] The European Society of Hypertension has also published recommendations on prevention, diagnosis, and treatment of high BP in children and adolescents.[2] Diabetes-specific guidelines are available from International Society for Pediatric and Adolescent Diabetes, and American Diabetes Association.[3,4]

EPIDEMIOLOGY

Hypertension in adults with type 1 diabetes mellitus (T1DM) is more frequent than in nondiabetic adults. The major drivers of this occurrence are essential hypertension and diabetic nephropathy. In children, too, a similar situation is expected. In a large study conducted in Germany and Austria, children with diabetes had elevated nocturnal blood pressure, with reduced dipping of systolic blood pressure (SBP), diastolic BP (DBP), and mean arterial pressure (MAP). The presence of microalbuminuria was associated with nocturnal DBP and diastolic dipping. In this study, 9.2% of all registered children aged 5–18 years were found to be on antihypertensive therapy. Hypertension was associated with high insulin dosage, female gender, body mass index, glycosylated hemoglobin and duration of diabetes in children with diabetes. The presence of microalbuminuria was associated with nocturnal DBP and diastolic dipping. Lack of nocturnal dipping can therefore be used as an early marker of hypertension.[5]

While age-related changes in vascular regulation occur in all individuals, children with T1DM seem to experience "accelerated vascular aging" 15–20 years earlier.[6] Hence, one must keep a close watch on vascular health, including BP, in children with diabetes.

BLOOD PRESSURE EVALUATION

All children above 3 years of age should have their BP measured in the diabetic clinic. While this can be done at every visit, it is mandatory to measure and document BP at least once a year. Children with heart disease or nephropathy should be monitored for hypertension more frequently, and from an earlier age. This should be done by auscultation, using a stethoscope placed over the brachial artery pulse, 2 cm above the cubital fossa, along with a clinical sphygmomanometer. While the head of the stethoscope is used by most clinicians, the bell can be used for auscultation in very small children.

Blood pressure should be checked when the child has avoided stimulant drugs and foods; after having sat quietly for 5 minutes; with his/her back supported; with feet on the floor and right arm supported; with cubital fossa at heart level. Blood pressure is usually measured using the right arm, to ensure consistency and comparison, and to avoid a false low reading that may occur in the left arm with coarctation of aorta.

The sphygmomanometer cuff should be appropriate for the child's age and size (Table 1). An appropriate cuff must be used. This implies a cuff with an inflatable bladder width that is at least 40% of the mid-arm circumference, and a bladder length that should cover 80–100% of the arm circumference without overlapping; and the bladder width to length ratio should be at least 1:2. Recommended BP cuff bladder dimensions are listed in table 1. A small cuff leads to overestimation of BP to a greater extent than a large cuff underestimates BP. Therefore, in case of doubt, a relatively larger cuff size should be used.[1]

Systolic blood pressure is recorded as the BP levels when tapping Korotkoff sounds appear (K1). Diastolic blood pressure is the level when Korotkoff sounds disappear (K5). In some

TABLE 1: Recommended blood pressure cuff bladder dimensions[1]

Age	Width (cm)	Length (cm)	Maximum arm circumference (cm)
Newborn	4	8	10
Infant	6	12	15
Child	9	18	22
Adolescent	10	24	26
Adult	13	30	44
Thigh	20	42	52

children, however, K5 may occur at 0 mmHg, even if the head of the stethoscope is applied very gently. In such cases, K4 (muffling of Korotkoff sound) can be used to determine DBP.

In India, mercury manometers or aneroid manometers can be used to measure BP. Regular calibration is advised. Automated devices or oscillometric devices can also be used, but must be calibrated and validated. They are preferred only in newborns, infants, and in intensive care settings.

Blood pressure is highly variable, even within the same child. A recent study demonstrated that assessment of BP using oscillometric devices should include at least three measurements in the same sitting to avoid inaccurate assessment.[7] Ambulatory blood pressure monitoring (ABPM) is measured with a wearable oscillometric BP device usually placed on the nondominant arm, which automatically measures and records BP at prescribed frequent intervals (e.g., every 20 minutes when awake and every 30 minutes during sleep) over an entire 24-hour period. Ambulatory blood pressure monitoring allows evaluation of BP throughout the day in the patient's own environment to reduce anxiety-induced elevations in blood pressure. It may be needed to confirm the diagnosis, rule out white coat hypertension, masked hypertension (hypertension not picked up by office measurements but only by ABPM) and thus helps in evaluation of nature and degree of hypertensive morbidity. However, recently it could be shown that office BP measurements are also higher when masked hypertension is present.[8]

Blood pressure tables[1] provided by the Fourth Report on the Diagnosis, Evaluation, and Treatment of High Blood Pressure in Children and Adolescents are used in India. There is a strong need to have India-specific tables for evaluation of BP in our children and adolescents.

DEFINITIONS OF HYPERTENSION

- Hypertension, in children, is defined as an average SBP and/or DBP that is greater than or equal to the 95th percentile for sex, age, and height on three separate occasions
- Prehypertension, in children, is defined as average SBP or DBP levels that are greater than or equal to the 90th percentile, but less than the 95th percentile
- Prehypertension, in adolescents, is defined as a BP greater than or equal to 120/80 mmHg, even if this value is less than the 90th percentile. SBP crosses the 90th percentile at 12 years of age, while DBP does so at 16 years
- Stage 1 hypertension includes BP levels that range from the 95th percentile to 5 mmHg above the 99th percentile
- Stage 2 hypertension implies BP levels that are higher than 5 mmHg above the 99th percentile
- Stage 2 hypertension can be classified as symptomatic and asymptomatic, to help plan further evaluation and treatment.

The separation of pediatric BP levels into "hypertension" and high normal" mirrors the terms "hypertension" and prehypertension" used in adults (Joint National Commission 7). The concept of high normal BP allows the institution of prevention and therapeutic lifestyle measures, without creating a need for pharmacotherapy (Table 2).

TABLE 2: Management of high blood pressure in children with diabetes

Category	Follow-up	Nonpharmacological	Pharmacological
Normal	Recheck at next scheduled visit	Healthy diet, sleep, physical activity	None
Prehypertension	Recheck in 6 months	As above; weight management if needed	Only if compelling indications exist
Stage 1 hypertension • Symptomatic	Recheck in 1–2 weeks Recheck sooner than 1 week	As above; stress management	Initiate therapy with ACE inhibitor
Stage 2 hypertension • Symptomatic	Evaluate or refer within 1 week	As above if needed	Initiate therapy with ACE inhibitor

ACE, angiotensin converting enzyme.

CLINICAL EVALUATION

Clinical evaluation in children includes a detailed history taking and comprehensive physical examination. This should cover sleep history, family, dietary recall, history of drug use (such as tobacco, narcotics, and alcohol) and a history over-the-counter drug intake. Physical examination must cover the cardiovascular system, and assess peripheral pulses, stigmata of metabolic syndrome (xanthomas, xanthelasma, skin tags, and arcus senilis) and a retinal examination.

LABORATORY INVESTIGATIONS

All hypertension in children with diabetes cannot be attributed to diabetes or diabetic nephropathy. A workup should be able to exclude or identify other causes of hypertension, and evaluate for target organ damage. Common causes of pediatric hypertension include white coat hypertension, renal parenchymal disease, and cardiovascular and adrenal hypertension. These can be identified by ABPM, renal function tests, plasma renin activity, renovascular imaging, echocardiography, plasma and urine steroid, and catecholamine levels. Comorbidity and target organ damage is assessed by renal function tests, lipid profile, polysomnography, electrocardiogram, and echocardiogram.

One should remember to do a thorough endocrine assessment, as Cushing syndrome (moon facies), Williams syndrome (elfin facies), Turner syndrome (short stature, webbed neck), and hyperthyroidism (goiter) may coexist with diabetes and hypertension.

MANAGEMENT: GENERAL PRINCIPLES

In children with diabetes and/or evidence of end organ damage, the goal BP should be less than the 90th percentile for age, sex, and height. This goal differs from that for children with uncomplicated primary hypertension, where a BP less than 95th percentile is deemed adequate.

Blood pressure management includes screening and monitoring for comorbid conditions, target organ damage and concomitant causes of elevated blood pressure. It also includes monitoring of BP and pharmacovigilance for possible drug side effects. Counseling regarding mitigation of other cardiovascular risk factors, including avoidance of smoking and alcohol, is an important aspect of BP care.

MANAGEMENT

Nonpharmacological

Nonpharmacological intervention is an important component of hypertension therapy. Diet and physical activity are essential for BP normalization, while stress management and weight reduction may be necessary in some children.

While dietary advice is already provided to all children with diabetes, it focuses only on glucose management. Those with hypertension are advised to restrict salt intake and follow a DASH (Dietary Approach to Stop Hypertension) diet[9] as much as possible, within the framework of a diabetes-friendly diet. The Indian kitchen is rich in salt substitutes: spices such as asofoetida (*heeng*), black pepper (*kali mirch*) and oregano, or condiments like ginger and onions can be used to improve flavor.[10] Acute caffeine intake may increase central BP by increasing catecholamine release and vascular resistance. Though this rise may not be reflected in peripheral blood pressure, caffeine should be avoided in children.

Physical activity is necessary for good cardiovascular health. Aerobic exercises (30–45 min/day) should be encouraged, and the need for adequate sunlight exposure must be emphasized. Stress management must be discussed with the child as well as family. Many children (and families) living with diabetes face a significant amount of diabetes distress.[11] This may contribute to hypertension, and should be tackled by appropriate means. Referral to a qualified mental health professional may be indicated.

Weight reduction and maintenance must be included in all hypertension management strategies. While dietary intervention and exercise form the bedrock of weight reduction, orlistat,[12] and liraglutide may be indicated in select pediatric or adolescent patients. Table 3 shows the impact of lifestyle modification in reduction of SBP.

TABLE 3: Lifestyle modification and approximate reduction in systolic blood pressure (mmHg) (obtained from adult studies)

Lifestyle modification	Reduction in systolic blood pressure (mmHg)
Exercise/limit television and other sedentary activities	4–9
Weight reduction (smaller portions/exercise)	5–20/10 kg weight loss
Consume more fresh vegetables and fruits, low-fat dairy products and low content of saturated fats	2–8
Reduce sodium intake	2–8
Avoid alcohol	2–4
Limit caffeine	–
Avoid tobacco (cigarettes/chewing)	–

MANAGEMENT: PHARMACOLOGIC

Pharmacologic management is indicated in children with diabetes in whom nonpharmacologic measures have failed. The aim is twofold: to achieve normotension, and to prevent or limit target organ damage.

Angiotensin converting enzyme (ACE) inhibitors are the drugs of choice in diabetic hypertension. The other drugs commonly used in India, and their doses, are listed in Table 4.

There is relatively less data to support the use of angiotensin receptor blockers (ARBs) in children with hypertension. Any drug that is to be started should be initiated in the lowest recommended dose. Up titration is done until the desired BP goal is reached. If the child is unable to tolerate the drug, or if the highest recommended dose appears inadequate, a second drug can be added. A drug combination should contain molecules of action, such as an ACE inhibitor and diuretic. It is irrational to combine two drugs with similar mechanism of action, such as an ACE inhibitor and ARB. If ACE inhibitor/ARB and/or diuretics are used, serum creatinine/estimated glomerular filtration rate (modified Schwartz formula) and serum potassium levels should be monitored.

BLOOD PRESSURE AND NEPHROPATHY

Effective control of BP slows the progression of diabetic nephropathy, and delays onset of end-stage renal disease. The contribution of BP control is more significant than that of glucose control and cessation of tobacco intake. ACE inhibitors are beneficial in every reno-phenotype. They reduce progression from microalbuminuria to macro albuminuria, enhance the chances of reversal to normoalbuminuria, increase taken for doubling of serum creatinine, and reduce all-cause mortality. ARBs achieve the same effects, but have not shown any mortality benefits.

TABLE 4: Antihypertensive drugs for children

Class	Drug	Dose (Initial)	Dose (Maximum)
Angiotensin converting enzyme inhibitor	Captopril	0.3–0.5 mg/kg/dose (tid)	6 mg/kg/day
	Enalapril	0.08 mg/kg/day (bid)	0.6 mg/kg/day
	Lisinopril	0.07 mg/kg/day (qd)	0.6 mg/kg/day
Angiotensin receptor blocker	Losartan	0.7 mg/kg/day (qd)	1.4 mg/kg/day
α, β-blocker	Labetalol	1–3 mg/kg/day (bid)	10–12 mg/kg/day
β blocker	Metoprolol	1–2 mg/kg/day (bid)	6 mg/kg/day
	Bisoprolol	2.5/6.25 mg/day (qd)	10 g/day
Calcium channel blocker	Amlodipine	2.5–5 mg (7–17 y) (od)	
Central α agonist	Clonidine	0.2 mg/day (>12 y) (bid)	2.4 mg/day
Diuretic	HCTZ	1 mg/kg/day (qd, -bid)	3 mg/kg/day
	Chorthalidone	0.3 mg/kg/day (qd)	2 mg/kg/day
	Furosemide	0.5–2.0 mg/kg/dose (qd, -bid)	6 mg/kg/day
	Spironolactone	1 mg/kg/day (qd, -bid)	3.3 mg/kg/day

Do not exceed adult doses.

od, once a day; bid, twice a day; tid, thrice a day; qd, four times a day.

A vascular legacy effect has been demonstrated in adults[8] using perindopril + indapamide fixed dose combination: use of this ACE inhibitor + diuretic lowers the risk of long-term vascular complications, even after the initial intensive BP lowering effect (as compared to placebo) has ceased. Such a vascular legacy may be operative in children. There is no consensus regarding the utility of ACE inhibitor in normotensive, nonalbuminuric or microalbuminuric children with diabetes.

HYPERTENSION: SYMPTOMATIC

Severe, symptomatic hypertension may occur in some children with diabetes and advanced chronic renal failure. Prompt treatment is essential. A hypertensive emergency is accompanied by signs of hypertensive encephalopathy, with seizures. An intravenous BP lowering drug should be used to reduce BP by 25% within 8 hours, and normalize it over 26–48 hours. A hypertensive urgency is marked by less serious symptoms, such as vomiting and headache. Either oral or intravenous drugs can be used, depending on the clinical situation.

CONCLUSION

Our strategy for hypertension care in diabetes should be a comprehensive and proactive one. Regular screening for BP and associated risk factor is the primary intervention that all paediatric diabetes care providers must follow. Use of ABPM and microalbuminuria may be considered as screening tools in select settings and situations. An emphasis on healthy lifestyle, weight management, and cardiovascular risk factor mitigation must be practiced. Appropriate, and timely, use of antihypertensive therapy, aiming to control BP to less than 90th percentile, relieve symptoms, and prevent progression of nephropathy, is equally important.

As we move from a glucocentric to a vascular-oriented approach in diabetes, we must include comprehensive strategies, i.e., promotive, preventive, and therapeutic; nonpharmacological and pharmacological, in hypertension care as well.

REFERENCES

1. National High Blood Pressure Education Program Working Group on High Blood Pressure in Children and Adolescents. (2005). The fourth report on the diagnosis, evaluation, and treatment of high blood pressure in children and adolescents. NIH Publication No. 05–5267. Available from http://www.nhlbi.nih.gov/health/prof/heart/hbp/hbp_ped.pdf. Accessed January, 2017.
2. Lurbe E, Cifkova R, Cruickshank JK, Dillon MJ, Ferreira I, Invitti C, et al. Management of high blood pressure in children and adolescents: recommendations of the European society of hypertension. J Hypertens. 2009; 27:1719-42.
3. Standards of Medical Care in Diabetes—2016. Diabetes Care. 2016;39 (Suppl 1):S86-S93.
4. Donaghue KC, Wadwa RP, Dimeglio LA, Wong TY, Chiarelli F, Marcovecchio ML, et al. Microvascular and macrovascular complications in children and adolescents. Pediatric diabetes. 2014;15(S20):257-69.
5. Raile K, Galler A, Hofer S, Herbst A, Dunstheimer D, Busch P, et al. Diabetic Nephropathy in 27,805 Children, Adolescents, and Adults With Type 1 Diabetes Effect of diabetes duration, A1C, hypertension, dyslipidemia, diabetes onset, and sex. Diabetes care. 2007;30(10):2523-8.
6. Rönnback M, Fagerudd J, Forsblom C, Pettersson-Fernholm K, Reunanen A, Groop PH; Finnish Diabetic Nephropathy (FinnDiane) Study Group. Altered age-related blood pressure pattern in type 1 diabetes. Circulation. 2004;110(9):1076-82.

SECTION 6: Chronic Complications

7. Negroni-Balasquide X, Bell CS, Samuel J, Samuels JA. Is one measurement enough to evaluate blood pressure? A Blood pressure screening experience in more than 9000 children with a subset comparison of auscultatory to mercury measurements. J Am Soc Hypertens. 2016;10(2):95-100.
8. Mitsnefes MM, Pierce C, Flynn J, Samuel J, Dionne J, Furth S, et al; CKiD study group. Can office blood pressure readings predict masked hypertension? Pediatr Nephrol. 2016;31(1):163--6
9. Sacks FM, Svetkey LP, Vollmer WM, Appel LJ, Bray GA, Harsha D, et al. Effects on blood pressure of reduced dietary sodium and the Dietary Approaches to Stop Hypertension (DASH) diet. New Engl J Med. 2001;344(1):3-10.
10. Kalra S, Sahay M, Baruah MP. Reducing salt intake, for a healthier world. J Med Nutr Nutraceut. 2013;2(1):1.
11. Kalra S, John M, Baruah MP. The Indian family fights diabetes: Results from the second Diabetes Attitudes, Wishes and Needs (DAWN2) study. J Soc Health Diabetes. 2014;2(1):3.
12. Canadian Task Force on Preventive Health Care. Recommendations for growth monitoring, and prevention and management of overweight and obesity in children and youth in primary care. CMAJ. 2015;187(6):411-21.

CHAPTER 23

Microvascular Complications

Vijay Viswanathan

INTRODUCTION

Nowadays pediatricians were confronting many challenges because of the new epidemics which affect the physical and mental health of children. Infectious diseases like pneumonia, viral infections, chicken pox, diarrhea, mumps, and many nutritional deficiencies were predominant in childhood. Perhaps, nowadays, it has been replaced by noncommunicable disease such as diabetes and obesity.[1] Diabetes mellitus is the common endocrine metabolic disorder in childhood known as type 1 diabetes mellitus (T1DM). Its incidence was peak around the age of 10 and it is prevalent in Hispanic whites.[2] The prevalence of T1DM is high among the South-East Asia Region (SEAR), further it is estimated that 77,900 children were affected. According to the estimate of International Diabetes Federation, in 2013 alone, 12,600 children under the age of 15 was diagnosed as T1DM in SEAR region.[3]

Globally, there is an increasing phenomenon in the incidence of T1DM with the annual rate of 3–5%, predominantly seen in the children below the age of 5 years.[4,5] It is associated with a significant burden, mainly related to the development of vascular complications. The microvascular complication of diabetes includes long-term complications of diabetes such as retinopathy, neuropathy, and nephropathy which affects small blood vessels. Long-term microvascular and neurologic complications are responsible for major morbidity and mortality in T1DM.[6] In developed countries, diabetes is considered as the major cause for renal failure, amputation of the lower limb, and blindness, further it is also considered as the major cause of mortality due to cardiovascular disease (CVD).[7] The following section will focused on the microvascular complications in T1DM such as nephropathy, retinopathy, and neuropathy, respectively.

DIABETIC NEPHROPATHY

Diabetic nephropathy is the most common microvascular complication in T1DM with earlier onset. Proteinuria is a typical characteristic of diabetic nephropathy and it is found in 15–40%

patients with T1DM. The risk of CVD is tenfolds higher in T1DM patients with diabetic nephropathy than their counterparts without diabetic nephropathy, the risk increases with the severity of the renal involvement.[8]

Thus, diabetic nephropathy is considered as the major determinant of cardiovascular morbidity and mortality.[9] International Society for Pediatric and Adolescent (ISPAD) has recommended, that for T1DM patients, the routine screening of microalbuminuria have to be started from 11 years of age and after 2 years of the onset of diabetes.[10] The early kidney changes in T1DM patients include subclinical morphological changes, hyperperfusion, and hyperfiltration, within the normal range increase in albumin excretion rate values. In addition, raised albumin excretion between 30–300 mg/24 h, in a 24 hour or timed urine collection 20–200 µg/min shows microalbuminuria development, further may progress to overt protrinuria (>200 µg/min), and to end-stage renal disease if untreated.

Gross et al.[9] conducted 10-year follow-up study with 939 T1DM adults, the finding highlighted that the mortality rate was 15, 25, and 44% for normoalbuminuria, microalbuminuria, and macroalbuminria patients, respectively. Diabetic nephropathy is considered as the marker of other major microvascular complication like retinopathy, further it is also associated with the autonomic nervous system dysfunction. In a study conducted by Vijay et al.,[11] the occurrence of microalbuminuria in T1DM was only after 20 years of age and it is observed in a large percentage among south Indian population. The recent studies highlighted that the nocturnal blood pressure was higher in T1DM patients with microalbuminuria than their counterparts without microalbuminuria.[12,13] Thus, it can be concluded that the T1DM patients with early development of nephropathy were often associated with nocturnal hypertension.

In T1DM, when nephropathy is detected hypertension is usually absent, perhaps in T2DM, when the patient is first detected with microalbuminuria, hypertension is associated.[14-16] Thus for hypertension, if the conventional definition or the recent definition proposed for the persons with diabetes[17] is considered, it can be concluded that T1DM patients, who are susceptible to kidney disease, hypertension does not occur until or otherwise there is an established microalbuminuria. It is recommended that in T1DM patients, the routine screening for complications at regular interval has to be followed which provides information to both family and diabetes team, this serves to improvise the glycemic control and early precautions can be taken accordingly.

DIABETIC RETINOPATHY

Diabetic retinopathy is the leading cause for loss of vision among working age group in developed countries.[18] It is strongly associated with other microvascular complications, specifically diabetic nephropathy, and proliferative diabetic retinopathy is strongly associated with cardiovascular events.[19] It initially appeared as retinal abnormalities which is non-proliferative and characterized by capillary microaneurysms, hemorrhages, exudates, the development of vascular obstruction, and the infarction of the retinal nerve fibers causing cotton wool spots.[20] In diabetic macular edema, microvascular permeability is increased and hard retinal exudates are deposited, which complicates proliferative and nonproliferative retinopathy and these are the serious cause of vision loss in patients with diabetes.

The prevalence of diabetic retinopathy increases with the duration of the disease after 20 years.[21] Minimal diabetic retinopathy risk was observed in T1DM patients aged less than 10 years, however, in post pubertal patients, the rate of prevalence was increased after 5 years.[22] In 12% of the prepubertal T1DM patients, early retinopathy was recorded, when compared to 29% of adolescent with 6 years of T1DM duration in the incident cohort.[23] When compared to adults, T1DM adolescents had an increased risk of progression of diabetic retinopathy to eye sight threatening condition with rapid progression, when glycemic control is poor.[22] The ISPAD recommended that retinopathy screening should be started from 11 years of age to after 2 years of diabetes duration. The minimum assessment of the diabetic retinopathy should be done by ophthalmoscopy through dilating the pupils. In general, annual checking of retinopathy is recommended, but the frequency may vary based on the risk features for loss of vision. The rate of loss of vision can be reduced through laser therapy. Earlier studies have highlighted that the risk of retinopathy was increased when the blood pressure and glycemic condition is not under control.[24] Tight regulation of glycemic status and blood pressure, along with the prompt eye examination, diabetic retinopathy can be prevented and controlled. When required, diabetic retinopathy can be treated with laser photocoagulation and vitreoretinal surgery.[25]

DIABETIC NEUROPATHY

Diabetic neuropathy can be defined as the disorder which does not have any additional reasons for peripheral neuropathy other than diabetes, which can be autonomic or somatic.[22,26] At rare situation, temporary or poor metabolic control leads to acute sensory symptoms, whereas chronic distal symmetric polyneuropathy (DPN) is the commonest form of diabetic neuropathy. Distal symmetric polyneuropathy can be associated with or without any change in the autonomic nervous system. Many comprehensive epidemiological studies which includes both adult and pediatric population, emphasized that the DPN diagnosed subjects can range from 7 to 57%.[22] Approximately, 60–70% of the adult patients with persistent and progressive neuropathy can have certain degree of nerve damage. In a Diabetes Control and Complications Control trail study, 278 T1DM patients were enrolled and the finding showed that on careful examination 39% of the patients were detected with subclinical DPN and the patients were asymptomatic.[27]

The prevalence of lower joint mobility (LJM) in T1DM ranged between 9 and 58%.[28,29] The etiology of LJM is still unknown, but certain evidences showed that the accumulation of the soft tissue of advanced glycation end products may cause the stiffening. The joint mobility and plantar foot pressure in Asian Indian type 1 diabetic subjects showed that T1DM has limited joint mobility which decreased further with longer duration of diabetes with high planter pressure among T1DM.[30,31] These results, however, emphasizes the problem that, prevalence rates of diabetic neuropathy will vary depending on different cohorts of patients studied, different testing modalities, different criteria, and the cutoff values. The risk and the progression of the diabetic neuropathy can be prevented through the tight glycemic control. The contributing factors such as excess alcohol, uremia, and vitamin B12 deficiency have to be ruled out to teat diabetic neuropathy. Furthermore, based on the predominant symptoms, the pain relief can be recommended.[32] According to the recommendations of ISPAD, peripheral and autonomic neuropathy has to be accessed through history and by physical examination from the 11 years of age with 2 years of diabetes duration. The annual examination of feet of diabetic patients for neuropathy, infection, and ulcer, after 2 years of diabetes duration and annually thereafter.

RISK FACTORS ASSOCIATED WITH THE MICROVASCULAR COMPLICATIONS IN TYPE 1 DIABETES MELLITUS

There are several risk factors which are associated with the development of the microvascular complications among T1DM. The risk factors include both modifiable factors such as glycemic control, hypertension, dyslipidemia, and diet and nonmodifiable factors like diabetes duration, puberty, genes, and constitutional factors.[33-35] Apart from this, male gender, smoking, and high body mass index were considered as the additional risk factors for the development of diabetic nephropathy.[36] Furthermore, longer duration of diabetes increases the risk of complications, which increases significantly following puberty. The risk of developing complications may also be increased by modifiable factors and behavior such as smoking in addition to genetic factors.

Studies have shown that in T1DM, the actual risk of getting microvascular complications like microalbuminuria and retinopathy progression starts at glycosylated hemoglobin level of 7%.[37] The poor glycemic control plays a major role in the development of the complications. Hyperglycemia can promote many functional and structural changes in the microvasculature, through the activation of different mechanisms, including the polyol and hexosamine pathways, accumulation of nonenzymatic glycation end products, and activation of diacylglycerol-protein kinase C pathway.

PREVENTION STRATEGIES

In T1DM patients, the prevention strategies may vary and it depends on the onset of diabetes. Before the onset of T1DM, prevention can be possible through working out the risk factor such as use of antibodies, prediabetic conditions, and genetic risk. If the child is diagnosed with T1DM through appropriate intervention, further damage of β-cells can be prevented (Box 1).

Treatment for T1DM further highlighted the need of new methods such as "insulin replacement therapy" or "artificial pancreas," through which tight glycemic control can be achieved without any hypoglycemia. Management of T1DM also includes the development of new methods such as "biological cure" through transplantation or by regeneration for replacing the function of β-cells and in-depth knowledge on immune-pathogenesis or improvised understanding, leads to preventive therapies which are more effective. The early stage treatment for T1DM should focus on the effective therapeutic targets for immune modulation particularly on effector and native T cells and β-cell/antigen presenting cell.[38]

CHAPTER 23: Microvascular Complications

> **BOX 1: Recommendation for screening microvascular complication among type 1 diabetes mellitus**
>
> **When to start**
> - Three to five years after diagnosis
> - In children and adolescents at the age of 11 with 2 years type 1 diabetes mellitus duration/from age 9 with 5 years of duration
>
> **Frequency:** Annually
>
> **Screening methods**
> - Diabetic nephropathy: Albumin-creatine ratio in a spot urine sample or albumin excretion rate in 24 h or overnight urine collection
> - Diabetic retinopathy: Dilated fundus opthalmoscopy or fundal photography
> - Diabetic neuropathy: History of physical examination; nerve conduction and autonomic tests

CONCLUSION

Diabetes is a complicated and multidimensional condition, which requires a team approach with different focus, from compilations related to diabetes, marriage, and concern for reproduction. Starting the screening after the first 2 years of the diabetes appears to be an appropriate approach. In addition to good metabolic control to prevent and to delay microvascular complications in T1DM children and adolescents, early diagnosis and treatment of hypertension and dyslipidemia are also important. Integrated and individualized care is required for T1DM patients. Type 1 diabetes mellitus child will develop a long-term diabetic complications at early age, when they did not receive a proper medical care. Intensive therapy in T1DM children at an early age can prevent micro- and macrovascular complications. Thus, the main aim of the integrated treatment should be early diagnosis with an appropriate and prompt intervention.

REFERENCES

1. Brüne M, Hochberg Z. Secular trends in new childhood epidemics: insights from evolutionary medicine. BMC Med. 2013;11:226.
2. Imperatore G, Boyle JP, Thompson TJ, Case D, Dabelea D, Hamman RF, et al.; SEARCH for Diabetes in Youth Study Group. Projections of type 1 and type 2 diabetes burden in the US population aged <20 years through 2050: dynamic modeling of incidence, mortality, and population growth. Diabetes Care. 2012;35(12):2515-20.
3. International Diabetes Federation. IDF Diabetes Atlas. 6th ed. Brussels: International Diabetes Federation; 2013. Available from: http://www.idf.org/diabetesatlas.
4. Soltesz G, Patterson CC, Dahlquist G. Worldwide childhood type 1 diabetes incidence—what can we learn from epidemiology? Pediatr Diabetes. 2007;8(Suppl. 6):6-14.
5. Patterson CC, Dahlquist GG, Gyurus E, Green A, Soltesz G. Incidence trends for childhood type 1 diabetes in Europe during 1989–2003 and predicted new cases 2005–20: a multicentre prospective registration study. Lancet. 2009;373:2027-33.
6. Diabetes Control and Complications Trial Research Group. The effect of intensive treatment of diabetes on the development and progression of long-term complications in insulin-dependent diabetes mellitus. N Engl J Med. 1993;329:977-86.
7. International Diabetes Federation (IDF) Diabetes Atlas. 2007. Available from: http://www.eatlas.idf.org/.
8. Tuomilehto J, Borch-Johnsen K, Molarius A, , Forsén T, Rastenyte D, Sarti C, et al. Incidence of cardiovascular disease in Type 1 (insulin-dependent) diabetic subjects with and without diabetic nephropathy in Finland. Diabetologia. 1998;41:784-90.

SECTION 6: Chronic Complications

9. Gross JL, deAzevedo MJ, Silveiro SP, Canani LH, Caramori ML, Zelmanovitz T. Diabetic nephropathy: diagnosis, prevention, and treatment. Diabetes Care. 2005;2(8):164-76.
10. Global IDF/ISPAD guideline for diabetes in childhood and adolescence. Available from: www.ispad.org.
11. Vijay V, Snehalatha C, Shina K, Ramachandran A. Persistent microalbuminuria in type 1 diabetic subjects in South India. J Assoc Physicians India. 2002;50:1259-61.
12. Pecis M, Azevedo MJ, Moraes RS, Ferlin EL, Gross JL. Autonomic dysfunction and urinary albumin excretion rate are associated with an abnormal blood pressure pattern in normotensive normoalbuminuric type 1 diabetic patients. Diabetes Care. 2000;23:989-93.
13. Lafferty AR, Werther GA, Clarke CF. Ambulatory blood pressure, microalbuminuria, and autonomic neuropathy in adolescents with type 1 diabetes. Diabetes Care. 2000;23:533-8.
14. Sowers JR, Epstein M, Frohlich ED. Diabetes, hypertension, and cardiovascular disease: an update. Hypertension. 2001;37:1053-9.
15. Ritz E, Orth SR. Nephropathy in patients with type 2 diabetes mellitus. N Engl J Med. 1999;341:1127-33.
16. Parving HH, Lehnert H, Brochner-Mortensen J, Gomis R, Andersen S, Arner P. The effect of irbesartan on the development of diabetic nephropathy in patients with type 2 diabetes. N Engl J Med. 2001;345:870-8.
17. Bakris GL, Williams M, Dworkin L, Elliott WJ, Epstein M, Toto R, et al. Preserving renal function in adults with hypertension and diabetes: a consensus approach. National Kidney Foundation Hypertension and Diabetes Executive Committees Working Group. Am J Kidney Dis. 2000;36:646-61.
18. Ciulla TA, Amador AG, Zinman B. Diabetic retinopathy and diabetic macular edema: pathophysiology, screening, and novel therapies. Diabetes Care. 2003;26:2653-64.
19. van Hecke MV, Dekker JM, Stehouwer CD, Polak BC, Fuller JH, Sjolie AK, et al.; EURODIAB prospective complications study. Diabetic retinopathy is associated with mortality and cardiovascular disease incidence: the EURODIAB prospective complications study. Diabetes Care. 2005;28:1383-9.
20. Aiello LP, Gardner TW, King GL, Blankenship G, Cavallerano JD, Ferris FL 3rd, et al. Diabetic retinopathy. Diabetes Care. 1998;21:143-156.
21. Klein R, Klein BE, Moss SE, Cruickshanks KJ. The Wisconsin Epidemiologic Study of Diabetic Retinopathy: XVII. The 14-year incidence and progression of diabetic retinopathy and associated risk factors in type 1 diabetes. Ophthalmology. 1998;105:1801-15.
22. Trotta D, Verrotti A, Salladini C, Chiarelli F. Diabetic neuropathy in children and adolescents. Pediatr Diabetes. 2004;5:44-57.
23. Donaghue KC, Craig ME, Chan AK, Fairchild JM, Cusumano JM, Verge CF, et al. Prevalence of diabetes complications 6 years after diagnosis in an incident cohort of childhood diabetes. Diabet Med. 2005;22:711-8.
24. Chaturvedi N, Sjoelie AK, Porta M, Aldington SJ, Fuller JH, Songini M, et al. Markers of insulin resistance are strong risk factors for retinopathy incidence in type 1 diabetes. Diabetes Care. 2001;24:284-9.
25. Klein R, Klein BE, Moss SE. Relation of glycemic control to diabetic microvascular complications in diabetes mellitus. Ann Intern Med. 1996;124:90-6.
26. Boulton AJ, Vinik AI, Arezzo JC, Bril V, Feldman EL, Freeman R, et al. Diabetic neuropathies: a statement by the American Diabetes Association. Diabetes Care. 2005;28:956-62.
27. The Diabetes Control and Complications Trial Research Group. The effect of intensive treatment of diabetes on the development and progression of long-term complications in insulin-dependent diabetes mellitus. The Diabetes Control and Complications Trial Research Group. N Engl J Med. 1993;329:977-86.
28. Rosenbloom AL, Silverstein JH, Lezotte DC, Richardson K, McCallum M. Limited joint mobility in childhood diabetes mellitus indicates increased risk for microvascular disease. N Engl J Med. 1981;305:191-4.
29. Karavanaki K, Baum JD. Prevalence of microvascular and neurologic abnormalities in a population of diabetic children. J Pediatr Endocrinol Metab. 1999;12:411-22.
30. Viswanathan V, Madhavan S, Rajasekar S, Kumpatla S. Limited joint mobility and plantar pressure in type 1 diabetic subjects in India. J Assoc Physicians India. 2008;56:509-12.
31. Viswanathan V, Snehalatha C, Sivagami M, Seena R, Ramachandran A. Association of limited joint mobility and high plantar pressure in diabetic foot ulceration in Asian Indians. Diab Res Clin Pract. 2003;60:57-61.
32. The effect of intensive treatment of diabetes on the development and progression of long-term complications in insulin-dependent diabetes mellitus. The Diabetes Control and Complications Trial Research Group. N Engl J Med. 1993;329:977-86.

33. Raile K, Galler A, Hofer S, Herbst A, Dunstheimer D, Busch P, et al. Diabetic nephropathy in 27,805 children, adolescents, and adults with type 1 diabetes: effect of diabetes duration, A1C, hypertension, dyslipidemia, diabetes onset, and sex. Diabetes Care. 2007; 30(10):2523-8.
34. Salgado PP, Silva IN, Vieira EC, Simões e Silva AC Risk factors for early onset of diabetic nephropathy in pediatric type 1 diabetes. J Pediatr Endocrinol Metab. 2010; 23(12):1311-20.
35. Olsen BS, Johannesen J, Sjølie AK, Borch-Johnsen K, Hougarrdss P, Thorsteinsson B, et al. Metabolic control and prevalence of microvascular complications in young Danish patients with type 1 diabetes mellitus. Danish Study Group of Diabetes in Childhood. Diabet Med. 1999;16(1):79-85.
36. Harjutsalo V, Maric C, Forsblom C, Thorn L, Wadén J, Groop PH; FinnDiane Study Group. Sex-related differences in the long-term risk of microvascular complications by age at onset of type 1 diabetes. Diabetologia. 2011;54(8):1992-9.
37. The effect of intensive treatment of diabetes on the development and progression of long-term complications in insulin-dependent diabetes mellitus. The Diabetes Control and Complications Trial Research Group. N Engl J Med. 1993;329:977-86.
38. Bluestone JA, Herold K, Eisenbarth G. Genetics, pathogenesis and clinical interventions in type 1 diabetes. Nature. 2010;464:1293-300.

CHAPTER 24

Future Metabolic Risk among Subjects with Type 1 Diabetes Mellitus

SK Hammadur Rahaman, Mohd Ashraf Ganie

INTRODUCTION

Type 1 diabetes mellitus (T1DM) is classically described as absolute insulin deficiency secondary to autoimmune destruction of pancreatic β-cells. It affects mostly children and young adults. Usually, the disease presents with osmotic symptoms, weight loss, and/or diabetic ketoacidosis. The latter condition may sometimes be life-threatening. Subjects with T1DM are traditionally of low body mass index (BMI). Microangiopathic complications are fairly common while those of macrovascular and metabolic syndrome complications are less. With the pandemicity of obesity, T1DM subjects are not spared. The development of metabolic syndrome has been described in patients with T1DM as the disease progresses over time. Studies have shown 30–40% of T1DM are obese and satisfy the criteria of metabolic syndrome.[1,2]

DOUBLE DIABETES

Teupe and Bergis first coined the term 'double diabetes' in 1991. They observed that patients of T1DM with positive family history of type 2 diabetes mellitus (T2DM) tended to have more weight, obesity, and required higher insulin doses to achieve glycemic control.[3] This increased insulin requirement in this subgroup of T1DM was because of increased resistance to insulin mediated glucose disposal. Here, one must differentiate between double diabetes from accelerator hypothesis. Double diabetes is mere association of both T1DM and obesity/insulin resistance (IR), whereas accelerator hypothesis talks about increased BMI and IR as precipitating factors of autoimmune diabetes.[4]

There are several studies which showed clearly that patients with T1DM with positive family history of T2DM or IR were at significantly higher risk of developing both micro- and macrovascular complications. The European Diabetes Study Group which recruited 3,250 T1DM patients from 16 European countries showed higher risk of developing albuminuria in patients with positive family history of T2DM than those with negative family history [hazard ratio (HR) 1.36, p = 0.04].[5] Kilapatric et al.[6] studied whether IR and metabolic syndrome which are known risk factors for micro- and macrovascular complications in T2DM were also predictors of complications in T1DM patients participating in Diabetes Control and Complication Trial (DCCT). They found higher IR as estimated by estimated glucose disposal rate (eGDR) at baseline strongly predicted retinopathy, nephropathy, and cardiovascular disease (CVD) (HR 0.75, 0.88, and 0.70, respectively per mg/kg change p <0.001, p <0.005, p <0.002, respectively). Another study[7] involving 658 T1DM patients of whose family history (first degree) of T2DM was reported in 112 subjects and coronary artery disease (CAD) was in 119 subjects, found that the risk of having CAD was high in association with positive family history of T2DM (odds ratio 1.89, 95% CI 1.27-2.84). The authors concluded that presence of IR as evidenced by positive family history of T2DM was a risk factor for developing CAD in T1DM. These results relate that genetic IR in parents gets transmitted to type 1 diabetic offspring or shared parental-offspring lifestyle factors predisposing parents to T2DM and increasing the risk of metabolic complications in type 1 diabetic offspring.

ESTIMATED GLUCOSE DISPOSAL AND CARDIOVASCULAR DISEASE

The gold standard method of estimation of IR is hyperinsulinemic-euglycemic clamp technique. Due to invasiveness of hyperinsulinemic-euglycemic clamp study, people tried to use eGDR as a measure of IR. Estimated glucose disposal rate is derived from a 'best-fit' model:[8] eGDR = 24.31−12.22, waist-to-hip ratio (WHR) 3.29, (hypertension status) 0.57 glycosylated hemoglobin (HbA1c) where '0' for no hypertension and '1' for blood pressure (BP) more than 140/90 mmHg or antihypertensive drugs; HbA1c taken as value in %. Low eGDR represented as surrogate measure of IR both for clinical and epidemiological purposes.

Schauer et al.[9] studied 87 subjects (40 diabetics and 47 nondiabetics) to assess insulin action on peripheral glucose disposal and nonesterified fatty acid (NEFA) suppression as a marker of coronary artery calcification (CAC). Subjects of T1DM had poor peripheral blood glucose utilization rate compared to nondiabetic controls: glucose infusion rate (mg/kg fat-free mass/min) = 6.19 ± 0.72 versus 12.71 ± 0.66, mean ± SE, p <0.0001. Similarly, insulin induced NEFA suppression was lower in T1DM. There was also good correlation with lower glucose utilization and higher NEFA levels with CAC volume (r = -0.42, p <0.0001, and r = -0.41, p <0.0001, respectively) and these two parameters predicted the presence of CAC [odds ratio (OR) = 0.45, p = 0.03; OR = 2.4, p = 0.032, respectively] and indirectly CVD.

Orchard et al.[10] analyzed 10 year follow up data from the Pittsburgh Epidemiology of Diabetes Complications (EDC) study involving 603 T1DM patients. About 108 patients had CAD events during the 10 year follow up. The eGDR was inversely associated with CAD events. However, HbA1c was not associated with subsequent CAD events. In addition, they also showed conventional parameters of CAD like blood pressure, lipid levels, inflammatory markers, renal disease, and peripheral vascular disease independently associated with CAD in T1DM. Kalipatrick et al.[6] reported eGDR to be a significant predictor of CVD along with retinopathy and nephropathy in T1DM.

METABOLIC SYNDROME IN TYPE 1 DIABETES MELLITUS

The metabolic syndrome in adults is defined as constellation of some clinical and biochemical parameters that predicts the risk of having CVDs and development of diabetes. These risk factors include waist circumference, blood pressure, high density lipoprotein (HDL), triglycerides (TG), and fasting plasma glucose. There are clear cutoffs, although gender and ethnicity specific, for these parameters in at risk adults.[8] However, in children and adolescents, there are no such upper limits as the blood pressure, lipids, anthropometric parameters, and IR vary according to age and stages of puberty. Sex steroid surge during puberty causes significant changes in fat distribution causing increase in IR. Therefore, it is not possible to use single cutoff points to define abnormalities in children and adolescents. As a result, 90th, 95th, and 97th percentile values for age and sex are used as cutoffs. Again, there is no consensus on as to which level should be used for the criteria to define metabolic syndrome in children. Pittsburgh Epidemiology of Diabetes Complications cohort of T1DM study revealed variable prevalence of metabolic syndrome when different definitions were used.[11] It was 8%, 12%, and 21% according to International Diabetes Federation (IDF), National Center for Environmental Protection (NCEP), and World Health Organization (WHO) definitions, respectively. However, the prevalence of metabolic syndrome in T1DM in FinnDiane study was remarkably high 44%, 35%, and 36% using WHO, NCEP, and IDF definition, respectively.[12] An IDF defined criteria was used in DCCT/Epidemiology of Diabetes Interventions and Complications (EDIC) study where prevalence metabolic syndrome was 22%.[6]

TYPE 1 DIABETES MELLITUS AND CARDIOVASCULAR OUTCOME IN RELATION TO COMPONENTS OF METABOLIC SYNDROME

Pittsburgh EDC study[11] revealed that metabolic syndrome predicted adverse outcome in composite endpoint of CAD, renal failure, and diabetes related death [HR: NCEP = 5.8, (95% CI 3.9–8.6); WHO = 6.5, (95% CI 4.5–9.4). However, it could not predict better than its individual component (i.e., microalbuminuria = 6.3, (95% CI 3.8–10.5); BP = 4.5, (95% CI 3.1–6.6); triacylglycerol = 4.4, (95% CI 3.0–6.6). In FinnDiane study,[12] only WHO definition of metabolic syndrome predicted risk of cardiovascular events [HR 2.05, (95% CI 1.38–3.04)] in T1DM after adjustment for conventional risk factors and nephropathy, even in subjects with microalbuminuria [HR 1.44, (95% CI 1.06–1.96)]. The individual components of metabolic syndrome except for obesity also predicted cardiovascular events. In DCCT/EDIC study, type 1 diabetic patients were followed for 17 years but baseline metabolic syndrome could not predict any macro- or microvascular complications.

Therefore, in T1DM, the presence of metabolic syndrome, irrespective of its definition do not provide added risk of cardiovascular events over and above to its individual components.

TYPE 1 DIABETES MELLITUS AND LIPID HANDLING

Lack of physiological insulin secretion from pancreas in T1DM results decreased insulin in portal circulation. On top of this, exogenous insulin administration in subcutaneous tissues causes peripheral hyperinsulinemia. However, in subjects with metabolic syndrome or T2DM, there is endogenous hyperinsulinema characterized by significantly higher portal venous insulin compared to peripheral hyperinsulinemia. Both of these have significant effect on lipid metabolism. Hyperinsulinemia causes stimulation of sterol regulatory element binding protein 1c (SREBP1c) which promotes triacylglycerol accumulation in liver. Besides this, SREBP1c also activates fatty acid synthase and acetyl-coenzyme A carboxylase which are involved in *de novo* lipid synthesis. So, it is suggested that relative portal hypoinsulinemia in T1DM causes reduced fat accumulation in liver in contrast to nonalcoholic fatty liver disease or nonalcoholic steatohepatitis associated with T2DM or obesity. Perseghin et al.[13] studied 19 T1DM patients and 19 healthy matched subjects to assess insulin resistance alongwith whole body glucose metabolism, glucose and lipid oxidation, and intrahepatic lipid content by magnetic resonance spectroscopy. Insulin stimulated glucose clearance was significantly reduced in T1DM patients in comparison to controls (4.3 ± 1.3 vs. 6.0 ± 1.6 mL/kg/min; $p < 0.001$). Estimated portal venous insulin concentration was lower in diabetes group than the normal subjects. The intrahepatic fat content was significantly lower in diabetic group compared to controls (1.5 ± 0.7% and 2.2 ± 1.0%; $p < 0.03$) and favorably increased fasting lipid oxidation in diabetes group (1.5 ± 0.5 vs. 0.8 ± 0.4 mg/kg/min; $p < 0.01$). The reduced hepatic insulin concentration in T1DM promotes lipid oxidation in liver, resulting increased circulating NEFAs. This increased NEFA along with peripheral hyperinsulinemia from exogenous administration causes increased accumulation of lipid droplets in skeletal muscle causing peripheral insulin resistance similar to T2DM or metabolic syndrome subjects.[13,14] This is supported by Vethakkan et al. who demonstrated endogenous insulin secretion post-islet transplantation in liver normalized abnormal NEFA dynamics after 2-hour oral glucose tolerance test.[15] Thus, factors like abdominal adiposity, increased NEFA, increased exogenous insulin requirement predispose T1DM subjects to have more IR. This abnormal fat distribution may also result in accumulation of fat in epicardial and perivascular areas which are related to CVD. The correlation among epicardial adipose tissue (EAT) thickness, WHR, and eGDR was studied by Yazici et al.[16] in 36 T1DM patients and 43 matched healthy controls. Epicardial adipose tissue thickness measured by echocardiography was significantly higher in T1DM patients than controls (3.30 ± 1.06 vs. 2.30 ± 0.34 mm, $p < 0.0001$). There was positive correlation of EAT thickness with age, WHR, and daily insulin dose/kg body weight and negative correlation with eGDR.

It is well-known that high density lipoprotein-cholesterol (HDL-C) is higher in T1DM subjects with good glycemic control than in T2DM subjects. This is because of increased lipoprotein lipase in presence of peripheral hyperinsulinemia and reduced activity of hepatic lipase as a result of low portal venous insulin concentration. Type 2 diabetes mellitus subjects with increased portal hyperinsulinemia are associated with low HDL-C levels. When route of insulin administration is changed from subcutaneous to intraperitoneal, increased hepatic insulin exposure reversed the lipid parameters in T1DM[17] when T1DM subjects gained obesity and IR resulting in double diabetes because of lifestyle factors, or genetic predisposition or increased insulin dose for strict glycemic control, this atheroprotective high HDL-C was reduced and more atherogenic lipid profile emerged.[18]

TYPE 1 DIABETES MELLITUS, PROINFLAMMATORY CYTOKINE, AND METABOLIC SYNDROME

Adipose tissue is now considered as an endocrine organ because of its immense capacity for secreting variety of cytokines involved in cellular metabolism and inflammation. Tumor necrosis factor (TNF)-α and interleukin (IL)-6 impair insulin signaling by reduced expression of insulin receptor substrate 1.[19] Tumor necrosis factor-α plays an important role in linking obesity, inflammation, and IR. Free fatty acid impairs insulin mediated glucose uptake. The only adipocytokine favoring insulin mediated glucose uptake, reducing IR, and favoring lipid metabolism is reduced in obesity. It also has anti-inflammatory action.[20] Another adipokine, leptin, also catabolizes free fatty acids, reduces TG synthesis, and improves insulin sensitivity in both skeletal muscle and liver. However, there is leptin resistance in obesity.[21]

This altered adipocytokine profile in patients with metabolic syndrome is irrespective of presence of diabetes mellitus and type of diabetes mellitus. Timar et al.[22] studied T1DM patients with metabolic syndrome[22] and without metabolic syndrome (using American Heart Association and the National Heart, Lung, and Blood Institute 2009 criteria). They found significantly higher level of leptin (11.23 ± 2.37 vs. 7.36 ± 3.22 ng/mL, p <0.0001), TNF-α (7.5 ± 1.82 vs. 5.36 ± 1.89 pg/mL, p <0.0001), IL-6 (4.32 ± 0.84 vs. 3.36 ± 0.89 pg/mL, p <0.0001) and daily insulin doses, (0.93 ± 0.24 vs. 0.66 ± 0.12 IU/kg, p <0.001) and significantly lower level of adiponectin (7.64 ± 2.56 vs. 12.58 ± 4.73 µg/mL, p <0.0001) and eGDR (7.22 ± 1.91 vs. 8.13 ± 1.61, p = 0.037) in metabolic syndrome groups than absent metabolic syndrome groups. The higher IR as estimated by eGDR at baseline strongly predicted retinopathy, microalbuminuria, and CVD.

TYPE 1 DIABETES MELLITUS AND POLYCYSTIC OVARIAN SYNDROME

The most common endocrine disorder in adolescent and adult premenopausal women is polycystic ovarian syndrome (PCOS) with a prevalence of 6–15% worldwide.[23] In a meta-analysis of 475 adolescent and young women with T1DM, Escobar-Morreale et al.[24] found 24% (95% CI 15–34) pooled prevalence of PCOS which is clearly higher than general population. Patients with PCOS are at increased risk of having IR, T2DM, dyslipidemia, and hypertension, and as a consequence micro-and macrovascular complications. In one study, it was revealed that T1DM patients with intensive insulin regime had significantly higher prevalence of PCOS than those with two doses of insulin.[25] Figure 1 depicts how IR, altered adipocytokine profiles,

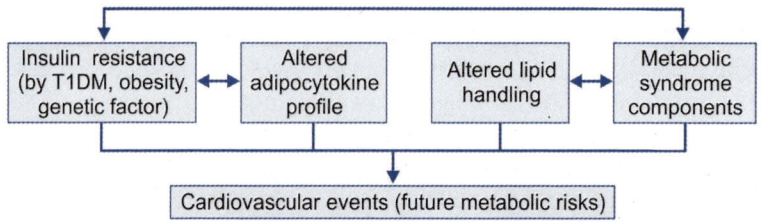

Fig. 1: Showing the factors involved in the pathogenesis of future metabolic risk in type 1 diabetes mellitus.

abnormal lipid metabolism, and components of metabolic syndrome are interrelated and progress to future metabolic risk in T1DM.

CONCLUSION

Type 1 diabetes mellitus subjects, who tend to be obese are at equal risk of having metabolic complications as subjects without T1DM. Individuals having T1DM with positive family history of obesity and T2DM, are at increased risk of being overweight and obese. Besides, they have more IR and low insulin mediated glucose disposal, high normal blood pressure, and low HDL-C. Obesity, IR, altered adipocytokine profile, and altered lipid handling in individuals with T1DM may attenuate the vascular benefit of glycemic control in long run, predisposing them to future micro- and macrovascular complications.

REFERENCES

1. Chillarón JJ, Flores-Le-Roux JA, Goday A, Benaiges D, Carrera MJ, Puig J, et al. Metabolic syndrome and type-1 diabetes mellitus: prevalence and associated factors. Rev Esp Cardiol. 2010;63(4):423-9.
2. Thorn LM, Forsblom C, Fagerudd J, Thomas MC, Pettersson-Fernholm K, Saraheimo M, et al. Metabolic syndrome in type 1 diabetes: association with diabetic nephropathy and glycemic control (the FinnDiane study). Diabetes Care. 2005;28:2019-24.
3. Teupe B, Bergis K. Epidemiological evidence for "double diabetes". Lancet. 1991;337:361-2.
4. Wilkin TJ. The accelerator hypothesis: a review of the evidence for insulin resistance as the basis for type 1 as well as type II diabetes. Int J Obes. 2009;33:716-26.
5. Roglic G, Colhoun HM, Stevens LK, Lemkes HH, Manes C, Fuller JH. Parental history of hypertension and parental history of diabetes and microvascular complications in insulin-dependent diabetes mellitus: the EURODIAB IDDM Complications Study. Diabet Med. 1998;15:418-26.
6. Kilpatrick ES, Rigby AS, Atkin SL. Insulin resistance, the metabolic syndrome, and complication risk in type 1 diabetes: "double diabetes" in the Diabetes Control and Complications Trial. Diabetes Care. 2007;30(3):707-12.
7. Erbey JR, Kuller LH, Becker DJ, Orchard TJ. The association between a family history of type 2 diabetes and coronary artery disease in a type 1 diabetes population. Diabetes Care. 1998;21:610-4.
8. Alberti KG, Zimmet P, Shaw J. Metabolic syndrome –a new world-wide definition. A Consensus Statement from the International Diabetes Federation. Diabet Med. 2006:23:469-80
9. Schauer IE, Snell-Bergeon JK, Bergman BC, Maahs DM, Kretowski A, Eckel RH, et al. Insulin resistance, defective insulin-mediated fatty acid suppression, and coronary artery calcification in subjects with and without type 1 diabetes: The CACTI study. Diabetes. 2011;60:306-14.
10. Orchard TJ, Olson JC, Erbey JR, Williams K, Forrest KY, Smithline Kinder L, et al. Insulin resistance related factors, but not glycemia, predict coronary artery disease in type 1 diabetes. Diabetes Care. 2003;26:1374-9.
11. Pambianco G, Costacou T, Orchard TJ. The prediction of major outcomes of type 1 diabetes: a 12-year prospective evaluation of three separate definitions of the metabolic syndrome and their components and estimated glucose disposal rate: the Pittsburgh Epidemiology of Diabetes Complications Study experience. Diabetes Care. 2007;30:1248-54.
12. Thorn LM, Forsblom C, Fagerudd J, Thomas MC, Pettersson-Fernholm K, Saraheimo M, et al.; the FinnDiane Study Group. Metabolic syndrome in type 1 diabetes association with diabetic nephropathy and glycemic control (the FinnDiane Study). Diabetes Care. 2005;28:2019-24.
13. Perseghin G, Lattuanda G, De Cobelli F, Esposito A, Costantino F, Canu T, et al. Reduced intrahepatic fat content is associated with increased whole-body lipid oxidation in patients with type 1 diabetes. Diabetologia. 2005;48:2615-21.
14. Heptulla RA, Stewart A, Enocksson S, Rife F, Ma TY, Sherwin RS, et al. In situ evidence that peripheral insulin resistance in adolescents with poorly controlled type 1 diabetes is associated with impaired suppression of lipolysis: a microdialysis study. Pediatr Res. 2003;53:830-5.
15. Vethakkan SR, Walters JM, Gooley JL, Boston RC, Kay TW, Goodman DJ, et al. Normalized NEFA dynamics during an OGTT after islet transplantation. Transplantation. 2012;94:e49-51.

16. Yazici D, Ozben B, Yavuz D, Deyneli O, Aydın H, Tarcin Ö, et al. Epicardial adipose thickness in type 1 diabetic patients. Endocrine. 2011;40:250-5.
17. Ruotolo G, Parlavecchia M, Taskinen MR, Galimberti G, Zoppo A, Le NA, et al. Normalization of lipoprotein composition by intraperitoneal insulin in IDDM. Role of increased hepatic lipase activity. Diabetes Care. 1994;17:6-12.
18. Sibley SD, Palmer JP, Hirsch IB, Brunzell J. Visceral obesity, hepatic lipase activity, and dyslipidaemia in type 1 diabetes. J Clin Endocrinol Metab. 2003;88:3379-84.
19. Hotamisligil GS. Inflammation and metabolic disorders. Nature. 2006;444:860-7.
20. Weyer C, Funahashi T, Tanaka S, Hotta K, Matsuzawa Y, Pratley RE, et al. Hypoadiponectinemia in obesity and type 2 diabetes: close association with insulin resistance and hyperinsulinemia. J Clin Endocrinol Metab. 2001;86:1930-5.
21. Havel PJ. Control of energy homeostasis and insulin action by adipocyte hormones: leptin, acylation stimulating protein, and adiponectin. Curr Opin Lipidol. 2002;13:51-9.
22. Timar R, Timar B, Degeratu D, Serafinceanu C, Oancea C. Metabolic syndrome, adiponectin and proinflammatory status in patients with type 1 diabetes mellitus.J Int Med Res. 2014 Oct;42(5):1131-8.
23. Asuncion M, Calvo RM, SanMillan JL, Sancho J, Avila S, Escobar-Morreale HF. A prospective study of the prevalence of the polycystic ovary syndrome in unselected Caucasian women from Spain. J Clin Endocrinol Metab. 2000;85:2434-8.
24. Escobar-Morreale HF, Roldán-Martín MB. Type 1 diabetes and polycystic ovary syndrome: systematic review and meta-analysis. Diabetes Care. 2016;39(4):639-48.
25. Codner E, Soto N, Lopez P, Trejo L, Avila A, Eyzaguirre FC, et al. Diagnostic criteria for polycystic ovary syndrome and ovar- ian morphology in women with type 1 diabetes mellitus. J Clin Endocrinol Metab. 2006;91:2250-6.

SECTION 7

Special Situations

Editor

Nikhil Tandon

CHAPTER 25

Sick Day Management

Banshi D Saboo

INTRODUCTION

Diabetes is fast gaining the status of a potential epidemic in India with more than 69 million diabetic individuals currently diagnosed with the disease. Having diabetes which is under control, especially does not mean that one is likely to fall ill more often than anyone else. However, there are some precautions one should take when one is sick in order to avoid acute complications of diabetes. Any kind of sickness, simple like cold, flu, sore throat, and infections of ear, teeth, or bladder, gastroenteritis, or more serious illnesses like pneumonia or a foot infection can affect diabetes. Any acute illness or infection can alter blood glucose levels in many ways. An infection or illness can lead to high blood sugar levels or appearance of ketones even when the child is eating less. It can also lead to hypoglycemia or low blood sugar levels. All these changes mean that diabetes is more difficult to control when one is sick. These changes in blood sugar levels if detected early and managed properly along with acute illness can prevent acute complications and hospitalization.[1-4]

REASONS OF HIGH BLOOD SUGAR LEVELS

Many illness or infections especially those associated with fever can cause high blood glucose levels. Any type of illness, infection, surgery, dental problem, or injury can cause stress to body. To "fight" this stress, body needs more energy and for that it releases hormones (they are called "counterregulatory hormones"). These hormones lead to gluconeogenesis and release of extra glucose from liver to provide with the energy. These hormones also inhibit the effect of insulin which means a person having any infection may become somewhat insulin resistant. As a result, blood glucose rises. Whenever there are constantly high blood sugar levels, it adds to the infection, delays healing, and the vicious cycle begins.

SECTION 7: Special Situations

REASONS OF LOW BLOOD GLUCOSE LEVELS

Gastrointestinal symptoms like diarrhea and vomiting associated with any illness may lead to hypoglycemia due to decreased food intake, poor absorption of food, and changes in intestinal motility. In such cases, ketones are produced by the liver from free fatty acids that are mobilized as an alternative energy source when there is lack of glucose for intracellular metabolism. These ketones accumulate because of increased lipolysis, increased ketogenesis, and decreased ketone body utilization leading to ketoacidosis.[5]

During any acute illness children or people with diabetes face four main risk factors:
1. High blood sugar levels or hyperglycemia
2. Diabetic ketoacidosis
3. Dehydration
4. Low blood sugar levels or hypoglycemia.

MANAGING BLOOD GLUCOSE LEVELS DURING SICKNESS

Check sugars more often, at least 3–4 hours (and more frequently if glucose level fluctuates) and test your urine for ketones 1–2 times per day. Blood sugar should be less than 200 mg/dL. Whenever you visit any doctor, you must tell him or her about your diabetes. Recent record of blood sugar levels, medicines, temperature, and weight helps the doctor to give appropriate advice.[6] It is strongly recommended that some form of ketone testing be available, and urine strips are a relatively cheap investment. However, in some circumstances, no ketone testing may be available or affordable. In these situations, it must be emphasized that during intercurrent infections, blood glucose testing remains very important in helping to avoid worsening ketoacidosis and hospital admission. In practice, most patients depend on the less reliable urine ketone tests as the blood ketone strips are costly. Urine strips measure acetoacetate while blood strips measure beta-hydroxybutyrate. In acute ketoacidosis, the ketone body ratio rises from normal (1:1) to 10:1 or more. Blood beta-hydroxybutyrate more than 0.5 mmol/L is abnormal in children with diabetes.[7]

Diet during Sickness

To avoid dehydration and hypoglycemia when you are ill, it is very important to keep up your fluid and carbohydrate intake. Replacing meals with easily digestible food and sugar containing fluids provides energy (carbohydrates) and may help prevent further ketosis. If you are able to eat normally, do so and sip extra fluids each hour, about one-half to three-fourth cup, a little less for children. To prevent dehydration, drink unsweetened fluids such as water, diet soft drinks, diet cordial, weak tea, or broth. If you can not eat normally, have some easy to manage carbohydrate drinks, snacks, or small meals. Maintaining water and electrolyte balance is very important so as to avoid the precipitating factors for diabetic ketoacidosis (DKA). In conditions like diarrhea and vomiting, one should increase intake of salt and water, clear broths, soups, etc. Other essential sick day supplements include sweets, candies, jellies, glucose tablets, dry fruits, and sugar containing drinks like juices and colas.

If appetite is decreased or in cases of hypoglycemia blood glucose levels need to be elevated to a normal level. This is achieved by feeding the child with rapid-acting carbohydrates such as sweetened drinks, fruit juices, and glucose-containing sweets.[8,9]

Insulin during Sickness

The most common mistake made with caregivers who are unfamiliar with diabetes is to stop insulin as the child is not eating, which in turn increases the risk of DKA. Insulin is needed during fasting as well, and its requirement increases during illness, thus needing more frequent monitoring of blood glucose and ketones. Never omit your insulin. If you are on other medicines, consult your doctor as to what to do when you are sick: certain medicines should not be taken if you become dehydrated due to vomiting or diarrhea. Illnesses such as infections or fever can cause your blood sugars to increase. This may even last for a few days after you are feeling better. Decreased appetite, vomiting, and/or diarrhea may lower blood sugar levels but you will still need some insulin. Left untreated, illness and high blood sugars can quickly cause a serious and life threatening condition called DKA. Rest and stay warm. Do not exercise vigorously as physical activity can increase blood sugar and ketone levels. You may need to see a doctor to diagnose your illness and help you with treatment.

Ideally the type of insulin treatment is chosen according to the child's lifestyle. The treatment can include one, two, or more injections per day. Different types of insulin are: short-acting (duration 3-8 h), intermediate/long-acting (duration 10-18 h), and new, very long-acting insulins (duration up to 24 h). Additional doses of short/rapid-acting insulin are required with careful monitoring to reduce blood glucose in order to prevent ketoacidosis, and avoid hospital admission. The dose and frequency of insulin injection will depend on the level and duration of hyperglycemia as well as the severity of ketosis. When only hyperglycemia is there with no or small ketones; it is recommended to give an additional 5-10% of total daily dose (basal plus bolus together) approximately 0.05-0.1 U/kg short/rapid-acting insulin to be given on urgent basis and this can be repeated every 2-4 hours based on blood glucose values. When hyperglycemia is associated with moderate to high ketonuria; the recommendation is to give an additional 10-20% of total daily dose (basal plus bolus together) approximately 0.1 U/kg short/rapid-acting insulin. This can be repeated every 2-4 hours based on blood glucose values.[10,11]

The general recommendation for additional dose is of 0.05-0.1 U/kg for children with standard insulin requirements of approximately 1 U/kg/day.

However, for children who have low requirements or adolescents with insulin resistance and high insulin requirements the percentage calculations should be used rather than the 0.1 U/kg empiric additional dose. During illness it also may be necessary to increase basal insulin doses whether by multiple injection therapy or when using an insulin pump. With a pump, temporary basal rate increases of 20% to as high as 50 or 100% may be used until the blood glucose begins to normalize and the ketones clear based upon ongoing blood glucose, ketone monitoring, and clinical response. If you are an insulin pump user and are finding that you are having to do repeated correction doses when you are ill, you should consider temporarily increasing your basal rate by 30% and continue to test blood glucose every 2 hours (Table 1).

TABLE 1: Calculating extra insulin on sick days

Ketones		Blood glucose values (mg/dL)					Comments
Blood ketones (mmol/L)	Urinary ketones	<100	100–180	180–250	250–400	>400	
<0.6	–ve/Trace	No extra insulin/ mini dose glucagon	No action needed	Increase insulin for next meal if BG is high	Give extra 5% of TDD or 0.05 U/kg	Give extra 10% of TDD or 0.1 U/kg	Monitor BG and Ketones in two hours
0.6–0.9	Trace/small	Extra carbohydrate and fluids to be given	Extra carbohydrate and fluids to be given	Give extra 5% of TDD or 0.05 U/kg	Give extra 5–10% of TDD or 0.05–0.1 U/kg.	Give extra 10% of TDD or 0.1 U/kg	Repeat if needed
1.0–1.4	Small/moderate	Extra carbohydrate and fluids to be given	Extra carbohydrate and fluids to be given	Give extra 5–10% of TDD or 0.05–0.1 U/kg.	Give extra 10% of TDD or 0.1 U/kg	Give extra 10% of TDD or 0.1 U/kg	Repeat if needed
1.5–2.9	Moderate/large	Extra carbohydrate and fluids to be given	Extra carbohydrate and fluids to be given Give extra 5% of TDD or 0.05 U/kg	Give extra 10% of TDD or 0.1 U/kg	Give extra 10–20% of TDD or 0.1 U/kg.	Give extra 10–20% of TDD or 0.1 U/kg	Repeat dose after 2 hours if ketones do not decrease
>3.0	Large	Extra carbohydrate and fluids to be given	Extra carbohydrate and fluids to be given Give extra 5% of TDD or 0.05 U/kg	Extra carbohydrate and fluids to be given plus 10% of TDD or 0.1 U/kg	Give extra 10–20% of TDD or 0.1 U/kg	Give extra 10–20% of TDD or 0.1 U/kg	Repeat dose after 2 hours if ketones do not decrease. These patients are at immediate risk of ketoacidosis and should be evaluated in an emergency department

CHAPTER 25: Sick Day Management

Treatment of the underlying illness is necessary as it would be for a child or adolescent without diabetes (i.e., antibiotics for bacterial infections but not viral infections). Clinical manifestations of the underlying illness may be complicated in diabetes patients. Treating fever, malaise, and headache with antipyretics or pain medications such as paracetamol, acetaminophen, or ibuprofen is acceptable but not mandatory. Consult your doctor for sugar-free over-the-counter drugs for treatment of symptoms like cough and nasal congestion. Mention your diabetes, as well as any other conditions you may have (high blood pressure etc.) and any other medications (prescription and over-the-counter) that you are currently taking. Do not take any nonprescription medicines without consulting your doctor. Vomiting may be caused by the illness itself (i.e., gastroenteritis, unclean food or food poisoning, surgical condition, or other illness), resulting in low blood glucose levels, and lack of insulin resulting in high blood glucose and ketosis. If food poisoning is suspected, the treatment of vomiting with single injection or rectal administration of anti-emetics to help oral intake of carbohydrate is accepted. However, in the case of high blood glucose and an excess of ketones, priority should be given to administering extra insulin as well as sufficient salt and water solutions. In this situation, the vomiting often stops once extra insulin has been given to reverse ketosis.

A sick day kit should include:
- Sick day plan
- For monitoring: Thermometer, blood glucose monitor/meter, lancets and strips, ketone testing strips (blood or urine)
- For hygiene: Hand sanitizer
- For management:
  o Sugar-free and regular pop such as ginger ale, soups
  o Insulin (rapid or short-acting insulin) and insulin supplies
  o Glucagon (ask your doctor for a prescription)
  o Some over the counter medicines for general ailments: Like acetaminophen, sugar-free cough drops and syrup, dimenhydrinate, loperamide, glucose or dextrose tablets, etc.

Sick day plan should include:
- To test blood sugar levels every 2 hours (levels to be kept 100–160 mg/dL)
- Insulin dose adjustment guide
- Sick day meal (optimal proportion of carbohydrate/fat)
- Ketone testing every 4 hours
- Temperature monitoring every 3 hours
- To limit physical activity
- Some over-the-counter medicines for immediate care
- Seek immediate medical attention if there are symptoms of diabetic ketoacidosis.

Call doctor when blood sugar is more than 200 mg/dL for more than 3–4 hours.

Important phone numbers	
Family Member: _____	Friend: _____
Diabetes Educator: _____	Doctor: _____

Some guidelines to be followed:
- Create a "sick day plan" to help you keep track of everything when you are sick which would include; the doctor's guidelines including when to call, your diabetes care team's daytime and after-hours phone numbers, sick-day meal plans, list of over-the-counter medicines that do not interfere with insulin or blood glucose levels, record of blood glucose readings, insulin dosages, and carbohydrate counts of foods eaten
- Blood sugar levels to be checked every 4 hours
- In case of type 1 diabetes, check for ketone bodies and sugar levels above 240 mg/dL. Ketones are a form of waste that people with type 1 make when they are under stress (like an illness). Consult the doctor if in doubt
- Check your temperature regularly. If you are losing weight and your temperature, breathing rate, and pulse are increasing, contact a doctor. You may be getting worse
- Drink liquids if you are unable to eat. Have one cup of liquid every hour while you are awake to prevent dehydration. If you are unable to take liquids you may need to go to the emergency room or hospital
- Do not miss your insulin dose. You may need to eat or drink something with sugar so that your blood sugar does not drop too low in case if you cannot eat anything solid
- Rest and do not exercise
- Consult your doctor for sugar-free over-the-counter drugs for treatment of symptoms like cough and nasal congestion. Do not take any nonprescription medicines without talking with your doctor.

Additional care is required for sick children:
- They are likely to need extra insulin
- They will need to check blood glucose as often as every 2–3 hours
- They will need to check blood or urine ketones as often as every 4 hours
- They should drink lots of clear liquids—no caffeine
- They should continue taking regular medicine.

Consult a doctor if the child has:
- Had a fever for two days
- Been vomiting or having diarrhea for 6 hours
- Unable to take liquid, even in small amount
- High blood sugar levels
- Moderate or large urine ketones
- Symptoms of dehydration or ketoacidosis including in difficulty breathing, chest pains, fruity smelling breath, or dry lips.

CONCLUSION

In any underlying illness metabolic derangement should be identified and treated appropriately. Some people may be at risk of hypoglycaemia rather hyperglycaemia and or associated dehydration. Prevention of ketoacidosis should be the key. In order to provide optimum healthcare, the facility should have updated sick day management information, telephonic consultation, emergency transportation, laboratory and bedside blood glucose, blood ketones urinary ketones monitoring & supplies, intravenous fluids, surgical and intensive care support.

REFERENCES

1. IDF Diabetes Atals. Seventh Edition. 2015.
2. Joshi SR, Parikh RM. India—diabetes capital of the world: now heading towards hypertension. J Assoc Physicians India. 2007;55:323-4.
3. Kumar A, Goel MK, Jain RB, Khanna P, Chaudhary V. India towards diabetes control: Key issues. Australas Med J. 2013;6:524-31.
4. Muller LM, Gorter KJ, Hak E, Goudzwaard WL, Schellevis FG, Hoepelman IM. Increased risk of infection in patients with diabetes mellitus type 1 or 2. Ned Tijdschr Geneeskd. 2006:150:549-53.
5. ISPAE. (2011). Diabetic Ketoacidosis. Clinical PracticeGuidelines. [Online] Available from: http://www.ispae.org.in/download_docs/Diabetes_guideline_for_Web.pdf [Accessed March, 2017].
6. ISPAE. (2011). Sick Day Management. Clinical Practice Guidelines. [Online] Available from: http://www.ispae.org.in/download docs/Diabetes_guideline_for_Web.pdf [Accessed March, 2017]
7. Laffel LM, Wentzell K, Loughlin C, Tovar A, Moltz K, Brink S. Sick day management using blood 3 hydroxybutyrate compared with urine ketone monitoring reduces hospital visits in young people with T1DM: a randomized clinical trial. Diabet Med.2006:23: 278-84.
8. American Diabetes Association. Living With Diabetes: Sick Days. [online] Available from: http://www.diabetes.org/living-withdiabetes/parents-and-kids/everyday-life/sick-days.html. [Accessed March, 2017].
9. American Diabetes Association. Living with Diabetes: When You're Sick. [online] Available from: http://www.diabetes.org/livingwith-diabetes/treatment-and-care/whos-on-your-health-care-team/when-youre-sick.html. [Accessed March, 2017].
10. Stuart J. Brink, Lori Laffel et al. Sick Day Management. Global IDF/ISPAD Guideline for Diabetes in Childhood and Adolescence. IDF 2011;91-7.
11. Brink S, Laffel L, Likitmaskul S, Liu L, Maguire AM, Olsen B, et al. Sick day management in children and adolescents with diabetes. Pediatric Diabetes. 2009;10 (Suppl. 12):146-53.

CHAPTER 26

Managing Diabetes in Neonates and Toddlers

Aashima Dabas, Rajesh Khadgawat

INTRODUCTION

Type 1 diabetes mellitus (T1DM) is a common endocrine illness in childhood which has shown increasing trends in incidence over last few years.[1] Of interest is the alarming increase in incidence of T1DM in preschool age group.[1] The incidence of T1DM in children younger than 2 years of age in United Kingdom is about 1:15,000. The proportion of children with diabetes, younger than 2 years of age was approximately 4% among total children with diabetes.[2]

Neonatal diabetes mellitus (NDM) has emerged as a distinct subgroup of diabetes which unlike T1DM, is not linked to autoimmunity. Neonatal diabetes mellitus will be discussed separately in the chapter, followed by diabetes in toddlers.

NEONATAL DIABETES MELLITUS

Neonatal diabetes mellitus is recognized as diabetes presenting in initial few months of life, generally first 6 months of life, though some authors agree to 9 months as age limit.[3] The disease occurs due to single gene defect involving the β-cell structure or function. Thus, it is distinct from T1DM as is not associated with autoimmunity. The term 'monogenic diabetes of infancy' has been thus suggested. It may be classified as transient or permanent, depending on whether symptoms get resolve or persist after 18 months of birth.[4] Neonatal diabetes mellitus has an incidence of 1 in 300,000 to 500,000 live births, and approximately over half (57%) of the cases are transient [transient neonatal diabetes mellitus (TNDM)].[5] Data from India is limited and the incidence of TNDM was reported as only 5% from Chennai.[6]

Genetic Basis

The insulin release from β-cells is governed by adenosine triphosphate (ATP)-sensitive potassium (K-ATP) channels over the surface. These channels consist of an octameric assembly of four pore-forming Kir and four regulatory sulfonylurea receptor (SUR) subunits. *KCNJ11* gene encodes Kir6.2, the pore-forming subunit of the K-ATP channel and *ABCC8* gene codes for SUR. The most common genetic locus which cause the disease are heterozygous gain-of function mutations in *KCNJ11*, seen in 30% cases, followed by mutations in insulin gene (*INS*) (20%), *ABCC8* (19%), and *GCK* (4%). In addition, there are few other genetic loci which are implicated in syndromic associations of NDM like *FOXP3, PTF1A, GLIS3, NEUROD1, RFX6, EIF2AK3, GATA6, SLC19A2, HNF1B, PAX6,* and *WFS1*.[7] All mutations associated with NDM are heterozygous.

The mutations in *KCNJ11* gene manifest in heterozygous state. Thus, the ATP sensitivity of any individual potassium channel in a population depends on the number of mutant subunits it contains and the extent to which each subunit contributes to the overall ATP sensitivity. There are various polymorphisms which exist for Kir6.2 mutations which determine the clinical severity of diabetes. The K-ATP channels mediate potassium efflux which maintains the hyperpolarized state of cell membrane of β-cells and keeps the calcium channels closed. Increase in blood glucose levels increases cytosolic nucleotide concentration to cause closure of K-ATP channels which in turn leads to opening of calcium channels. The increase in cytosolic calcium triggers exocytosis of insulin from β-cells which regulates blood glucose. The K-ATP channel closure is thus the central step in glucose-stimulated insulin release. The K-ATP channels are also the target for sulfonylurea drugs which are commonly used to treat type 2 diabetes mellitus (T2DM). These drugs act by stimulating closure of K-ATP channel to cause insulin release. Apart from the role of K-ATP channels in islet cells, these channels also mediate glucagon-like peptide-1 secretion from intestinal L-cells, glucose uptake in skeletal muscle, and counter-regulatory response to glucose via effects on hypothalamic neurons. Under physiological conditions, the activity of K-ATP channel is determined by the balance between ATP, which blocks the channel, and MgADP, which reverses channel inhibition by ATP. Their role in NDM is confirmed by studies on genetically modified mice which have shown that targeted overactivity of K-ATP channels induces profound NDM whereas their targeted suppression leads to hyperinsulinism.[8] Few forms of Kir6.2 mutations can cause transient NDM due to partial compensation by β-cells or increase in turnover in β-cells.[8]

The other subunit which forms part of K-ATP channels assembly is SUR encoded by *ABCC8* gene.[9] Mutations in this locus are also detected in neonates with transient diabetes mellitus (TDM) and permanent diabetes mellitus. A higher prevalence of Kir6.2 mutations are reported in PND while SUR mutations may be seen in both PND and TND.

The second most common cause of PNDM is heterozygous autosomal dominantly inherited mutations in the *INS*.[10] *INS* mutations may also be found in patients with a diagnosis of type 1B (antibody-negative) diabetes and in a few patients with maturity onset of diabetes in the young subtype. Certain mutations which are recessively inherited can also cause large deletions in *INS* gene and result in complete insulin deficiency. Children who inherit *INS* mutations from their fathers have an earlier onset of disease than those who inherit from their mothers, suggesting the preferential silencing of maternally inherited mutant allele by imprinting effects at the *INS-IGF2* locus.[10]

The genetic basis for TNDM has been related to overexpression of associated paternally imprinted genes at chromosome 6q24. This is due to uniparental paternal disomy, a paternally inherited duplication causing relaxation of genomically imprinted *ZAC1* (zinc-finger protein 1 regulating apoptosis and cell cycle arrest) or a maternal methylation defect, such as from recessive mutations in *ZFP57*.[5,10]

Clinical Features

Around 80% of children with PNDM will manifest with hyperglycemia in first 6 weeks of life. Most of them also have ketoacidosis. The mean age of diagnosis from India was 3.75 months and 67–83% neonates had ketoacidosis at presentation.[6] However, children with NDM due to glucokinase mutations or pancreatic aplasia due to homozygous *IPF1* mutations have a more severe insulin deficiency, with lower birth weight and a younger age at diagnosis.[4] Neonates with transient diabetes mellitus may have severe intrauterine growth restriction. This form, being transient, will usually resolve over next few months of life, but carries a high propensity to recur again in adolescence.

Some neonates may present with developmental delay, muscle weakness, and epilepsy, which are associated with some Kir6.2 mutations. The neurological features are consistent with the tissue distribution of Kir6.2 in muscle, nerve, and brain, proposing this occurrence as a syndrome of developmental delay, epilepsy, and neonatal diabetes (DEND) syndrome.[8] A milder phenotype may occur where patients manifest with motor delay but no epilepsy. Certain subtypes associated with *ABCC8* mutations also manifest with developmental delay and dyspraxia. Table 1 enlists the genotypic and phenotypic correlations of syndromes associated with NDM. A close follow-up is advised for neonates who outgrow of their transient diabetic state as they are more prone to develop T2DM later in life.[6] Data from India found Wolcott Rallison syndrome (NDM with liver/renal failure, epiphyseal dysgenesis, growth failure, and hypothyroidism) as most common type of monogenic diabetes.[6] These neonates also had greater risk of mortality. The mortality reported among NDM varies from 16–32%, being higher in developing countries. Few causes attributed to mortality include cerebral edema, sepsis, acute respiratory distress syndrome, disseminated intravascular coagulation, hypoglycemia, refractory cardiac failure, septic shock, renal failure, and hepatic failure.

Investigations

The diagnosis of NDM is based on evidence of persistent hyperglycemia (plasma glucose concentration >150–200 mg/dL) in infants younger than age 6 months. Autoantibodies are generally negative in NDM, except mutations caused by *FOX3* gene resulting in immuno-dysregulation polyendocrinopathy enteropathy X-linked syndrome (IPEX).[3,10] Other typical laboratory findings of diabetes mellitus (e.g., glucosuria, ketonuria, hyperketonemia) may be present. The measurement of glycosylated hemoglobin (HbA1c) is not suitable for diagnosing diabetes mellitus in infants younger than age 6 months because of the higher proportion of fetal hemoglobin compared to hemoglobin A. Thus, these neonates need to be monitored with premeal blood glucose. Imaging of the pancreas with ultrasound, computed tomography, or magnetic resonance imaging may be done to determine its presence and size.

Genetic testing would confirm the genetic defect. The most common mutation to be tested is K-ATP channel defect followed by *INS* gene. The other specific loci should be ordered depending on clinical phenotype.

Therapy

Parental support and counseling is of chief concern in this age as they need to cope up with the child's disease. The physician should encourage sharing of disease responsibility among the parents and family. Calorie and glucose restriction at this age is strongly discouraged as infancy is the most crucial period to grow and most children with NDM are growth restricted.

During acute decompensation, neonates with diabetes may require more fluids for restoration of body hydration than an older child. This is because they have larger proportion of body as water. Insulin is required in infants for control of hyperglycemia and prevention of further complications. The initial choice of insulin would be intermediate or long-acting insulin, while short or rapid insulin is avoided in view of risk of hypoglycemia. The starting dose could be as little as 0.35–0.5 U/kg/day. In early life when the baby is on predominant breastfeeds, a single basal insulin dose would suffice. Later as the child grows up and develops meal timings, small premeal insulin can be administered as bolus. Insulin dosage needs close titration to prevent hypoglycemia as that is detrimental to the growing brain. Insulin pens which dispense 0.5 units of insulin may be preferred. Continuous subcutaneous insulin is emerging as a safer and better alternative even in this age group. It carries a significant advantage of delivering very small doses of both bolus and basal accurately.

Sulfonylurea group of drugs is the promising alternative to insulin therapy in NDM which results due to mutations in K-ATP channels. The SUR1-selective sulfonylurea (gliclazide and tolbutamide) close the islet cells K-ATP channels, and not bind to the SUR2 receptors of muscle and brain, making them a better choice when attempting to alleviate neurological symptoms.[8]

DIABETES IN TODDLERS

The occurrence of T1DM at this age is a result of autoimmune attack on the pancreas. The clinical features and course resembles any other child with T1DM. However, certain points of concern in this age group like lack the fine motor control, cognitive development, and impulse control, makes diabetes management in this age challenging.

Clinical Features

There are subtle variations in clinical presentation of young children with diabetes. An increased risk of diabetic ketoacidosis and cerebral edema is reported among them, signifying rapid and severe decompensation. This severity is postulated to more severe form of disease at presentation than delay in diagnosing.[11] This hypothesis is corroborated by the reduced duration of partial remission or honeymoon phase in younger children, who need higher insulin requirements in first 6 months after diagnosis.[12] Similar findings have been reported in other studies where duration of partial remission was significantly lower in toddlers than school age children with diabetes.[13]

SECTION 7: Special Situations

TABLE 1: Genetic syndromes associated with neonatal diabetes mellitus[3,10]

S. No.	Genetic locus	Clinical phenotype
Abnormal pancreatic development		
1	PLAGL1	Syndrome of diabetes, macroglossia and umbilical hernia
2	RFX6	Syndrome of diabetes, intestinal atresia, gallbladder hypoplasia, and diarrhea
3	IER3IP1	Syndrome of neonatal diabetes with microcephaly and infantile seizures
4	NEUROG3	Syndrome of intractable diarrhea from birth with early-onset diabetes
5	NEUROD1	Syndrome of diabetes with cerebellar hypoplasia without pancreatic exocrine dysfunction
6	PTF1A	Syndrome of diabetes with cerebellar and pancreatic hypoplasia with exocrine dysfunction
7	GLIS3	Syndrome of diabetes and congenital hypothyroidism
8	PDX1	Syndrome of congenital diabetes with pancreatic hypoplasia and exocrine dysfunction
9	HNF1B	Neonatal diabetes with renal anomalies
10	PAX6	Syndrome of neonatal diabetes with brain malformations, microcephaly, and microphthalmia
Abnormal β-cell function		
11	SLC19A2	Diabetes as part of thiamine-responsive megaloblastic anemia syndrome
12	KCNJ11, ABCC8	Developmental delay, epilepsy, neonatal diabetes
Destruction of β-cells		
13	EIF2AK3	Syndrome of diabetes with epiphyseal dysplasia and episodic liver or renal dysfunction, hypothyroidism (Wolcott Rallison syndrome)
14	FOXP3	Immunodysregulation, polyendocrinopathy, enteropathy, X-linked (IPEX) syndrome
15	WFS1	Syndrome of diabetes with optic atrophy, diabetes insipidus, and/or deafness

Toddlers have an increased propensity to infection as rate of acute infection at the time of presentation in them is reported to be twice than rate of infection in those between 5 and 19 years of age.[14] Therefore, infection needs to be investigated for and treated at presentation. It should also form a part of workup during acute deterioration or repeat episodes of diabetic ketoacidosis in toddler age group.

The more challenging aspect of clinical care is extreme variability in food quantity, meal patterns, and daily activities. The children show variable sensitivity to insulin provoking wide glucose fluctuations. In addition, younger children are more likely to suffer from minor ailments which can disturb glucose homeostasis. Rapid growth during this period also impacts their insulin control.

Toddlers with diabetes are predisposed to frequent nocturnal or early morning hypoglycemic episodes, which can be devastating. Almost half of the diabetics younger than 2 years of age had suffered from hypoglycemia compared to 10–15% of older diabetics.[15] Another study reported variable periods of nocturnal hypoglycemia of 10–480 minutes during continuous glucose monitoring in toddlers.[16] Various factors which influence this include variable insulin sensitivity, irregular meal patterns, and delay in detecting hypoglycemia due to nonspecific clinical features. Hypoglycemic episodes were initially thought to carry risk of neurocognitive defects, which has now been refuted by current evidence.

Long-term Complications

Most of the long-term complications in diabetes mellitus are attributed to hyperglycemia. In addition, there are other molecular mechanisms which contribute to disease morbidity and complications.[17] The risk of diabetic complications is thus directly dependent on the disease duration and severity of hyperglycemia. However, few authors have shown that the prepubertal disease duration does not have harmful, if not protective, effect on diabetic complications like retinopathy.[17,18] Even if the risk for diabetic retinopathy exists, the risk increment per year is smaller for prepubertal duration than pubertal disease duration. Similar results were reported by Salardi et al. on comparison of 53 prepubertal and 52 pubertal children with diabetes after 19 years follow-up.[19] They also found similar HbA1c between both groups, precluding poor glycemic control as the only factor to contribute to diabetic complications. A small proportion of prepubertal subjects with poor metabolic control, however, manifested with severe retinopathy. The other factor which could have contributed to risk during pubertal years was hypertension, which was reported among pubertal diabetics. The risk for microalbuminuria was reported to be same in both groups.

Investigations

The basic workup of a toddler diabetic is similar to any childhood diabetic. The following points need to be kept in mind while interpreting investigations in this age group.

The fasting blood glucose values at presentation are usually higher than children in older age group. Likewise, the mean HbA1c is also higher in this age group. This is explained by a greater severity of disease among toddlers, which is validated by lowest serum C-peptide levels in toddlers at diagnosis than those in older age group.[14] It is equally important to note that younger children also have low C-peptide values by the virtue of their low β-cell mass.[20] However, Komulainen et al. demonstrated that despite low serum C-peptide levels in toddlers at diagnosis, there was no substantial increase in endogenous insulin secretion on follow-up in this age group. This was in contrast to older diabetics where partial improvement in insulin secretion was seen after 6 months of follow-up.[14]

Since the disease pathogenesis in this age group is classified as type 1a disease, these children demonstrate raised autoantibodies in the blood, similar to the older diabetics. The majority of toddler diabetics show raised levels of glutamic acid decarboxylase autoantibody (GADA), islet cell antibody (ICA), insulin autoantibody (IAA), or insulinoma-2-associated autoantibodies (IA-2A). The proportion of children being tested positive for one of these antibodies is nearly 100% as compared to 85–95% in older age groups. However, the youngest of the diabetics showed significantly raised levels of IAA and ICA than GADA, while levels of IA-2A were the lowest in this age group.[14]

With the advances in molecular genetics, there is evidence to support the role of genes and major histocompatibility locus antigens (human leukocyte antigen) in determining genetic susceptibility to diabetes. These probably determine and govern the level of autoantibody production and susceptibility of pancreatic damage.[21] In a study which compared the genotype of 35 young diabetics (<2 years) to 766 older diabetic children, it was seen that younger diabetics carried the high-risk genotype of DQB1*02/*0302 more often than their older counterparts. The older diabetics had higher propensity of carrying the protective genotype (DQB1z/z).[14]

Management

An important aspect of patient care is maintenance of adequate growth and nutrition during these crucial growing years. Addressing feeding issues is the biggest challenge in managing toddler diabetes. Children in this age group, including nondiabetics, are fussy eaters. This age is also when children learn food refusal and eating behaviors. Unjustified demand of high calorie density food and sweetened beverages has to be curbed. The parents have to be watchful to avoid development of such behaviors. The toddler with diabetes have to be addressed likewise, insisting parents to first adopt a regular meal pattern for the child. The meals should consist of complex carbohydrate-based foods and snacks like yoghurt, cereals, and fruits. Fruit juices should be discouraged. Parents should assume more responsibility and avoid food bribes in preschool age. A coercive feeding regimen is discouraged and instead a flexible schedule should be promoted.

Dietetics professionals should educate parents of infants and toddlers about the importance of nutrient content and texture of foods to promote healthy eating habits and adequate nutrition. They should be encouraged to avoid relying on fortified foods and supplements to meet nutrient needs. Nutrient and mineral intake should be accounted for by consumption of fruits and vegetables with minimizing intake of juices or supplements.

The American Diabetes Association (ADA) initially suggested that an HbA1c reading of 7.5–8.5% was acceptable and recommended for children with diabetes younger than 6 years. This was based on the increased propensity of hypoglycemia in this age group. However, the recent ADA guideline now emphasizes on uniform goal of HbA1c less than 7.5% across all age groups.[22] Self-monitoring of blood glucose (SMBG) is recommended frequently in this age group as most toddlers are on multiple dose insulin regime. There is extensive literature which supports the utility of SMBG in improving glycemic control and achieving reduction in HbA1c.[22] The targets indicators for optimal glucose control in this age are shown in table 2.

Insulin Therapy

Managing insulin therapy in toddler diabetic is demanding by the virtue of their eating patterns and body sensitivity to insulin. Each toddler will behave differently with respect to meal timings and insulin requirement. Most clinicians would now prefer the multiple injection regimen or continuous subcutaneous insulin therapy. The use of single daily long-acting insulin is no longer practiced. The other alternative option used to be split mix regime. This regime is

TABLE 2: Targets for optimal glycemic control in toddler diabetic[22,23]

	ISPAD[23]	ADA[22]
Self-monitoring of blood glucose		
Pre-prandial or fasting	90–145 mg/dL	90–130 mg/dL
Postprandial	90–180 mg/dL	Not mentioned
Bedtime	120–180 mg/dL	90–150 mg/dL
Nocturnal	80–162 mg/dL	90–150 mg/dL
Glycosylated hemoglobin	<7.5%	<7.5%

ISPAD, International Society for Pediatric and Adolescent Diabetes; ADA, American Diabetic Association.

TABLE 3: Pediatric cutoffs for various insulin analogs

Insulin	Pediatric cutoff
Aspart	• ≥1 year
Lispro	• ≥2 years (EU) • ≥3 years (US)
Glulisine	• ≥4 years (US) • ≥6 years (EU)
Glargine	• ≥2 years
Detemir	• ≥1 year (US and EU)
Degludec	• ≥1 year both USFDA and EU

discouraged as mixing insulin in small doses is difficult and prone to errors. It does not achieve a comparable glucose control than the former regimen and is difficult to titrate in small doses to prevent hypoglycemia.

Multiple daily insulin injections should be administered taking into account the meal timings and carbohydrate counting. Few children may have hypoglycemia with short-acting insulin. In such children, intermediate-acting insulin may be administered as once or twice daily bolus at 0.3–0.5 U/kg/day. There is enough published literature which supports the use of newer insulin analogues in toddlers.[24-27] The fast-acting analogs offer more flexible insulin injection timing with regard to meals and activities, whereas the long-acting analogs have a more predictable action profile and lack a peak effect. They offer significant benefits in terms of reduced frequency of nocturnal hypoglycemia, better postprandial blood glucose control, and improved quality of life when compared with traditional insulins. In addition, insulin detemir is unique in that patients may benefit from reduced risk of excessive weight, particularly during adolescence.

Table 3 shows pediatric cutoffs for various insulin analogs.

The longer acting analog can be combined with rapid-acting insulin. In contrast to older children who receive premeal insulin shot before meals, rapid-acting insulin should be administered after meals to toddlers. The dose of rapid-acting insulin can thus be titrated to the amount of meal consumed which promotes flexibility for the toddler and prevents hypoglycemia.

The insulin pump therapy is emerging as an equally effective and safer option.[28] The pump allows flexibility in meal quantity and amount. The average blood glucose and HbA1c was shown to decrease significantly while on subcutaneous insulin pump therapy.[29] It also reduces the episodes of hypoglycemia. The incidence of lipodystrophy also reduces on insulin pump therapy. The concerns of it use are cost, limited availability, and logistics of maintenance by the family.

Support Group

Management of toddler with diabetes needs combined team effort. The children have to be empowered to cope up with their disease without feeling guilt or burden. The parents have to be counseled to responsibly handle children's food tantrums and fuss over injectable therapy. The daycare and kindergarten team should also be involved in the following responsibilities like blood glucose testing, insulin administration, detecting signs of hypoglycemia, timing and quantity of meal and snacks, and participation in physical exercise. The parents should provide with necessary information about the child and any supplies needed to manage the children with diabetes at school.

DO'S AND DON'TS WITH TODDLERS WITH DIABETES

- Promote physical activity
- Prefer to administer short-acting insulin after meals in younger children or fussy eaters
- Do titrate short-acting insulin dose according to meals
- Maintain regular blood glucose log and bring it for review to child's physician on regular basis
- Do monitor glucose, ketones, and hydration on 'sick day'. Maintain adequate hydration. Offer clear liquids if child uncooperative to eat
- Do not restrict calorie and nutrients which are essential for growth
- Do not discontinue insulin if report low or normal blood sugars. Dosage will need adjustment
- Maintain strong family and school support and involvement regarding plan of care.

CONCLUSION

Neonatal diabetes mellitus, or monogenic diabetes of infancy, is an entity which needs to be diagnosed and managed timely. Since half of the cases are transient, the disease may self-abort in these cases. However, the other neonates who are detected with PNDM, will require lifelong therapy. Parental support and counseling is the prime responsibility of the treating physician. Adequate therapy includes monitoring growth and weight in these infants and close titration of insulin to prevent hypoglycemia.

Managing diabetes during preschool and toddler age group is challenging and requires a dedicated team effort. Most of these children require multiple daily insulin injections, frequent dietary adjustments, adjustments of insulin administration with meal timings, home blood glucose monitoring, family education, and support groups to achieve good metabolic control. Care should also be taken to prevent and manage hypoglycemia in the preschool child. To conclude, the children with diabetes need an extra care and support from his/her family, school, and community to help him/her cope up with burden of disease and continue to live freely.

REFERENCES

1. Cody D. Infant and toddler diabetes. Arch Dis Child. 2007;92:716-9.
2. Gardner SG, Bingley PJ, Satwell PA, Weeks S, Gale EA. Rising incidence of insulin dependent diabetes in children aged under 5 years in the Oxford region: time trend analysis. The Barts-Oxford Study Group. BMJ. 1997;315:713-7.
3. Rubio-Cabezas O, Ellard S. Diabetes mellitus in neonates and infants: genetic heterogeneity, clinical approach to diagnosis, and therapeutic options. Horm Res Paediatr. 2013;80:137-46.
4. Polak M, Cave H. Neonatal diabetes mellitus: a disease linked to multiple mechanisms. Orphanet J Rare Dis. 2007;2:12.
5. Hoffman A, Spengler D. Role of ZAC1 in transient neonatal diabetes mellitus and glucose metabolism. World J Biol Chem. 2015;6(3):95-109.
6. Varadarajan P. Infantile onset diabetes mellitus in developing countries-India. World J Diabetes. 2016;7(6):134-41.
7. Temple IK, Mackay DJG, Docherty LE. Diabetes mellitus, 6q24-related transient neonatal. Gene Reviews. [online] Available from: http://www.ncbi.nlm.nih.gov/books/NBK1534/.
8. Hattersley AT, Ashcroft FM. Activating Mutations in Kir6.2 and Neonatal Diabetes- new clinical syndromes, new scientific insights, and new therapy. Diabetes. 2005;54:2503-13.
9. Vaxillaire M, Dechaume A, Busiah K, Cavé H, Pereira S, Scharfmann R, et al. New ABCC8 mutations in relapsing neonatal diabetes and clinical features. Diabetes. 2007;56:1737-41.
10. Greeley SA, Naylor RN, Philipson LH, Bell GI. Neonatal Diabetes: an expanding list of genes allows for improved diagnosis and treatment. Curr Diab Rep. 2011;11(6):519-32.
11. Paul P, Ghatak A, Kerr S, et al. Severe metabolic decompensation at presentation of diabetes mellitus in children aged 2 years. Arch Dis Child. 2005;90:A19-22.
12. Muhammad BJ, Swift PGF, Raymond NT, Botha JL. Partial remission phase of diabetes in children younger than age 10 years. Arch Dis Child. 1999;80:367-9.
13. Bowden SA, Duck MM, Hoffman RP. Young children (<5 yr) and adolescents (>12 yr) with type 1 diabetes mellitus have low rate of partial remission: diabetic ketoacidosis is an important risk factor. Pediatr Diabetes. 2008;9(3):197-201.
14. Komulainen J, Kulmala MP, Savola MK, Lounamaa R, Ilonen J, Reijonen H, et al. Clinical, autoimmune, and genetic characteristics of very young children with type 1 diabetes. The Childhood Diabetes in Finland (Dime) study group. Diabetes Care. 1999;e22:1950-5.
15. Lteif AN, Schwenk WF. Type 1 diabetes mellitus in early childhood: glycemic control and associated risk of hypoglycaemic reactions. Mayo Clin Proc. 1999;74:211-6.
16. Deiss D, Kordonouri K, Meyer K, Denne T. Long hypoglycaemic periods detected by subcutaneous continuous glucose monitoring in toddlers and pre-school children with diabetes mellitus. Diabetic Med. 2001;18:333-8.
17. Svensson M, Nyström L, Schön S, Dahlquist G. Age at onset of childhood onset type 1 diabetes and the development of end-stage renal disease: a nationwide population-based study. Diabetes Care. 2006;29:538-42.
18. Donaghue KC, Fairchild JM, Craig ME, et al. Do all prepubertal years of diabetes duration contribute equally to diabetes complications? Diabetes Care. 2003;26:1224-9.
19. Salardi S, Porta M, Maltoni G, Rubbi F, Rovere S, Cerutti F, et al. Infant and Toddler Type 1 Diabetes Complications after 20 years' duration. The Diabetes study group of the Italian society of paediatric endocrinology and diabetology (ISPED)*. Diabetes Care. 2012;35:829-33.

20. Rahier J, Wallon J, Henquin J-C: Cell populations in the endocrine pancreas of human neonates and infants. Diabetologia. 1981;20:540-6.
21. Caillat-Zucman S, Garchon HJ, Timsit J, Assan R, Boitard C, Djilali-Saiah I, et al. Age-dependent HLA genetic heterogeneity of type 1 insulin dependent diabetes mellitus. J Clin Invest. 1992;90:2242-50.
22. American Diabetic Association (ADA)-Standards of Medical care in diabetes 2016-Children and adolescents. Diabetes Care. 2016;39(1):S86-93.
23. Global IDF/ISPAD guideline for diabetes in childhood and adolescence. 2011. [online] Available from: https://www.idf.org/sites/default/files/Diabetes-in-Childhood-and-Adolescence-Guidelines.pdf. Accessed June, 2016.
24. Hathout EH, Fujishige L, Geach J, Ischandar M, Maruo S, Mace JW. Effect of therapy with insulin glargine (lantus) on glycemic control in toddlers, children and adolescents with diabetes. Diabetes Technol Ther. 2003;5(5):801-6.
25. Danne T, Aman J, Schober E, Deiss D, Jacobsen JL, Friberg HH, et al. A comparison of postprandial and preprandial administration of insulin aspart in children and adolescents with type 1 diabetes. Diabetes Care. 2003;26(8):2359-64.
26. Thalange N, Bereket A, Larsen J, Hiort LC, Peterkova V. Treatment with insulin detemir or NPH insulin in children aged 2-5 yr with type 1 diabetes mellitus. Pediatr Diabetes. 2011;12(7):632-41.
27. Thalange N, Deeb L, Iotova V, Kawamura T, Klingensmith G, Philotheou A, et al. Insulin degludec in combination with bolus insulin aspart is safe and effective in children and adolescents with type 1 diabetes. Pediatr Diabetes. 2015;16(3):164-76.
28. Eugster EA, Francis G. Lawson-Wilkins Drug and Therapeutics Committee. Position statement: Continuous subcutaneous insulin infusion in very young children with type 1 diabetes. Pediatrics. 2006;118(4):e1244-9.
29. Berhe T, Postellon D, Wilson B, Stone R. Feasibility and safety of insulin pump therapy in children aged 2 to 7 years with type 1 diabetes: a retrospective study. Pediatrics. 2006;117(6):2132-7.

Psychiatric Management

Yatan PS Balhara, Sathya Prakash

INTRODUCTION

Diabetes in children and adolescents presents a significant challenge—both from a clinical as well as a public health perspective. Various aspects related to childhood and "growing up" bring in associated challenges that are unique to this population group. Moreover, these are in addition to those encountered in management of diabetes in general adult population. The rates of diabetes in children have seen an alarming increase in the recent years.[1] There is a dearth of literature providing guidance on treating this unique population of patients, especially from India. The present chapter aims to distill the available information to provide guidance on various aspects of management of psychological issues commonly encountered with children and adolescents diagnosed with diabetes. Besides the presence of comorbid psychiatric disorders, psychological interventions are potentially beneficial in many other aspects of diabetes care such as improving treatment adherence, obesity management, enhancing quality of life, stress reduction and family coping, which are also the focus of this chapter. The goals of psychiatric management are summarized in box 1.

OVERVIEW OF PSYCHIATRIC COMORBIDITY WITH DIABETES IN CHILDREN AND ADOLESCENTS

The prevalence of psychiatric disorders in children and adolescents diagnosed with diabetes has been estimated to vary between 19 and 48%.[2,3] While retrospective studies typically found

---

BOX 1: Goals of psychiatric management in children and adolescents diagnosed with diabetes

- Management of psychiatric comorbidity
- Improving treatment adherence
- Facilitating lifestyle modifications
- Enabling better coping with illness—both patient and family
- Improving quality of life—both patient and family

lower rates, the prospective studies tended to report higher rates. Apart from regional variations, other factors such as nature and size of sample could also account for such variations.

Depression and diabetes share a bidirectional causal association. While depression has been postulated to play a causal role in emergence of diabetes, diabetes has been recognized as a "depressogenic" condition.[4] Depression is commonly associated with diabetes in children and adolescents and rates of up to 23% have been reported for the same. Girls are more likely to suffer from depression compared to boys.[5] The rates of recurrence and recovery were not adversely affected in studies among children and adolescents as compared to adults. However, children and adolescents diagnosed with diabetes tended to spend longer durations of time in depression. Compounding the problem are lower rates of diagnosis and treatment when compared to control groups. Several of the physical complaints such as fatigue, sleep disturbances, and somatic symptoms associated with depression may be misconstrued as a part of physical manifestation of diabetes, thus delaying diagnosis and treatment.[6] Family stress, poor glycemic control, and maternal depression are some of the other important risk factors for depression among children and adolescents diagnosed with diabetes. Depression tends to be higher in the initial years post diagnosis, decreasing between 4 and 9 years before rising again. This may be related to the initial problems with adjustment and later development of complications.[6]

A second group of disorders commonly associated with diabetes in children and adolescents are eating disorders. Onset of diabetes in adolescence and preadolescence, particularly in girls, are important risk factors for development of eating disorders.[7-9] More often than not, patients do not fulfill all the criteria for a given eating disorder. Binge eating, driven exercise, and sometimes decreased food intake have been reported. Presence of eating disorders places children at increased risk for poor glycemic control, obesity, depression, and poorer quality of life.[10] Anorexia nervosa, when associated with type 1 diabetes mellitus (T1DM), results in increased mortality. Exploration of cognitions related to body shape and weight may help in early identification of risk groups.

Substance use disorders are considered to be relatively less common or at the most comparable to that of general population.[11,12] However, in those who do use substances, significant adverse influences on diabetes management have been observed. Comorbid psychiatric problems such as depression, poor diet, and cognitive problems may also be compounded by such comorbid substance use.[13,14]

A number of studies have reported neurocognitive impairments in children and adolescents with diabetes. However, several of these findings have remained controversial. Although most studies agree that cognitive deficits do occur, the extent and clinical significance of the same is controversial.[13,14] While some authorities believe that the cognitive deficits adversely impact school performance and diabetes management, others are of the opinion that the deficits are too subtle to have impact on these aspects. Some studies have also suggested the presence of cognitive deficits before the onset of diabetes.[15] Verbal intelligence, phonological processing, spelling accuracy, reading ability, mathematics, processing speed, new learning ability, and visuospatial processing are some of the domains that have been frequently reported as impaired in this population group. An earlier age of onset of diabetes, longer illness duration, poor glycemic control, and frequent hypoglycemic

> **BOX 2: Psychiatric morbidity in children and adolescents diagnosed with diabetes**
>
> - Depressive disorders
> - Eating disorders
> - Adjustment disorders
> - Neurocognitive impairment
> - Post-traumatic stress disorders
> - Nocturnal enuresis
> - Sleep disorders
> - Attention deficit hyperactivity disorder
> - Phobic disorders including fear of needles
> - Others such as psychotic disorders, bipolar disorders, obsessive compulsive disorders

spells including seizures have been reported as predictors of cognitive deficits. Although such findings are also controversial, with contradictory findings in other studies.[15]

Adjustment disorder, post-traumatic stress disorder (PTSD) like symptoms (related to hypoglycemic spells), attention deficit hyperactivity disorder, sleep disturbances, and nocturnal enuresis are some other problems encountered along with diabetes in children and adolescents.[16-20]

Fear of needles (also known as trypanophobia) is another important issue that gains relevance specifically in context of children and adolescent diagnosed with diabetes. This fear can make children and adolescents reluctant to adhere administered insulin and can impact therapeutic adherence. It is important to understand the genesis of such fear as the contributory factors may extend way beyond the perceived experience of pain. The possible underlying reasons, besides apprehension about the pain, could include a perceived loss of control over life, lack of confidence that one could handle the demands of therapy, equating insulin therapy with personal failure, and a perceived lack of personal gain.[21]

The commonly encountered psychiatric problems in diabetic children and adolescents are summarized in box 2.

DIABETES AND PSYCHIATRIC DISORDERS: NATURE OF INTERACTION

Diabetes and psychiatric disorders have been shown to share a multifaceted interface. Literature from adult population suggests while co-occurrence of diabetes and psychiatric disorders could be a mere chance association, at least in a subgroup of such population the two share causal associations. Additionally, the two can share clinical manifestations and the medications used for management of either can have clinically meaningful interactions.[4] There is support to some of these hypotheses from studies among children and adolescents as well.[22] A brief summary of this interface of diabetes and psychiatric disorders has been presented in table 1.

MANAGEMENT OF PSYCHIATRIC PROBLEMS

General Considerations

Irrespective of the nature of underlying psychiatric diagnosis, either syndromal or subsyndromal, certain issues and management strategies may be seen as cross cutting and

TABLE 1: Multifaceted interface of interaction between diabetes and psychiatric disorders and its clinical consequences

Interaction	Possible mechanisms/examples
Possible causal association (bidirectional)	• Biochemical factors (neuroendocrinal such as hypercortisolemia, leptin activity in limbic system, altered glucose transportation, proinflamatory cytokines) • Psychological factors (stress associated with living with diabetes, poor treatment adherence) • Behavioral factors (sedentary lifestyles, smoking, overeating) • Medications such as antipsyhcotics
Overlapping clinical presentation	• Panic attacks and episodes of hypoglycemia • Delirium during episodes of diabetic ketoacidosis
Altered metabolism of medications	• Tobacco smoking
Poor treatment adherence	• Patients with psychotic disorders with limited insight • Phobia of needles
Interaction of medications	• Various

common. Foremost among such concepts is the conceptualization of diabetes in this age group. Diabetes in children and adolescents is best viewed as a family disorder.[23] As much of the responsibility of caring for the child is placed on family members, they automatically become a key role player. Also, a number of aspects of diabetes care, such as proper diet, ensuring glucose monitoring, medication use and regular hospital follow-up, place significant demands on the family members. It follows from the above observations that psychological health of the entire family should be given equal importance as that of the child or adolescent diagnosed with diabetes. Psychological problems in the family members can influence the care of the child or adolescent diagnosed with diabetes.[23]

A number of key factors have been identified that are crucial to the health of family as a unit, which in turn, influences the care of the child or adolescent diagnosed with diabetes. Family communication, conflict resolution, responsibility sharing, and problem solving are among the most important of such factors.[23,24] Families choosing to actively communicate the problem with each other, having designated roles to play in order to solve a given problem, using adaptive strategies to solve problems, and resolve conflicts tend to report better psychological health of the patient as well as of the entire family. Such families also tend to garner appropriate social support, approach the problem with empathy and warmth, clearly define the goals that are to be achieved and anticipate and expect the possibility of falling short of the said goals. This also translates into superior glycemic control and quality of life of the child or adolescent diagnosed with diabetes. On the contrary, families with maladaptive coping often chose not to discuss the problem or discuss it in a manner that is not productive or involves blaming one another. Responsibility sharing is not clear and problems often precipitate mutual conflict in such families. The approach to solving problems also tends to haphazard and emotionally driven rather than rational.[24]

While for ease of communication, the diabetes of children and adolescents has been covered together in the current chapter, one must remember that children and adolescents are different from each other in many ways. Growing up is a period of active changes, both physical and psychological, with consequent influences on identity, self-esteem and outlook towards life among others. Therefore, with increasing age, there is an ever-changing array of psychological challenges the child and the adolescent is faced with. This is best exemplified by the differences in management issues between a younger child vis-à-vis an adolescent. Whereas, in the younger child, the treatment aspects are almost entirely managed by the parents (or caregivers), in the adolescent, an expectation often arises that he or she should now take over his or her treatment needs. It was believed that such a transfer of responsibility is welcomed or needed, however one needs to guard against the premature or excessive transfer of responsibility, as it could be detrimental to diabetes management. Also, the hormonal changes in adolescence often decrease insulin responsiveness leading to further management challenges. These observations highlight the complexity and heterogeneity of the psychological problems encountered when treating this population group.[25]

With this background, management of specific issues shall be discussed further.

Improving Treatment Adherence

A number of studies have focused on improving treatment adherence as this is an area of concern and many different techniques have been used.[26,27] Simplest among them is self-monitoring.[28] The very fact that one is regularly recording and monitoring one's behavior tends to improve the awareness and understanding into the nature of problem. This along with other factors improves overall management of diabetes. Such self-monitoring can include monitoring of behavior such as exercise, amount and nature of food, medication administration, and blood and urine testing among others.

Another technique that has been relatively well studied is behavioral contracting.[28] It essentially involves moderating an agreement between the parents (or caregivers) and the child. For instance, a permission to indulge in a favorite hobby for an additional hour is contracted for monitoring blood glucose twice a day. Care is to be taken to see that the bargain is both of interest to the child and reasonable. It must be made in an empathic fashion by making the child a partner in decision-making process and must not appear as if the child is being threatened or manipulated. When carefully done, behavioral contracting has been shown to significantly improve diabetes management related behaviors.[28]

Positive reinforcement has been the psychological principle behind psychotherapeutic interventions for various disorders. It has been tried in various forms to improve adherence to diabetes management as well.[29] In its simplest form, it involves praise for desirable behavior such as monitoring blood glucose and taking insulin by family members or caregivers at home and by the clinician at the hospital. The latter, besides improving the patient behavior, also encourages the family members and caregivers.[28,30] However, for such an intervention to be effective, it is important to be consistent and accurate. Such simple strategies may be particularly useful in younger children.[30] More detailed versions include a point based reward system. In this format, a predefined "point list" is prepared that consists of desirable and undesirable behaviors along with the number of points that would be added or deducted from the tally in case of a desirable and undesirable behavior, respectively. Also, a certain reward is prefixed on achieving a certain tally of points. The tally is displayed at a prominent place in the home so as to be readily visible to the child. The changes to the "scorecard" are made in close temporal proximity to the behavior so as to establish the relationship between reward and behavior.[28] The total tally at which the reward is fixed must also be reasonable, again, not to be reached easily, while at the same time, not frustratingly difficult to achieve. The reward must be of interest to the child, should not be harmful in itself, and be within the economic reach of the family. Depending on age and stage of development of the child, certain modifications can be made to this format such as replacing the points with "stars". A common mistake that is often made is that of offering reward without the child having to perform the desirable behavior. This could be detrimental to the success of the approach and should be avoided.[31]

Teaching problem solving skills is another important psychological intervention used to enhance adherence to diabetes care.[32] Self-monitoring of glucose as an aid to solving diabetes management problems has been empirically tested and found to be effective as evidenced by favorable glycemic control. Problem solving has also been combined with aforementioned behavior therapy paradigms with favorable outcomes.

It is important to address the fear of needles, if any. Patient's personal obstacles should be identified and acknowledged. Additionally, a sense of personal control should be re-established with a brief trial of insulin therapy. In case a syndromal diagnosis of phobic disorder is established, formal psychiatric consultation should be sought.[33]

Family based therapies and multisystemic therapies are some of the other psychological techniques that have been studied and found to be useful.[34] As the name suggests, multisystemic therapies targets multiple systems influencing diabetes related behaviors. It is an intensive, home based therapy targeting not just family environment but also that of school, hospital, and neighborhood. Studies suggest that multisystemic therapy is efficacious in improving multiple aspects of diabetes management such as glucose testing, glycemic control and rates of need for hospitalization.[34] The various psychological methods of improving treatment adherence are summarized in box 3.

Preventing/Treating Psychological Problems in Diabetes

Coping skills training is an important strategy to improve psychological health in diabetes.[35] Children are educated regarding common maladaptive coping styles and behaviors and how to replace these with more adaptive ones. Adaptive coping increases a sense of mastery, reduces stress, and decreases problems. Studies have shown superior glycemic control, quality

BOX 3: Strategies to improve treatment adherence in children and adolescents diagnosed with diabetes	
• Behavioral contracting	• Family therapy
• Self-monitoring	• Multisystemic therapy
• Behavior therapy	• Integration of peers
• Problem solving	

of life, and self-efficacy among those receiving coping skills training. Social skills training and integration of peers into diabetes care is another important area. Making a close friend a partner in diabetes care and teaching skills to face challenging situations such as peer teasing have been shown to significantly enhance quality of life and glycemic control.[36] As discussed earlier, family interventions and problem solving skills training are other important intervention modalities. Other modalities that have been used to reduce stress include biofeedback assisted relaxation and progressive muscular relaxation.[37]

Unique Challenges in Type 2 Diabetes Mellitus in Children and Adolescents

Type 2 diabetes mellitus (T2DM) is, in many ways, considered more challenging than T1DM.[38,39] One of the most important reasons for this is the association of obesity with T2DM and the need for lifestyle modifications. Moreover, T2DM often begins in adolescence, a period of life when one is already faced with various physiological and psychological challenges including struggle for autonomy and defiance. This can create problems with adherence to advice and treatment. There is also some evidence to suggest that T2DM more often affects resource poor families. Also, T2DM is more likely to be associated with family history, leading to frustration in families, upon discovery of diabetes in yet another family member.[39]

Psychological Measures to Aid Obesity Management

Obesity in children has many risk factors. However, from a management perspective, it is useful to consider the causative influences under three headings—overeating, lack of physical activity, and genetic influences. Overeating can be further broken down into eating excessive food or choice of high calorie/high fat foods, or a combination of both. Genetic influences also shape the obesity to a significant extent. Some component of this influence may be mediated by tendency to overeat and be physically inactive. As genetic components are not amenable to intervention, diet, and exercise are the two key factors on which interventions are focused.[38]

Management of food habits plays a key role in the prevention and management of obesity. An ideal diet to lose weight must be one that can be followed over long periods of time. Best results are obtained when such a diet is combined with regular exercise. Very low calorie diets taken for short durations almost invariably are followed by periods of overeating. Also, the body's compensatory mechanisms shift to a "conserve energy" mode, sensing lack of adequate calories, favoring calorie accumulation. Similar principles apply to exercise as well.[40]

Besides the nature of food itself, behavior during meals and management of cues are windows of opportunity to intervene.[38] These opportunities can be targeted in various ways and are a focus of this discussion. Postponing a desire to have a snack for 10 minutes is a good starting point. It is often the case that what one perceives as "hunger" is actually "boredom" and 10 minutes later, the desire to have a snack is gone! If one is indeed settling for a meal, chose to serve it on a smaller plate and to serve the intended portion in half so as to permit another portion. These strategies provide a sense of having eaten more with lesser amount of food being actually consumed. In between bites, take small (micro) breaks, put the spoon down and talk. It is quite common to gulp down a large amount of food when hungry and to realize later that one had probably overeaten. This is attributable to the slight delay in body's satiety sensing mechanisms discovering that adequate food has been consumed and the actual ingestion of food. Each mouthful must be chewed repeatedly, savored, and not gulped down in a hurry. This serves to maximize the pleasure or reward associated with eating food, which is a motivation for many to eat. This can help mimic the effects of larger amount of food by smaller amounts.[38]

Reduction of cues related to food is another important target for intervention.[38] First and foremost is to stock the house with healthier food stuff so that in the event of an urge to overeat, only healthy food is available. Shopping for food must be done on a full stomach, not when one is hungry. Substitution of snacking by other activities also helps to address the urge to eat, particularly those eating episodes that are in response to boredom rather than true hunger. It is useful to maintain a food diary recording eating behaviors including their relation to hunger and non-hunger (also referred to as emotional eating) episodes. The diary can later be used to plan meal timings and content. The place of eating must be designated beforehand, and eating must take place only at that place. One must leave the designated place as soon as the eating is done and not combine eating with other activities such as watching television or reading books. Food stuffs must not be placed on tables where they are readily visible and induce desire to eat.[38]

Besides the above described relatively simple measures, more advanced techniques include use of cognitive behavioral techniques. A referral to a psychiatrist/psychologist is usually needed. Basic principles involved are targeting the maladaptive cognitions related to eating and cognitive restructuring. Identifying triggers for excessive eating and devising alternative strategies to handle emotional stress are also part of such techniques.[41]

The psychological management of obesity is summarized in figure 1.

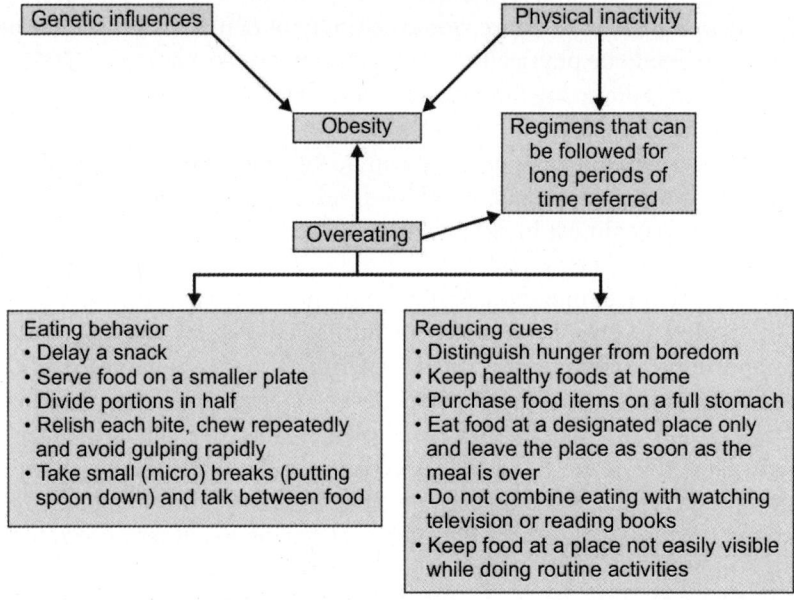

Fig. 1: Obesity management

Treatment of Specific Psychiatric Disorders

This section shall address the management of three specific psychiatric conditions—adjustment disorder, depressive disorder, and eating disorders.

Depression and Adjustment Disorders

Besides the above described general strategies, specific forms of therapy such as cognitive behavioral therapy can be useful in older children and adolescents. Age appropriate modifications in therapy may be needed, such as the use of dolls and toys.[42] Being a chronic condition since childhood, diabetes significantly influences the perception of self, and encourages formation of negative "core beliefs" that need to be corrected. Such core beliefs include ones such as "I am an ill person" or "I am not normal" or "I am different and not one among the rest". Cognitive distortions validating such beliefs are common and also need to be corrected. Diabetes related health events may provoke automatic thoughts in line with such beliefs and distortions leading to maladaptive behavior. For instance, experience of weakness during a sporting event may bring about automatic thoughts of "I can never play, I am useless" associated with distortions of overgeneralization and black and white thinking. Such thoughts are in line with the core beliefs suggested above. Cognitive behavioral therapy aims to correct all three levels of abnormalities in the thought processes and thereby improve mood and behavior.

Pharmacotherapy for syndromal depression with antidepressants must be initiated when necessary. Tricyclic antidepressants are not preferred as they may increase appetite and cause hyperglycemia. Additionally, the safety of tricyclic antidepressants in pediatric population in general is little established. Selective serotonin reuptake inhibitors (SSRIs) are preferred but can decrease appetite, increase insulin secretion, and cause hypoglycemia. The SSRI with the largest experience in pediatric population is fluoxetine. Lithium must be used with caution as its effects are unpredictable. Lithium can both mimic the effects of insulin while also stimulating the release of glucagon.[42] Diabetes may compound the long-term adverse effects of lithium (e.g., nephropathy). As depression is itself associated with change in food habits, physical activity, and treatment adherence, both onset of depression as well as recovery may significantly influence blood sugar levels necessitating adjustment of antidiabetic medications.[42]

Eating Disorders

The primary modalities of interventions for eating disorders in children and adolescents belong to the psychosocial realm. Pharmacological interventions have limited role and there is a paucity of studies that have explored its effectiveness and safety in this population group.[43] The SSRIs, particularly fluoxetine, have been used in both anorexia nervosa and bulimia nervosa. However, the results in case of anorexia nervosa have been disappointing whereas in case of bulimia nervosa, weak to moderate effects have been reported. Specific individual, group, and family therapies have been designed for the treatment of eating disorders in child and adolescent diabetes. Failure of outpatient treatment, markedly disturbed eating behaviors, and poor glycemic control may indicate necessity for hospitalization. Cognitive behavioral strategies have been used either in the group or individual setting. However, there is paucity of data on effects of such therapies on some unique diabetes related behaviors such as insulin omission.[44,45] Therapies are designed to target the excessive preoccupation with weight and food. Dietary management is of paramount importance and healthy planned diets may be given in a hospitalized patient in keeping with the exposure and response prevention paradigm. Such strategies usually require consultation with a psychiatrist or a psychologist having experience in managing eating disorders.

While psychoeducation can be an important component of a comprehensive management plan, it may not be sufficient as a standalone intervention sufficient to change eating disorder related behaviors.[44,45] Insulin pumps have come up as an important measure in both reducing disturbed eating behaviors as well as better glycemic control. Insulin pumps are said to ensure better physiological delivery of insulin leading to lesser requirement of insulin and therefore, lesser weight gain.[42,44,45] However, the core cognitions related to food and weight, obviously remain unchanged.

CONCLUSION

Psychiatric comorbidity is common in children and adolescents with diabetes mellitus. Psychotherapeutic and psychopharmacological treatments are not only beneficial in alleviating the burden of comorbid psychiatric problems, but also improve the overall management of diabetes. Psychotherapeutic interventions are immensely helpful in enhancing various aspects of diabetes care as well. Depression, adjustment disorder, and eating disorders are among the most commonly associated psychiatric disorders in children and adolescents with diabetes. Neurocognitive deficits, PTSD, and nocturnal enuresis have also been reported. Diabetes in this population is best approached as a family disorder and hence treatment should be focused at the family rather than only the individual diagnosed with diabetes. Family communication, conflict resolution, responsibility sharing, and problem solving are among the most crucial factors in management. Strategies targeting treatment adherence and obesity management have also been described and are useful. Specific treatment strategies have also been described for syndromal psychiatric disorders co-occurring with diabetes in children and adolescents. Besides psychotherapeutic measures, judicious use of pharmacotherapy is also useful, particularly in the more severe cases. However, one must be cautious to look into the effects of drugs on glycemic control, other metabolic parameters, potential synergistic effects on diabetes related complications, and drug interactions.

REFERENCES

1. Nelson RA, Bremer AA. Insulin resistance and metabolic syndrome in the pediatric population. Metab Syndr Relat Disord. 2010;8:1-14.
2. Levitt Katz EL, Swami S, Abraham M, Murphy MK, Jawad FA, McKnight-Menci H, et al. Neuropsychiatric disorders at the presentation of type 2 diabetes mellitus in children. Pediatr Diabetes. 2005;6:84-9.
3. Kovacs M, Goldston D, Obrosky SD, Bonar KL. Psychiatric disorders in youths with IDDM: rates and risk factors. Diabetes Care. 1997;20:36-44.
4. Balhara SYP. Diabetes and psychiatric disorders. Indian J Endocrinol Metab. 2011;15(4):274-83.

5. Lawrence MJ, Standiford AD, Loots B, Klingensmith JG, Williams ED, Ruggiero A, et al. Prevalence and correlates of depressed mood among youth with diabetes: the SEARCH for Diabetes in Youth study. Pediatrics. 2006;117:1348-58.
6. Kovacs M, Obrosky SD, Goldston D, Drash A. Major depressive disorder in youths with IDDM: a controlled prospective study of course and outcome. Diabetes Care 1997;20:45-51.
7. Grylli V, Hafferl-Gattermayer A, Wagner G, Schober E, Karwautz A. Eating disorders and eating problems among adolescents with type 1 diabetes: Exploring relationships with temperament and character. J Pediatr Psychol. 2005;30:197-206.
8. Pollock M, Kovacs M, Charron-Prochownik D. Eating disorders and maladaptive dietary/insulin management among youths with childhood-onset insulin-dependent diabetes mellitus. J Am Acad Child Adolesc Psychiatry. 1995;34:291-6.
9. Bryden KS, Neil A, Mayou RA, Peveler RC, Fairburn CG, Dunger DB. Eating habits, body weight, and insulin misuse. A longitudinal study of teenagers and young adults with type 1 diabetes. Diabetes Care. 1999;22:1956-60.
10. Nielsen S, Emborg C, Mølbak A-G. Mortality in concurrent type 1 diabetes and anorexia nervosa. Diabetes Care 2002;25:309-12.
11. Gold AM, Gladstein J. Substance use among adolescents with diabetes mellitus: preliminary findings. J Adolesc Health. 1993;14:80-4.
12. Martínez-Aguayo A, Araneda CJ, Fernandez D, Gleisner A, Perez V, Codner E. Tobacco, alcohol, and illicit drug use in adolescents with diabetes mellitus. Pediatr Diabetes. 2007;8:265-71.
13. Holmes SC, Fox AM, Cant CM, Lampert LN. Disease and demographic risk factors for disrupted cognitive functioning in children with insulin-dependent diabetes mellitus (IDDM). Sch Psychol Rev. 1999;28.
14. Northam AE, Anderson JP, Jacobs R, Hughes M, Warne LG, Werther AG. Neuropsychological profiles of children with type 1 diabetes 6 years after disease onset. Diabetes Care. 2001;24:1541-6.
15. Wysocki T, Harris AM, Mauras N, Fox L, Taylor A, Jackson CS, et al. Absence of adverse effects of severe hypoglycemia on cognitive function in school-aged children with diabetes over 18 months. Diabetes Care. 2003;26:1100-5.
16. McCarthy MA, Lindgren S, Mengeling AM, Tsalikian E, Engvall CJ. Effects of diabetes on learning in children. Pediatrics. 2002;109 (1):E9.
17. Estrada LC, Danielson KK, Drum LM, Lipton BR. Insufficient sleep in young patients with diabetes and their families. Biol Res Nurs. 2012;14:48-54.
18. Chen H-J, Lee Y-J, Yeh CG, Lin H-C. Association of attention-deficit/hyperactivity disorder with diabetes: a population-based study. Pediatr Res. 2013;73:492-6.
19. Şişmanlar ŞG, Demirbaş-Çakir E, Karakaya I, Çizmecioğlu F, Yavuz CI, Hatun Ş, et al. Posttraumatic stress symptoms in children diagnosed with type 1 diabetes. Ital J Pediatr. 2012;38:1-6.
20. Ferrara P, Rigante D, D'Aleo C, Schiavino A, Emmanuele V, Marrone G, et al. Preliminary data on monosymptomatic nocturnal enuresis in children and adolescents with type 1 diabetes. Scand J Urol Nephrol. 2006;40:238-40.
21. Tandon N, Kalra S, Balhara SYP, Baruah PM, Chadha M, Chandalia BH, et al. Forum for Injection Technique (FIT), India: The Indian recommendations 2.0, for best practice in Insulin Injection Technique, 2015. Indian J Endocrinol Metab. 2015;19(3):317-31.
22. Bobo VW, Cooper OW, Stein MC, Olfson M, Graham D, Daugherty J, et al. Antipsychotics and the risk of type 2 diabetes mellitus in children and youth. JAMA Psychiatry. 2013;70:1067-75.
23. Northam AE, Todd S, Cameron JF. Interventions to promote optimal health outcomes in children with Type 1 diabetes—are they effective? Diabet Med. 2006;23:113-21.
24. Kovacs M, Feinberg LT, Paulauskas S, Finkelstein R, Pollock M, Crouse-Novak M. Initial coping responses and psychosocial characteristics of children with insulin-dependent diabetes mellitus. J Pediatr. 1985;106:827-34.
25. Wysocki T. Parents, teens, and diabetes. Diabetes Spectr. 2002;15:6-8.
26. Hanson LC, De Guire JM, Schinkel MA, Kolterman GO. Empirical validation for a family-centered model of care. Diabetes Care. 1995;18:1347-56.
27. Wysocki T, Harris AM, Greco P, Bubb J, Danda EC, Harvey ML, et al. Randomized, controlled trial of behavior therapy for families of adolescents with insulin-dependent diabetes mellitus. J Pediatr Psychol. 2000;25:23-33.
28. Carney MR, Schecheter K, Davis T. Improving adherence to blood glucose testing in insulin-dependent diabetic children. Behav Ther. 1983;14:247-54.
29. Carney RM, Schecheter K, Davis T. Improving adherence to blood glucose testing in insulin-dependent diabetic children. Behav Ther. 1983;14:247-54.
30. Anderson B, Loughlin C, Goldberg E, Laffel L. Comprehensive, family-focused outpatient care for very young children living with chronic disease: Lessons from a program in pediatric diabetes. Child Serv Soc Pol Res Pract. 2001;4:235-50.

31. Anderson B, Loughlin C, Goldberg E, Laffel L. Comprehensive, family-focused outpatient care for very young children living with chronic disease: Lessons from a program in pediatric diabetes. Child Serv Soc Pol Res Pract. 2001;4:235-50.
32. Cook S, Herold K, Edidin DV, Briars R. Increasing problem solving in adolescents with type 1 diabetes: the choices diabetes program. Diabetes Educ. 2002;28:115-24.
33. Tandon N, Kalra S, Balhara PSY, Baruah MP, Chadha M, Chandalia HB, et al. Forum for Injection Technique (FIT), India: The Indian recommendations 2.0, for best practice in Insulin Injection Technique, 2015. Indian J Endocrinol Metab. 2015;19(3):317-31.
34. Ellis DA, Naar-King S, Frey M, Templin T, Rowland M, Greger N. Use of multisystemic therapy to improve regimen adherence among adolescents with type 1 diabetes in poor metabolic control: a pilot investigation. J Clin Psychol Med Settings. 2004;11:315-24.
35. Grey M, Boland EA, Davidson M, Li J, Tamborlane WV. Coping skills training for youth with diabetes mellitus has long-lasting effects on metabolic control and quality of life. J Pediatr. 2000;137:107-13.
36. Greco P, Pendley JS, McDonell K, Reeves G. A peer group intervention for adolescents with type 1 diabetes and their best friends. J Pediatr Psychol. 2001;26:485-90.
37. Jacobson AM. The psychological care of patients with insulin-dependent diabetes mellitus. New Engl J Med. Mass Medical Soc. 1996;334:1249-53.
38. Vaidya V, Steele KE, Schweitzer M, Shermack MA. Obesity. In: Sadock BJ, Sadock VA, Ruiz P, editors. Comprehensive Textbook of Psychiatry. Lippincott, Williams and Wilkins, Philadelphia; 2009.
39. Rosenbloom A, Silverstein J. Type 2 diabetes in children and adolescents: A guide to diagnosis, epidemiology, pathogenesis, prevention, and treatment [Internet]. American Diabetes Association; 2003 [cited 2003]. Available from: https://scholar.google.co.in/scholar.ris?q=info:kPcVAdNBcFUJ:scholar.google.com&output=cite&scirp=0&hl=en.
40. Krebs NF, Jacobson MS. Prevention of pediatric overweight and obesity. Pediatrics. 2003;112:424-30.
41. Wilfley DE, Welch RR, Stein RI, Spurrell EB, Cohen LR, Saelens BE, et al. A randomized comparison of group cognitive-behavioral therapy and group interpersonal psychotherapy for the treatment of overweight individuals with binge-eating disorder. Arch Gen Psychiatry. 2002;59:713-21.
42. Wysocki T, Buckloh LM, Lochrie AS, Antal H. The psychologic context of pediatric diabetes. Pediatr Clin North Am. 2005;52:1755-78.
43. Sigman GS. Eating disorders in children and adolescents. Pediatr Clin North Am. 2003;50:1139-77.
44. Olmsted MP, Daneman D, Rydall AC, Lawson ML, Rodin G. The effects of psychoeducation on disturbed eating attitudes and behavior in young women with type 1 diabetes mellitus. Int J Eat Disord. 2002;32:230-9.
45. Battaglia MR, Alemzadeh R, Katte H, Hall PL, Perlmuter LC. Brief report: disordered eating and psychosocial factors in adolescent females with type 1 diabetes mellitus. J Pediatr Psychol. Soc Ped Psychology. 2006;31:552-6.

SECTION 8

Miscellaneous

Editor
Rakesh Sahay

CHAPTER 28

Diabetes Education Material

Archana S Sarda, Shuchy Chugh

INTRODUCTION

Diabetes education and counselling are integrated as a part of the Changing Diabetes in Children (CDiC) program, to make it comprehensive in real terms. To be effective, diabetes education has to be carried out in a child-friendly way. Many innovative child friendly patient education tools have been created to help the child with type 1 diabetes mellitus (T1DM) know about basics of diabetes and its management. These allow children to gain maximum opportunity to control and understand diabetes and medical procedures while remaining a child. These also help parents and guardians of children with T1DM help their children manage diabetes.

Diabetes education is the very soul for creating awareness and management of diabetes. There can be many methods which may be used alone or in combination for imparting diabetes education based on culture and needs of community, person, and their understanding. Here is a list of few education materials we have been designed based on needs of the Indian community (Table 1).

TABLE 1: List of tools used for diabetes education

Educative tools	Materials
Mishti (story books)	Series of 4 story books (English and 9 Indian languages)
Video	Mishti educative video (English, Hindi, and Kannada)
Educative toys	NOTTI doll/snakes and ladders/hypo kit/healthy plate/diet snack box
Educative posters	Know the symptoms, hypoglycemia, hyperglycemia, insulin and glucose monitoring, make your own plate, foot door hanger
Educative visual aids	Type 1 diabetes education, Novo aid booklet, make a healthy change folder
Educative leaflets/newsletter	CDiC newsletter, Mishti Guardian, know about carbohydrates, diets leaflet, do and do not series
Educative monitor	HbA1c wheel, BMI chart

NOTTI, Novo Nordisk Teaches to Take Insulin; CDiC, Changing Diabetes in Children; HbA1c, glycosylated hemoglobin; BMI, body mass index.

SECTION 8: Miscellaneous

STORY BOOK

Mishti (Story Book)

Mishti is a story of a little girl with diabetes who shares her journey with T1DM. Four booklets of the series have been released so far (Fig. 1).
- Mishti-1 speaks about basic understanding of T1DM
- Misthi-2 is a story about Mishti participating in sports day and attending Christmas party. These includes instructions for the child with diabetes while doing any exercise or participating in any sports activity
- In Mishti-3, the story revolves around Misthi going to school trip. This includes instructions for the child with diabetes to be followed while travelling
- In Mishti-4, Mishti talk about things to be followed during any acute illness.

Mishti offers multiple benefits, namely:[1]
- Helping the child to be a friend with another child with diabetes
- Understanding what diabetes is
- Planning for diabetes self-management in various situations of life
- Keep the learning with themselves to reread and relearn.

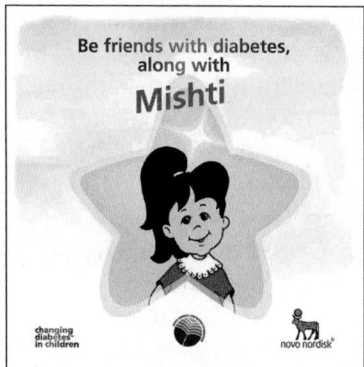 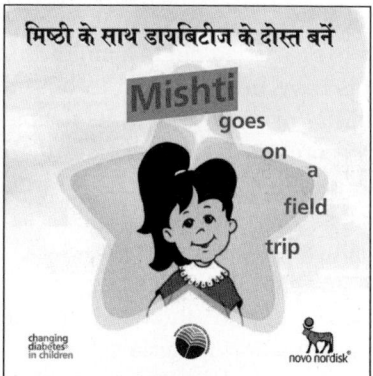

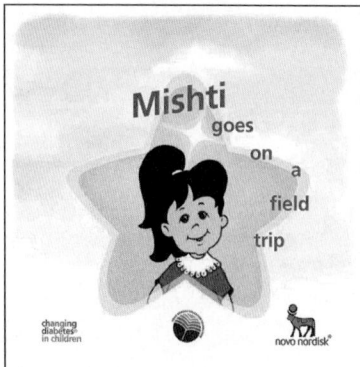 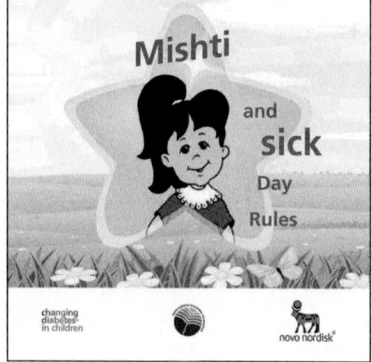

Fig. 1: Mishti story book *(For color version, see Plate 1)*

CHAPTER 28: Diabetes Education Material

VIDEO

Mishti (Video)

This video gives the journey of Mishti and her parents after being diagnosed with diabetes (Fig. 2). The little girl explains in simple and plain words her understanding of diabetes and its management. This video is animation which is liked by both children and adults alike and is useful for all people with diabetes but especially children with T1DM and T2DM. It comes with disclaimer—Mishti is a fictitious character. The content is meant for educational purpose and is not to be used as a substitute for professional medical advice.

While watching this animated video, children not only find a friend with diabetes but also will learn:
- How diabetes happens
- Basics of T1DM, insulin, and blood glucose
- Four pillars of diabetes management—diet, exercise, insulin, and monitoring
- How to take insulin
- Hypoglycemia and its management
- Myths and misconceptions about T1DM.

Mishti video offers multiple benefits, namely:
- Helping very small children and illiterate patients and their parents
- Teaching of children while they are waiting to meet doctor
- Dispelling myths and misconceptions about T1DM.

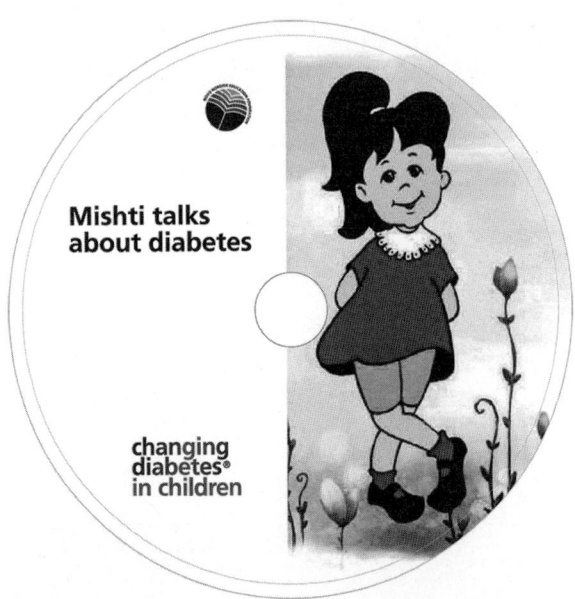

Fig. 2: Cover of Mishti video *(For color version, see Plate 1)*

SECTION 8: Miscellaneous

EDUCATIVE TOYS

Novo Nordisk Teaches to Take Insulin (NOTTI) Doll

Novo Nordisk Teaches to Take Insulin Doll is a soft, unbreakable, easy to carry educational toy, designed as a diabetes education tool to teach about correct insulin taking technique. It is being given to all the children with diabetes participating in the CDiC India program. The purpose is to help the children learn how to take insulin and how to rotate the site of injection. Nordisk teaches to take insulin doll also helps the physician to initiate conversation, to practice taking injection, and become well versed in self-injection.

Novo Nordisk teaches to take insulin doll has many uses, namely it helps to:[1]
- Initiate conversation
- Understand about taking insulin injection
- Understand sites for taking insulin (Fig. 3)
- Understand rotation of insulin site
- Practice taking injection
- Encourage self-injection
- Understand basic anatomy of human body
- Express symptomatology (e.g., child: "I have a pain in my tummy". Dr: "tell me where in the tummy. Show me on your doll")
- Encourage good self-care practices (take care of NOTTI, take care of yourself)
- As a gift to the child, since all children love toys.

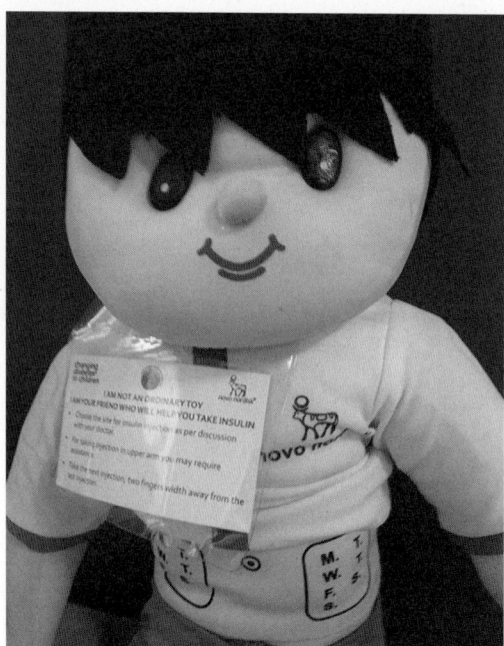

Fig. 3: NOTTI doll presenting sites of injection
(For color version, see Plate 2)

Snake and Ladder Game

It is another diabetes education tool which is designed from the old conventional board game. While playing this board game, the child learns the basic do's and don'ts of diabetes. In this game, each square represents a habit, some of them are applicable for all children and few are applicable specifically for children with T1DM. The square at the base of a ladder is represented by a good habit/the do's, which, like ladders will take you higher/ahead in life (Fig. 4). On the contrary, the square at the head of a snake is represented by a bad habit/the don'ts, like snakes bad habits create hindrance in moving ahead.

Snakes and ladders game offers multiple benefits, namely:[1]
- Motivating the child for self-care
- Reinforcing correct diabetes care essentials

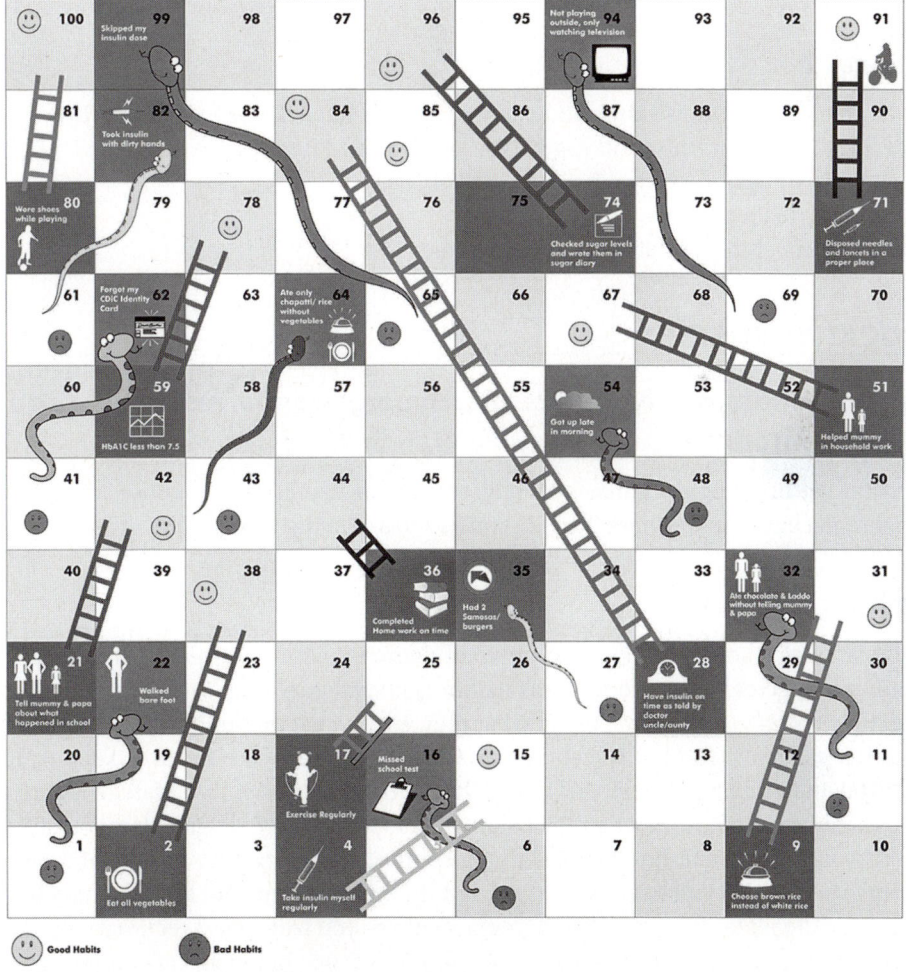

Fig. 4: Snake and ladder game *(For color version, see Plate 2)*

- Help them see the consequences of their various actions
- Influence friends and siblings to understand diabetes
- Creating a bond between, doctor, child, and society

HYPOKIT

This help the child prevent hypos and consists a snack box and water bottle to help them carry something to eat and water to drink everywhere they go.

Healthy Plate

It is a small plate with separate section for vegetables and salad and a simple message that one should have at least three colors in their plate.

Diet Snack Box

To inculcate healthy eating habits and carry snacks, this snack box was made. This snack box had special sections for fruits and vegetables and carried three simple messages:
- Eat healthy to have super brain
- Eat on time to look good
- Take insulin before eating to have healthy body

EDUCATIVE POSTERS

Know the Symptoms, Hypoglycemia, Hyperglycemia, and Insulin and Glucose Monitoring

This poster set on hypoglycemia, hyperglycemia, and insulin and glucose monitoring is a pictorial representation for these 3 important aspects of living with T1DM.

Make Your Own Plate

This educational material is made on physical demonstration of a plate containing balance diet and exchange of various food items within each category (Fig. 5). It has been a great hit among the children as they can decide what they want to eat and in how much quantity they can eat that particular food. It is also perceived as a great tool by educators keeping in mind the cultural and culinary diversity of India. This is to demonstrate that plate of a person with diabetes is not different from a healthy balanced diet. Creating your plate lets you still choose the foods you want to eat, but changes the portion sizes. You can try variety of foods within each food category. All you need is an approximately 9-inch plate. Put an imaginary line down the middle of the plate. Then on one side, cut it again so you will have 3 sections on your plate.[2]
- Fill the largest section with nonstarchy vegetables such as spinach, carrots, lettuce, greens, cabbage, cucumber, green beans, broccoli, cauliflower, tomatoes, okra, mushrooms, peppers, and turnip

CHAPTER 28: Diabetes Education Material

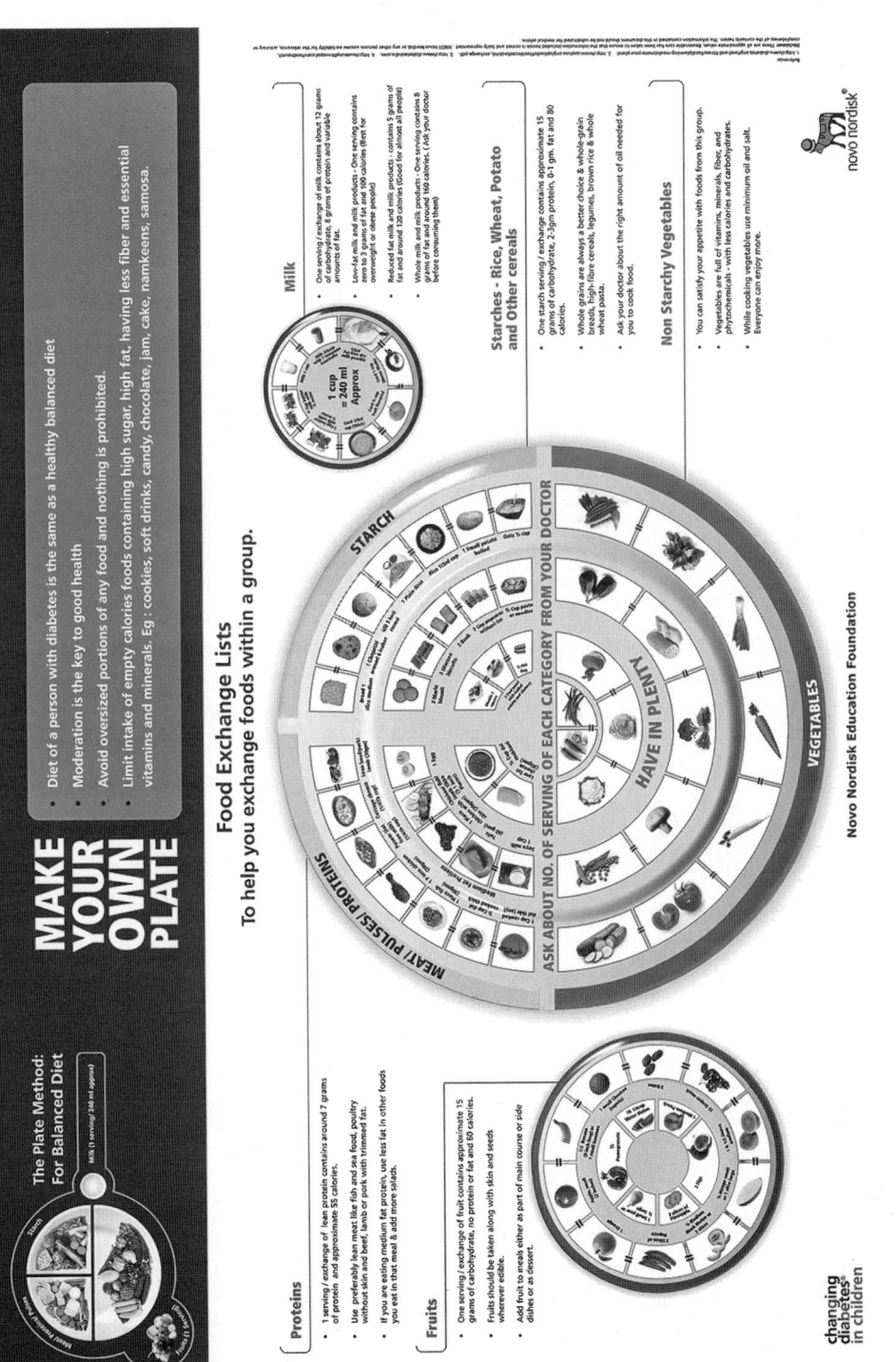

Fig. 5: Make your own plate poster (*For color version, see Plate 3*)

SECTION 8: Miscellaneous

- Now in one of the small sections, put starchy foods such as wheat chapatti, brown rice, whole grain breads, and cereal such as oatmeal or corn flakes, pasta, noodles, potatoes, green peas, corn, lima beans, and sweet potatoes. You can get the approximate idea of portion by looking into exchange list in that group
- On the other small section, put your proteins or meat such as whole pulses, grams, soybean, chicken, fish such as tuna, salmon, cod, or catfish, tofu, eggs, low-fat cheese/paneer
- Add a small bowl and/or glass for your fruit and dairy products
- Exchange list programs gives children a more structured system to control blood glucose along with flexibility to create their own menus. It contains group of measured foods of the same calorific value and similar proteins, fats, and carbohydrates and can be substituted for one another in a meal plan. A person is allowed a certain number of exchange choices from each food list per day (as directed by doctor or dietician). Foods can be substituted for each other within an exchange list[3] but not between lists even if they have the same calorie count, e.g., fruit exchange—1 small apple = 1/2 medium banana = 1/2 mango = 3 dates = 1 and 1/4 cup watermelon = 1 small chikoo = 1 and 1/2 guava = 15 grapes = 1 orange = 1/2 pomegranate = 1 kiwi = 2 figs = 2–3 slice of papaya = 3 plums = 2 slice pineapple.

Foot Door Knob Hanger

Foot Door Knob hangers emphasizes children to take care of their feet and get regular check-up (Fig. 6). When put at door of doctors' cabin, it reminds patient to remove footwear so that doctor can examine feet of a person with diabetes and also give easy tips to take care of feet. It is very important as most of foot complications occurring in people with diabetes can be prevented by timely examination and preventive care.

EDUCATIVE VISUAL AID

Diabetes in Children Visual Aid

It is a visual aid made out of International Society for Pediatric and Adolescent Diabetes posters to explain diabetes in children and its management.

Type 1 Diary

It is made to give basics of diabetes management for children with T1DM along with space to write their blood sugar levels.

Make a Healthy Change Folder

As the name suggest, this in an input consisting of healthy recipes, lifestyle tips on diet, exercise, insulin, and monitoring. It also contains insulin site rotation aid.

CHAPTER 28: Diabetes Education Material

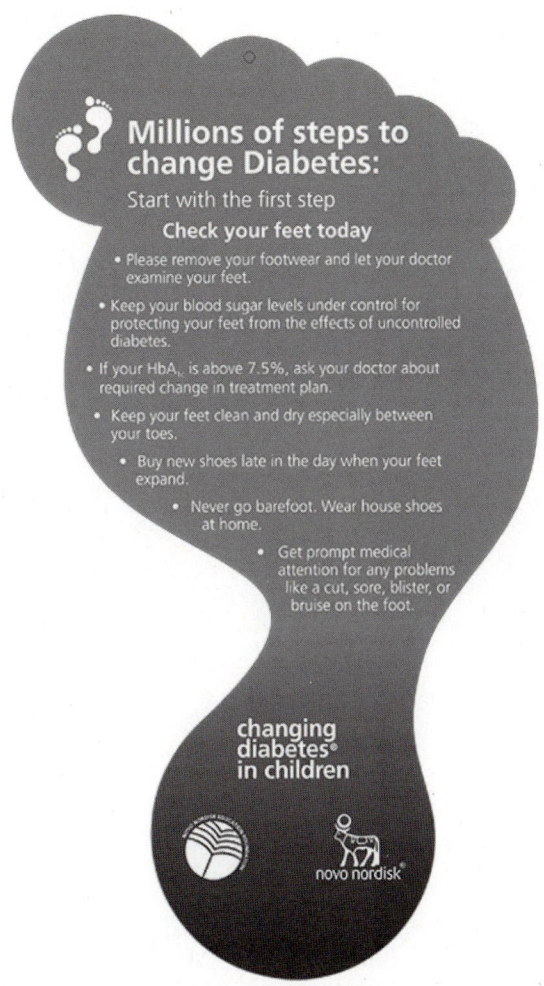

Fig. 6: Foot door knob hanger *(For color version, see Plate 4)*

EDUCATIVE LEAFLETS AND NEWSLETTERS

Changing Diabetes in Children Newsletter

Along with progress made by the project, the newsletter also shares useful tips and information to patients, parents, and diabetes educators for better management of T1DM. It showcases the useful patient education tools made for increasing the children's understanding of their diabetes and also enlists the programs undertaken for the healthcare providers across the country on management of children with T1DM (Fig. 7).

SECTION 8: Miscellaneous

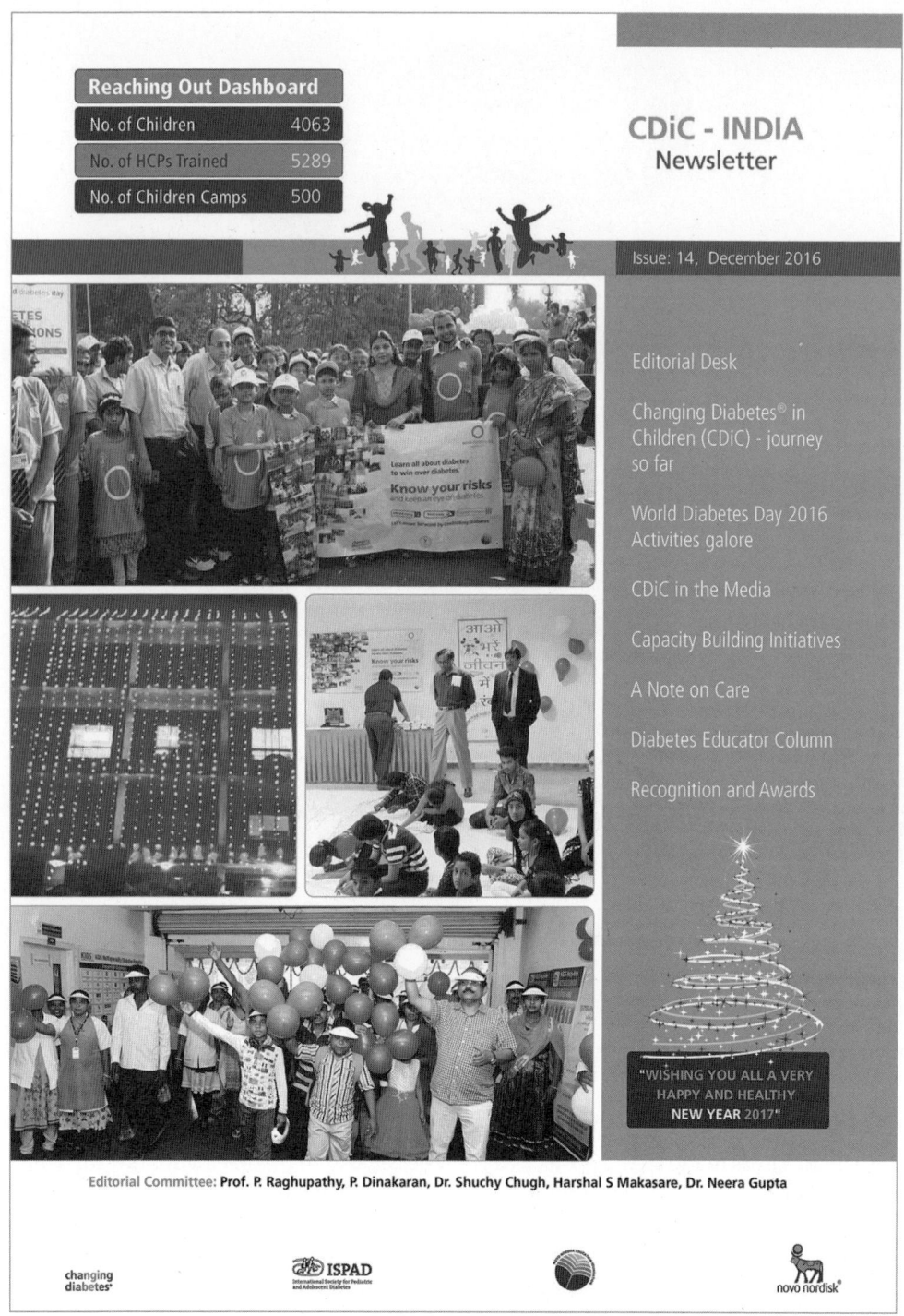

Fig. 7: CDiC newsletter; Table of contents *(For color version, see Plate 5)*

CHAPTER 28: Diabetes Education Material

Mishti Guardian

Twice in a year, a journal named Misthi Guardian, is released to address the awareness and understanding needs of parents and educators (Fig. 8). This is one of its kind newsletter focused on concerns of parents and guardians of children with diabetes in Indian scenario.

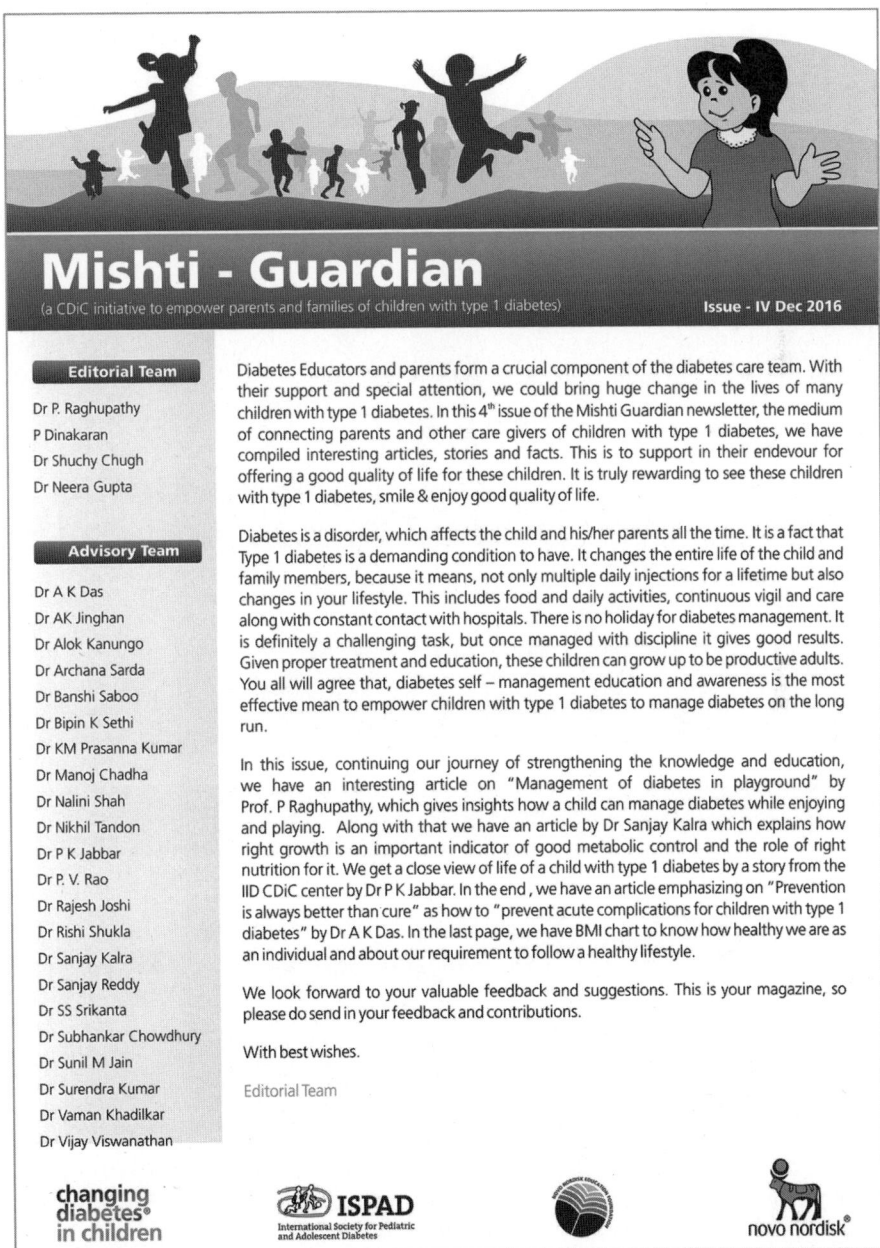

Fig. 8: CDiC newsletter; Editorial section *(For color version, see Plate 6)*

SECTION 8: Miscellaneous

Know About Carbohydrates

It is a leaflet prepared to give understanding about good and bad carbohydrates in Indian context (Fig. 9). There is one simple version which is for children less than 10 years. The complex version gives understanding about carbohydrate counting and adjustment of insulin dose also.

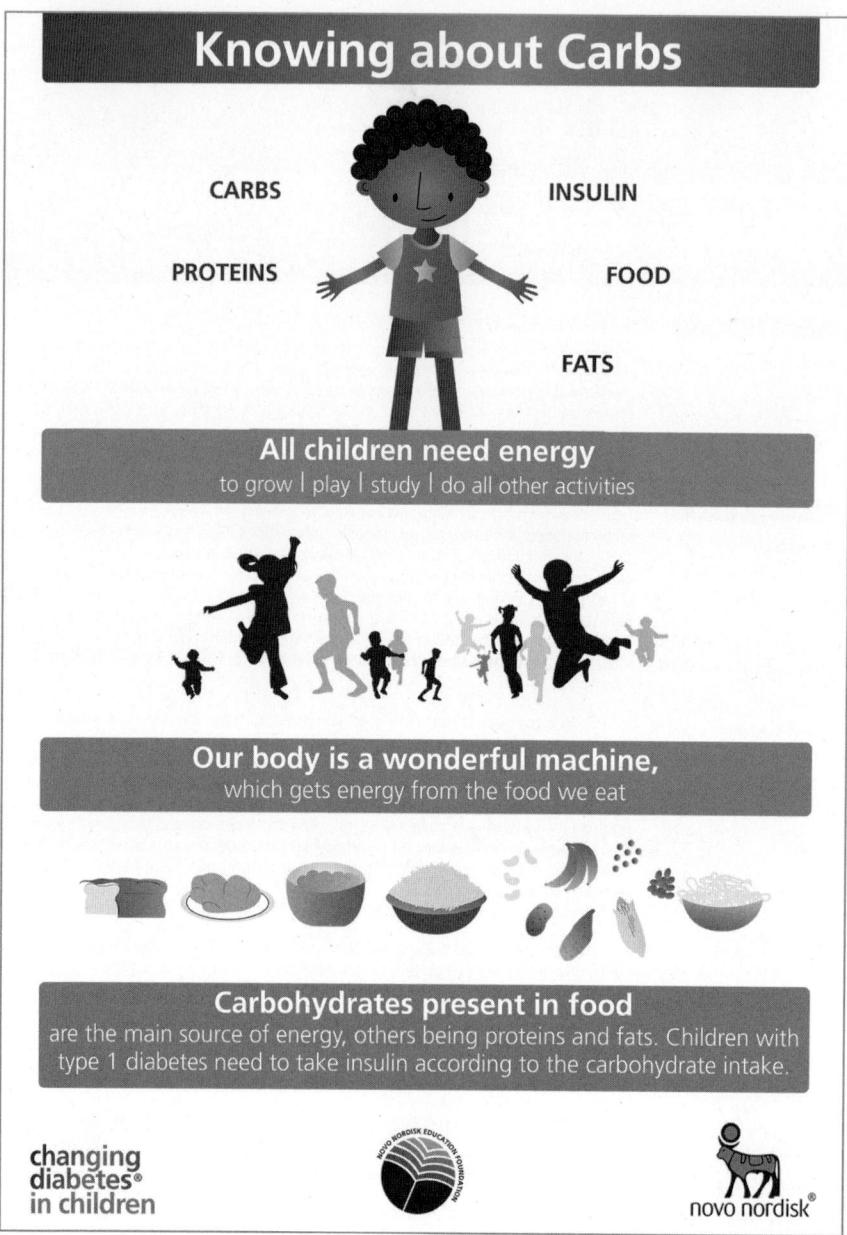

Continued

Continued

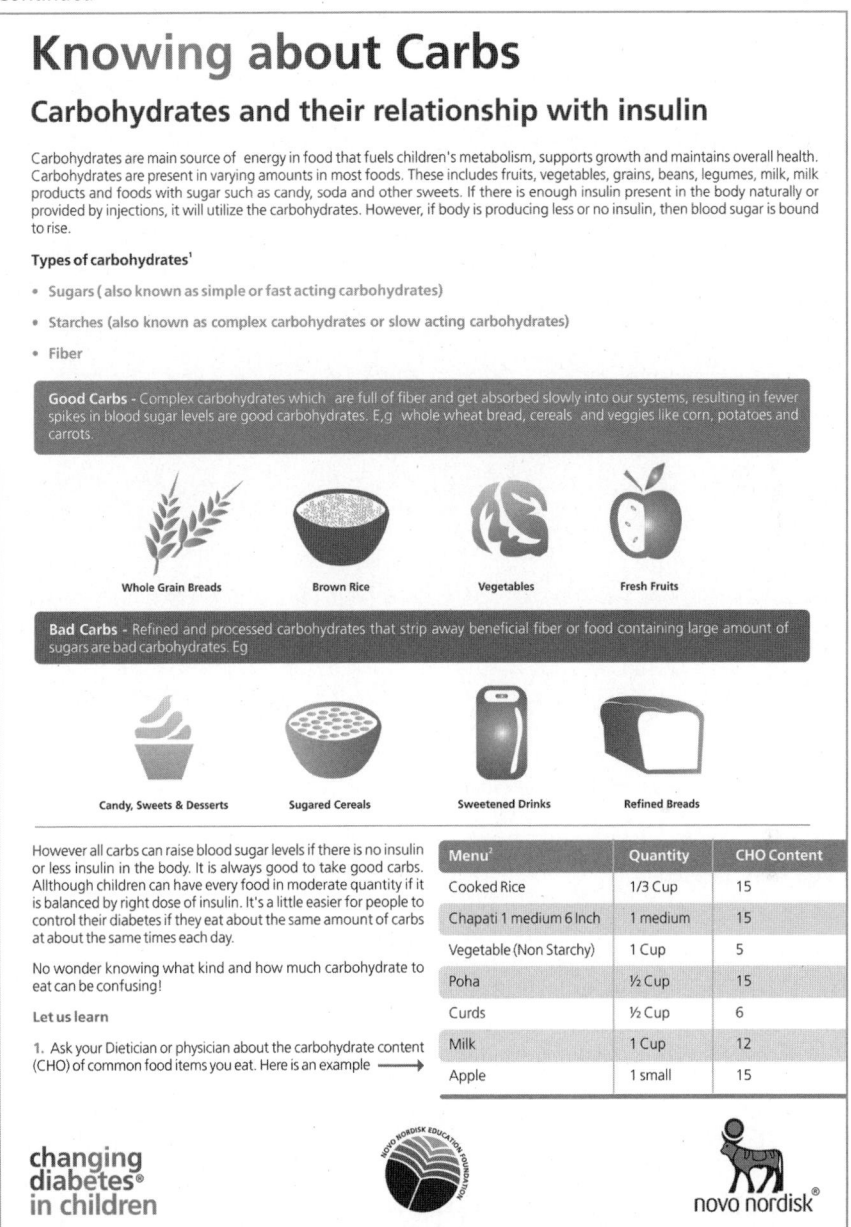

Fig. 9: Leaflet; knowing about carbohydrates *(For color version, see Plate 7)*

DIETS Leaflet

It explains multiple reasons which can affect diabetes management and can result in uncontrolled diabetes (Fig. 10).

SECTION 8: Miscellaneous

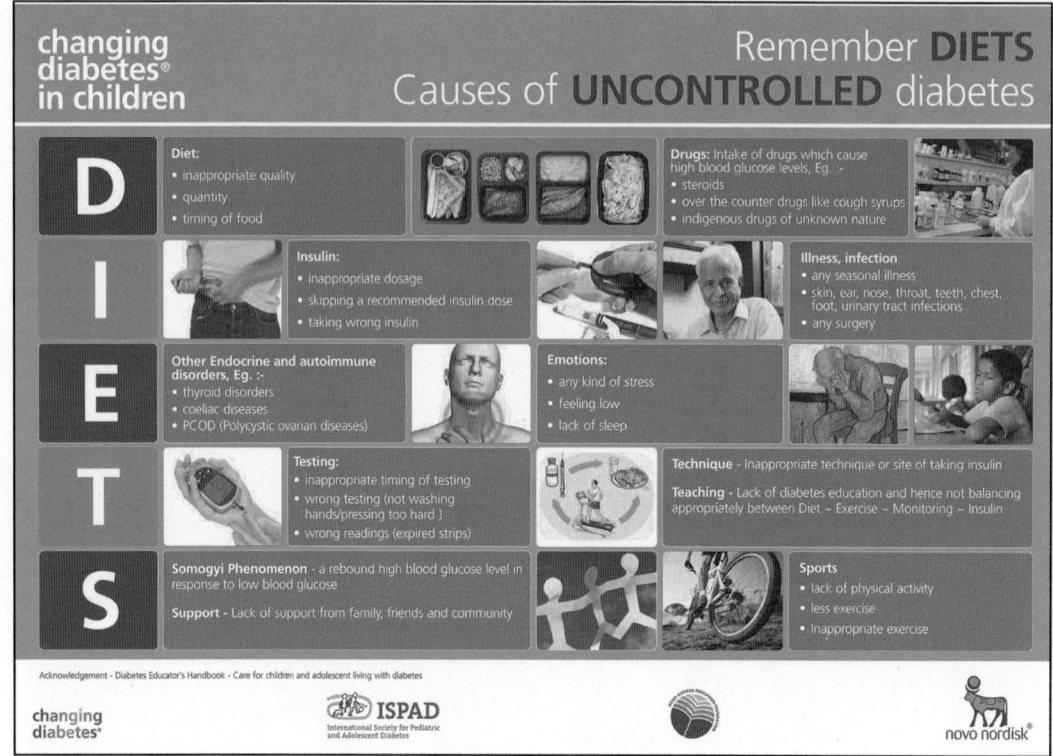

Fig. 10: DIETS leaflet *(For color version, see Plate 8)*

Do and Do not Series

One pager notes are created for improving understanding on T1DM for better management and avoid untoward complications. Three such notes were released currently in the form of an e-mailer: (i) T1DM, (ii) insulin, and (iii) monitoring. It is planned to be a continuous activity.
- It contains five correct and five incorrect notions about the subject along with infographics
- It also contains two socially relevant key facts about the topic.

EDUCATIVE MONITORS

Glycosylated Hemoglobin Calculator

This calculator helps child and their parents convert HbA1c readings in to average blood glucose (Fig. 11).

Body Mass Index Chart

Body mass index chart helps to evaluate right growth of the child according to his/her weight (Fig. 12).

Control Diabetes before it controls you

Average blood glucose (mg/dL)	HbA$_{1C}$
126	6
140	6.5
154	7
169	7.5
183	8
197	8.5
212	9
226	9.5
240	10
255	10.5
269	11
283	11.5
298	12
312	12.5
326	13
341	13.5
355	14
369	14.5
384	15
398	15.5
412	16
427	16.5
441	17
456	17.5
470	18
484	18.5
499	19

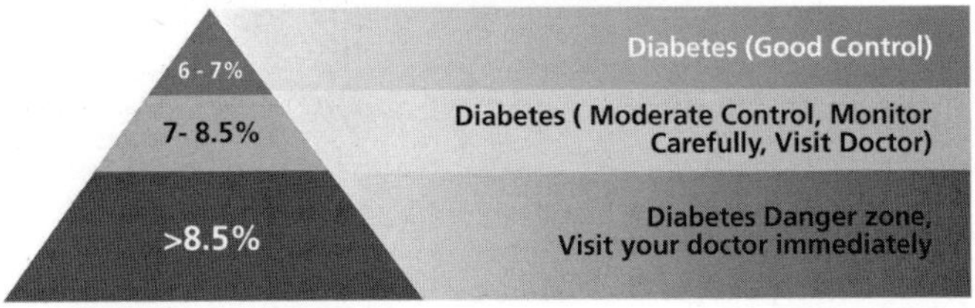

- 6 - 7%: Diabetes (Good Control)
- 7 - 8.5%: Diabetes (Moderate Control, Monitor Carefully, Visit Doctor)
- >8.5%: Diabetes Danger zone, Visit your doctor immediately

HbA$_{1c}$ calculations using the formula: 28.7 X A1C − 46.7 = eAG taken from http://professional.diabetes.org/glucosecalculator.aspx, * 2011 ADA guidelines.
*https://www.aace.com/files/dccwhitepaper.pdf **DCCT / UKPDS / Kumamoto*

changing diabetes® in children

novo nordisk®

Fig. 11: Glycosylated hemoglobin calculator *(For color version, see Plate 9)*

SECTION 8: Miscellaneous

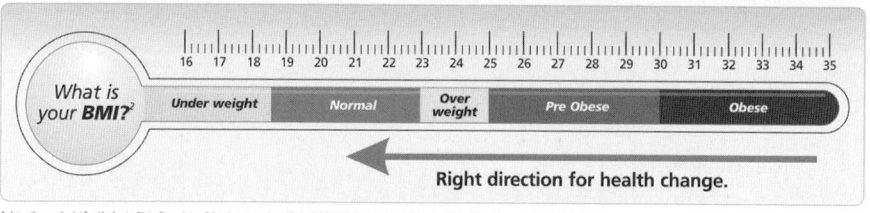

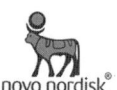

Fig. 12: Body mass index chart *(For color version, see Plate 10)*

Unique features and benefits:
- These educational toys have been made keeping in mind cultural and ethnic issues prevalent in India
- Most of these materials have been made in 10 Indian languages to cater to all the children across the country
- Helps in breaking the silence between child and doctor or educator
- Creating friendship rather than strict doctor patient relationship which has been taught knowingly or unknowingly to the child
- Reducing stress of unknown and being alone for the child
- Understanding what diabetes is
- Planning for diabetes self-management in various situations of life
- Keep the learning with them to reread and relearn
- Motivating the child for self-care
- Reinforcing correct diabetes care essentials.

This is made after keeping in consideration that these children are coming to doctors in remote areas, far from CDiC centers and cannot regularly come to attend CDiC diabetes education camps.

CONCLUSION

Type 1 diabetes mellitus is a lifelong disorder. Treatment of diabetes in children should aim at keeping blood glucose levels near normal and ensuring right growth for them. When a child is diagnosed with T1DM, to manage normal or near-normal blood sugar levels, child needs daily insulin and monitoring of blood glucose levels along with right diet and exercise. The management imposes a vast responsibility of learning about diabetes for both the child and parents. Education is the keystone of diabetes care and structured self-management, which ultimately leads to improved quality of life and successful treatment outcomes in child with T1DM.

REFERENCES

1. Kalra S, Chugh S, Dinakaran P. Diabetes and play therapy. J Soc Health Diabetes 2014;2:40-4.
2. Camelon KM, Hadell K, Jamsen PT, Ketonen KJ, Kohtamaki HM, Makimatilla S, et al. The Plate Model: A visual method of teaching meal planning. J Am Diet Assoc. 1998;98(10):1155-8.
3. American Diabetes Association, American Dietetic Association Exchange Lists for Meal Planning The American Diabetes Association and Chicago, Ill: The American Dietetic Association, Alexandria, Va (1986).

Genetics of Type 1 Diabetes Mellitus

Mudita Dhingra, J Jayannan, Ashok K Das, Sanjay Kalra

INTRODUCTION

Type 1 diabetes mellitus (T1DM) is an immunogenetic disorder which is called as "Geneticist's Nightmare". Type 1 diabetes mellitus is one among the chronic diseases that are more common in childhood. It is generally characterized by immune associated destruction of insulin producing β-cells of pancreatic islet cells. Type 1 diabetes mellitus is a complex disease resulting from the interplay of genetic, epigenetic, and environmental factors (Fig. 1). Worldwide, T1DM epidemic represents an increasing global public health burden, and the incidence of T1DM among children has been rising.[1] Historically, T1DM was largely considered a disorder in children and adolescents, but this opinion has changed over the past decade, so that age at symptomatic onset is no longer a restricting factor.[2]

GENETICS OF TYPE 1 DIABETES MELLITUS

Type 1 diabetes mellitus is a multifactorial polygenic disorder with nearly 40 loci known so far to affect the disease susceptibility. These includes human leukocyte antigen (HLA)-DQ alpha, HLA-DQ beta, HLA-DR, preproinsulin, the *PTPN22* gene, cytotoxic T-lymphocyte-associated antigen 4, interferon-induced helicase, interleukin-2 (IL-2) receptor, a lectin-like gene (*KIA0035*), ERBB3e, and undefined gene at 12q[3-9] and others like STAT4, CAPSL-IL7R, CLEC16A, PTPN2 ,MDA5/IFIH1 (Fig. 2).

There is also a difference in risk which is dependent on the parent with the disease. Mothers with T1DM have children with a risk of 2% for developing T1DM whereas fathers with T1DM have children with a risk of 7% for developing T1DM.

Human Leukocyte Antigen Genes

The human leukocyte antigen locus is located on short arm of chromosome 6.

CHAPTER 29: Genetics of Type 1 Diabetes Mellitus

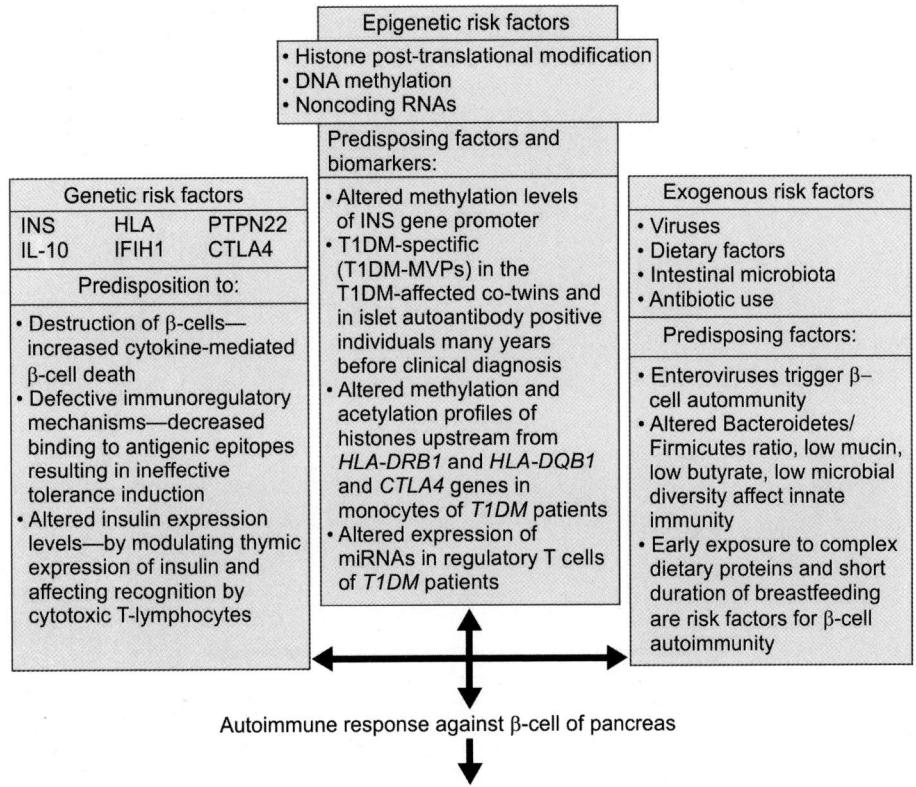

Fig. 1: Genetic, exogenous, and epigenetic predisposing factors and biomarkers in type 1 diabetes mellitus

HLA, human leukocyte antigen; CTLA4, cytotoxic T-lymphocyte-associated antigen 4; T1DM, type 1 diabetes mellitus; DNA, deoxyribonucleic acid; RNAs, ribonucleic acids; MPVs, mean platelet volume.

The concerned genes are classified as Class 1 (*HLA-A, HLA-B, HLA-C*) and class II (*HLADP,HLA-DQ, HLA-DR*). Amongst these, *HLA-A, HLA-B, HLA-C, HLA-DPA1, HLA-DPB1, HLADQA1, HLA-DQB1,* and *HLA-DRB1* are highly polymorphic .These polymorphic genes play a role in immune responses.

The high-risk HLA class II genes represent the strongest genetic association with almost 50% of total genetic contribution to disease. A 20-fold increase in risk for T1DM has been reported in those with *HLA-DR3-DQ2/DR4-DQ8* genotype.[10]

The mechanism of action of DR and DQ in the etiology of T1DM is the peptide binding activity of HLA Class II molecules in antigen presenting cells for the T-lymphocyte peptide recognition—CD4+ T Cells.. Several studies have reported that not all DRB1*03-DQ2 haplotypes predispose equally to disease.[11-15] Two conserved extended DRB1*03-DQ2 haplotypes or ancestral (AH) were associated with diabetes susceptibility, but the AH8.1 (also known as COX) and the AH18.2 haplotype confers significantly higher risk to T1DM according to the

SECTION 8: Miscellaneous

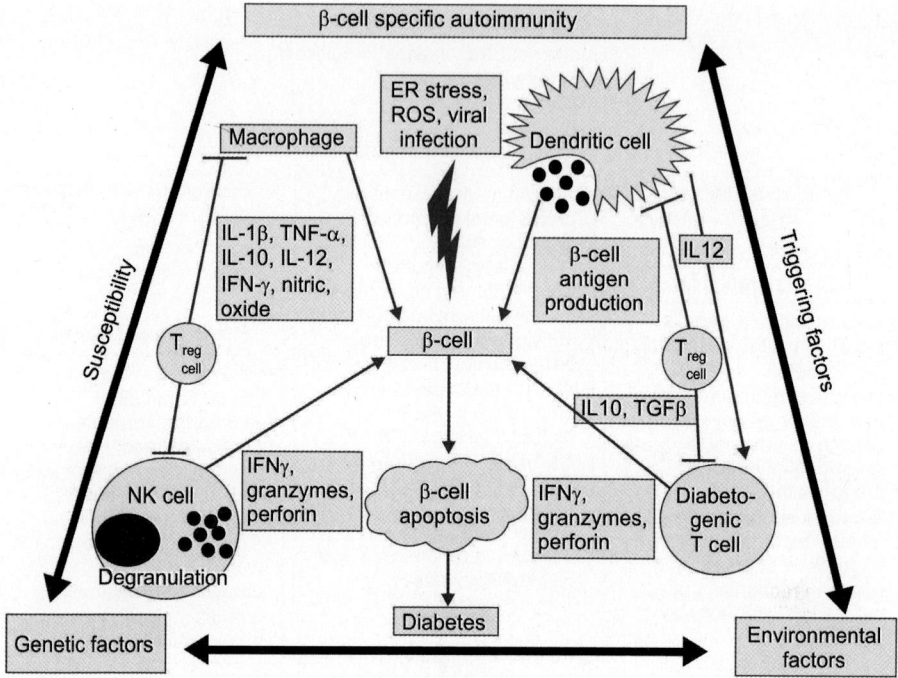

Fig. 2: Pathogenic mechanisms and environmental factors that trigger T1D onset in genetically susceptible people, resulting in β-cell apoptosis and diabetes

aforementioned studies. This increased susceptibility suggests the presence of an additional gene on AH18.2 different from classical MHC class II.

Association of HLA-B 39,57 and T1DM has been proved to be very strong. A probable mechanism for this is its role in antigen presentation to cytotoxic CD8+ lymphocytes.[16]

The HLA-A24 is also found to be strongly associated with T1DM along with rapid destruction of islet cells.[17] Whereas A03 allele is shown to have a protective role against T1DM in children with HLA DR3/DR4 genotype.[18]

Haplotypes of the MHC class II loci also confer the strongest protection from T1D. In Caucasian and Japanese populations the protective haplotype is DRB1*1501-DQ6.[19]

Non-human Leukocyte Antigen Genes

Association of over 40 non-HLA polymorphisms have been identified by genome-wide association studies.[20] But the risk added by them is much smaller as compared to HLA DR, DQ. The risk of islet cell autoimmunity increases 16-fold when family history of T1DM, the *HLA-DR3/4-DQB1 -0302* genotype, and the susceptibility variants of *PTPN22*, *UBASH2*, and *INS* occur in combination.[21,22] The increase in risk of T1DM is shown to be up to 40-fold in such cases. However, the effect of each individual gene is found to be small.

Insulin is a major β-cell auto antigen in T1DM. The insulin gene *INS* is located at chromosome 11p15.5. The insulin gene encodes for preproinsulin. This preproinsulin is converted to proinsulin, which is further converted to insulin. The *INS* gene is transcribed and translated in the thymus. The IDDM2 locus lies upstream to the *INS* promoter region. Variable number of tandem repeats (VNTR) of a consensus sequence at the 5' coding region are found in this region, which is one of the strongest risk factors for T1DM.

The number of repeats at this locus determines the class of proinsulin alleles. Class III has the highest repeats (141–209) followed by Class II (63–140), and Class 1 (26–63) respectively.[23-25] Mutation in VNTR region is associated with increased susceptibility to T1DM. Variable number of tandem repeats regulates insulin expression levels in the thymus by affecting promoter binding site. Variable number of tandem repeats type 1 promote lower transcription of insulin and its precursors in the thymus thereby reducing the tolerance which leads to the development of T1DM whereas VNTR type 3 destructs insulin reactive T cells by negative selection in the thymus thereby protecting against T1DM.

The *INS* disease-risk genotype is associated with lower levels of insulin expression in the thymus, leading to ineffective deletion of insulin-specific T cells. In addition, the *INS* disease-risk genotype has been associated with insulin autoantibody (IAA) which is usually the first autoantibody reactivity to be detected. The *INS* T1DM-risk genotype is likely to affect the initial breakdown of insulin-specific immunologic tolerance rather than to affect the immunoregulation leading to β-cell destruction.

On the other hand, *PTPN22* disease allele is shown to alter T cell and to some extent also β-cell function. A major hypothesis suggests that poor T cell receptor-mediated signaling in the thymus is associated with defective negative selection and maintenance of an autoreactive T cell repertoire. Substitution of arginine for tryptophan at position 620 disrupts binding between *PTPN22* and the intracellular kinase, Csk, altering responsiveness of T and β-cells to receptor stimulation. This leads to decreased inhibition of T cell activation, and promotes multiorgan autoimmunity. Among individuals with the high-risk HLA genotype for T1DM, the *PTPN22* 1858T allele is independently associated with diminished residual β-cell function with development of persistent islet autoimmunity and progression to T1DM.[26-28]

Interferon induced with helicase C domain 1 (IFIH1) activation has also been related to T1DM. It is a cytoplasmic helicase whose linkage disequilibrium block on long arm of chromosome 2 is associated with T1DM.

It plays a role in detection of intracellular dsRNA of picornavirus leading to activation of interferon pathways.[29] Infection of enterovirus (which belongs to picornavirus family) activates interferon pathways via IFIH1 in pancreatic β-cells which ultimately leads to cytotoxic $CD8^+$ T cell-induced β-cell death.

IMMUNOGENETICS

Type 1 diabetes mellitus is an autoimmune disease in which autoantibodies are produced which destroys β-cells of pancreas. Some of the autoantibiotics that plays an important role in the pathogenesis of T1DM includes islet cell autoantibodies, insulinoma antigen 2 autoantibodies, IAA, glutamic acid decarboxylase 65, imogen 38, and heat shock protein. Beta cell specific autoantibodies that are newly discovered includes zinc transporter-8, pancreatic duodenal homeobox factor-1, chromogranin A, and islet amyloid polypeptide.

The number of autoantibodies present and autoantibodies titer can be considered as independent predictors for T1DM. Insulin autoantibodies are highly specific and sensitive for detecting T1DM. However, due to the requirement of high serum volumes and the various subtypes of the autoantibody which have different capacities in predicting the disease, usage of IAA are difficult in diagnosis of T1DM.

Glutamic acid decarboxylase autoantibodies are seen in 60–70% of newly onset T1DM. In T1DM, epigenetic phenomena, such as deoxyribonucleic acid; methylation, histone modifications, and microRNA dysregulation, have been associated with altered gene expression.

CLINICAL IMPLICATIONS

Due to advances which were made to understand the pathogenesis of T1DM in recent years along with genetic and immunologic measurements, individuals who are not having diabetes can be identified at high risk of subsequent clinical T1DM. Identifying high risk subjects and to predict subsequent clinical T1DM with knowledge in pathogenesis set the stage for large scale intervention trials to test whether T1DM can be prevented. Risk groups for prediction and prevention of T1DM includes first-degree relatives of patients with T1DM, gestational diabetes mothers with autoantibody positivity, and children born to older mothers than general population.

Recently completed trials including diabetes prevention trial type 1 (DPT-1) and European Nicotinamide Diabetes Intervention Trial (ENDIT) and ongoing trials including Type 1 Diabetes Prediction and Prevention Project (DIPP), Finnish Diabetes Type 1 Prediction and Prevention Project, and Trial to Reduce T1DM in Genetically at Risk (TRIGR) aims to interrupt disease process and to prevent people from developing clinical T1DM.[30]

PREVENTIVE IMPLICATIONS-VACCINE STRATEGIES

The vaccine strategies tried to prevent T1DM are categorized into:
- Induction of tolerance
- Peptide based vaccine strategy
- Deoxyribonucleic acid; vaccine
- Adjuvants as vaccines and others.

Induction of Tolerance

One of the methods that is used to induce tolerance is administration of oral insulin conjugated to B subunit of cholera toxin[31] which effectively suppress systemic T cell reactivity. Cholera toxin B-subunit carries the insulin to the intestine and helps in the transfer of insulin molecule across the intestinal barrier. This helps in the reduction of the insulin dosage administered orally without causing hypoglycemia.

Peptide Based Vaccine Strategy

An immunomodulatory peptide called p277 (DiaPep277) vaccine strategy that has passed phase 2 acts by mechanism of glucagon mediated C-peptide production and Diamyd GAD65 vaccine acts by prevention of β-cell destruction are the two vaccines used in prevention of T1DM.

Deoxyribonucleic Acid Vaccine

Deoxyribonucleic acid vaccine is administering the GAD65 gene in a plasmid vector intramuscularly so that GAD65 protein is produced in the body that can induce tolerance has been tried in the prevention of T1DM.

Adjuvants as Vaccines and Others

Bacillus Calmette-Guérin vaccine has been tried in the prevention of T1DM by shifting T cell response from destructive to nondestructive.

CONCLUSION

Type 1 diabetes mellitus is a polygenic disease in which environmental factors triggers autoimmunity in genetically susceptible individuals, thus leading to β-cell apoptosis and hence insulin deficiency. Majority of patients with T1DM test positive for autoantibodies which destroys the β-cells of pancreas. These autoantibodies develop under the influence of HLA and non HLA genes and epigenetic modification leads to altered gene expression. Amongst non HLA gene (INS and *PTPN22*) have gene-environment interaction with enterovirus and cow's milk exposure in early life. Various strategies have been used in patients with islet cell autoimmunity to prevent development of T1DM or occurrence of DKA at diagnosis by modifying the natural course of autoimmunity with less promising results. Genetic testing although not routinely clinically indicated in these patients, may help in future for primary prevention trials in siblings or first degree relatives of T1DM with high risk HLA haplotypes (HLA-DR3/4,DQB1*0302) with exciting possibilities.

REFERENCES

1. Forlenza GP, Rewers M. The epidemic of type 1 diabetes: what is it telling us? Curr Opin Endocrinol Diabetes Obes. 2011; 18:248-51.
2. Leslie RD. Predicting adult-onset autoimmune diabetes: clarity from complexity. Diabetes. 2010;59:330-1.
3. Smyth DJ, Cooper JD, Bailey R, Field S, Burren O, Smink LJ, et al. A genome-wide association study of nonsynonymous SNPs identifies a type 1 diabetes locus in the interferon-induced helicase (IFIH1) region. Nat Genet. 2006;38:617-9.
4. Wellcome Trust Case Control Consortium. Genome-wide association study of 14,000 cases of seven common diseases and 3,000 shared controls. Nature. 2007;447:661-78.
5. Todd JA, Walker NM, Cooper JD, Smyth DJ, Downes K, Plagnol V, et al. Robust associations of four new chromosome regions from genome-wide analyses of type 1 diabetes. Nat Genet. 2007;39:857-864.

6. Hakonarson H, Grant SF, Bradfield JP, Marchand L, Kim CE, Glessner JT, et al. A genome-wide association study identifies KIAA0350 as a type 1 diabetes gene. Nature. 2007;448:591-4.
7. Lowe CE, Cooper JD, Brusko T, Walker NM, Smyth DJ, Bailey R, et al. Large-scale genetic fine mapping and genotype-phenotype associations implicate polymorphism in the IL2RA region in type 1 diabetes. Nat Genet. 2007;39:1074-82.
8. Concannon P, Onengut-Gumuscu S, Todd JA, Smyth DJ, Pociot F, Bergholdt R, et al. A human type 1 diabetes susceptibility locus maps to chromosome 21q22.3. Diabetes. 2008;57:2858-61.
9. Concannon P, Rich SS, Nepom GT. Genetics of type 1A diabetes. N Engl J Med. 2009;360:1646-54.
10. Noble JA, Valdes AM, Cook M, Klitz W, Thomson G, Erlich HA. The role of HLA class II genes in insulin-dependent diabetes mellitus:molecular analysis of 180 Caucasian, multiplex families. Am J Hum Genet. 1996;59:1134-48.
11. Johansson S, Lie BA, Todd JA, Pociot F, Nerup J, Cambon-Thomsen A, et al. Evidence of at least two type 1 diabetes susceptibility genes in the HLA complex distinct from HLA-DQB1, -DQA1 and -DRB1. Genes Immun. 2003;4:46-53.
12. Lie BA, Todd JA, Pociot F, Nerup J, Akselsen HE, Joner G, et al. The predisposition to type 1 diabetes linked to the human leukocyte antigen complex includes at least one non-class II gene. Am J Hum Genet. 1999;64:793-800.
13. Nejentsev S, Gombos Z, Laine AP, Veijola R, Knip M, Simell O, et al. Non-class II HLA gene associated with type 1 diabetes maps to the 240-kb region near HLA-B. Diabetes. 2000;49:2217-21.
14. Urcelay E, Santiago JL, de la Calle H, Martinez A, Mendez J, Ibarra JM, et al. Type 1 diabetes in the Spanish population: Additional factors to class II HLA-DR3 and -DR4. BMC Genomics. 2005;6:56.
15. Zavattari P, Lampis R, Motzo C, Loddo M, Mulargia A, Whalen M, et al. Conditional linkage disequilibrium analysis of a complex disease superlocus, IDDM1 in the HLA region, reveals the presence of independent modifying gene effects influencing the type 1 diabetes risk encoded by the major HLA-DQB1, -DRB1 disease loci. Hum Mol Genet. 2001;10:881-9.
16. Nejentsev S, Howson JM, Walker NM, Szeszko J, Field SF, Stevens HE, et al. Localization of type 1 diabetes susceptibility to the MHC class I genes HLA-B and HLA-A. Nature. 2007;450:887-92.
17. Honeyman MC, Harrison LC, Drummond B, Colman PG, Tait BD. Analysis of families at risk for insulin-dependent diabetes mellitus reveals that HLA antigens influence progression to clinical disease. Mol Med. 1995;1:576-82.
18. Lipponen K, Gombos Z, Kiviniemi M, Siljander H, Lempainen J, Hermann R, et al. Effect of HLA class I and class II alleles on progression from autoantibody positivity to overt type 1 diabetes in children with risk-associated class II genotypes. Diabetes. 2010;59:3253-6.
19. Ikegami H, Fujisawa T, Kawabata Y, Noso S, Ogihara T. Genetics of type 1 diabetes: Similarities and differences between Asian and Caucasian populations. Ann N Y Acad Sci. 2006;1079:51-9.
20. Bergholdt R, Brorsson C, Palleja A, Berchtold LA, Fløyel T, Bang-Berthelsen CH, et al. Identification of novel type 1 diabetes candidate genes by integrating genome-wide association data, protein-protein interactions, and human pancreatic islet gene expression. Diabetes. 2012;61:954-62.
21. Steck AK, Wong R, Wagner B, Johnson K, Liu E, Romanos J, et al. Effects of non-HLA gene polymorphisms on development of islet autoimmunity and type 1 diabetes in a population with high-risk HLA-DR, DQ genotypes. Diabetes. 2012;61:753-8.
22. Lempainen J, Hermann R, Veijola R, Simell O, Knip M, Ilonen J. Effect of the PTPN22 and INS risk genotypes on the progression to clinical type 1 diabetes after the initiation of -cell autoimmunity. Diabetes. 2012;61:963-6.
23. Todd JA, Walker NM, Cooper JD, Smyth DJ, Downes K, Plagnol V, et al. Robust associations of four new chromosome regions from genome-wide analyses of type 1 diabetes. Nat Genet. 2007;39:857-64.
24. Bennett ST, Lucassen AM, Gough SC, Powell EE, Undlien DE, Pritchard LE, et al. Susceptibility to human type 1 diabetes at IDDM2 is determined by tandem repeat variation at the insulin gene minisatellite locus. Nat Genet. 1995;9:284-92.
25. Lucassen AM, Julier C, Beressi JP, Boitard C, Froguel P, Lathrop M, et al. Susceptibility to insulin dependent diabetes mellitus maps to a 4.1 kb segment of DNA spanning the insulin gene and associated VNTR. Nat Genet. 1993;4:305-10.
26. Bottini N, Musumeci L, Alonso A, Rahmouni S, Nika K, Rostamkhani M, et al. A functional variant of lymphoid tyrosine phosphatase is associated with type I diabetes. Nat Genet. 2004;36:337-8.
27. Cho JH, Gregersen PK. Genomics and the multifactorial nature of human autoimmune disease. N Engl J Med. 2011;365:1612-23.
28. Steck AK, Zhang W, Bugawan TL, Barriga KJ, Blair A, Erlich HA, et al. Do non-HLA genes influence development of persistent islet autoimmunity and type 1 diabetes in children with high-risk HLA-DR,DQ genotypes? Diabetes. 2009;58:1028-33.

29. Liu S, Wang H, Jin Y, Podolsky R, Linga Reddy MV, Pedersen J, et al. IFIH1 polymorphisms are significantly associated with type 1 diabetes and IFIH1 gene expression in peripheral blood mononuclear cells. Hum Mol Genet. 2009;18:358-65.
30. Naik RG, Palmer JP. Pathophysiology and genetics of type 1 (insulin-dependent) diabetes. In: Porte DJ, Sherwen RS, Baron A, (Eds). Ellenberg and Rifkin's Diabetes Mellitus, 6th ed. New York: McGraw-Hill; 2003. pp. 301-30.
31. Bergerot I, Ploix C, Petersen J, Moulin V, Rask C, Fabien N, et al. A cholera toxoid-insulin conjugate as an oral vaccine against spontaneous autoimmune diabetes. Proc Natl Acad Sci U S A. 1997;94:4610-4.

30 CHAPTER

Type 2 Diabetes Mellitus in Children

Jabbar Khadar, Abilash Nair

INTRODUCTION

Till a few years back, diabetes in children was type 1 diabetes mellitus (T1DM) unless proved otherwise, or as it was earlier called insulin dependent diabetes mellitus (IDDM). With the global epidemic of obesity, there has been a trend of early occurrence of type 2 diabetes mellitus (T2DM) with the age of onset approaching up to the first decade of life.

Criteria for the diagnosis of diabetes mellitus in children are similar to those for adults. The criteria proposed by World Health Organization and American Diabetes Association include:[1]
- Classic symptoms of diabetes or hyperglycemic crisis, with plasma glucose concentration more than or equal to 11.1 mmol/L (200 mg/dL), or
- Fasting (for at least 8 h) plasma glucose more than or equal to 7.0 mmol/L (≥126 mg/dL)
- Two-hour post load glucose more than or equal to 11.1 mmol/L (≥200 mg/dL) during an oral glucose tolerance test (OGTT).

(The test should be performed using a glucose load containing the equivalent of 75 g anhydrous glucose dissolved in water or 1.75 g/kg of body weight to a maximum of 75 g), or
- Glycosylated hemoglobin (HbA1c) more than 6.5% (From National Glycohemoglobin Standardization Program certified lab standardized to the Diabetes Control and Complications Trial assay).

Glucose measurement to confirm the diagnosis should be based on laboratory values by glucose oxidase method and not by capillary blood glucose.

Hyperglycemia may occur in conditions of acute infective, traumatic, circulatory, or other stress, which may be transitory and should not be regarded as diagnostic of diabetes. In these situations, the diagnosis of diabetes should not be based on a single plasma glucose concentration and continued observation with fasting and 2-hour postprandial blood glucose levels and/or an OGTT may be required to confirm the diagnosis.

An OGTT is usually not required and should not be performed if diabetes can be diagnosed using fasting or random criteria, but is useful in diagnosing T2DM, monogenic diabetes, or cystic fibrosis related diabetes. If doubt remains, periodic retesting should be undertaken until the diagnosis is established or ruled out. Impaired glucose tolerance (IGT) and impaired fasting glucose (IFG) are intermediate stages in the natural history of disordered carbohydrate metabolism with relatively high risk for development of diabetes and cardiovascular disease. Impaired fasting glucose and IGT (collectively referred to as prediabetes) may be associated with the metabolic syndrome, the features of which include obesity (particularly abdominal or visceral obesity), dyslipidemia [high triglyceride and/or low high density lipoprotein (HDL)], and hypertension.

EPIDEMIOLOGY GLOBAL

Till about 10 years back, T2DM contributed to less than 3% of all children with diabetes globally. However, recent studies in developed countries has put the estimate to more than 45% of all cases of childhood diabetes. With the achievement of food sufficiency and increase in the number of affluent families, India has been no exception in this regard.[2]

INDIAN PERSPECTIVE

India is already at number two after China for adult diabetes but data about diabetes in children are scarce from India. However, considering factors in socioeconomic development in the last three decades with the change in nutrition pattern and lifestyle, the situation in India is one of a bomb waiting to explode. The factors include rapid urbanization causing the problems of overweight and obesity, the genetic predisposition of Indians, and higher prevalence of prenatal risk factors like small for gestational age, maternal obesity, and insulin resistance. Children who have a body mass index (BMI) equal to or exceeding the age and gender-specific 95th percentile are defined as obese and those with BMI equal to or exceeding the 85th but below 95th percentiles are defined overweight. In a recent study done at schools in Chennai by Jagadesan et al.[3] of the Madras Diabetes Research Federation, the prevalence of overweight/obesity was significantly higher in private compared to government schools [private schools: 21.4%, government schools: 3.6% (using International Obesity Task Force Criteria), p <0.001]. Similarly, a study from North India by Marwah et al.,[4] reported a prevalence of overweight and obesity in upper socioeconomic status children. It was 16.75% and 5.59% in boys and 19.01% and 5.03% in girls, respectively, in their study. The genetic predisposition of Indian children is attributed to the higher visceral to total fat ratio for the same BMI when compared to European people. The part of the problem in handling T2DM in children may also stem from misclassification of T2DM as T1DM, just based on the age at presentation. In addition, a greater problem is under diagnosis of T2DM in children as is evidenced by a study by Ramachandran et al., involving 18 children (5 boys and 13 girls) with T2DM diagnosed, aging less than 15 years. Of these 18 patients, 9 patients were asymptomatic and picked up on screening done due to strong family history of diabetes mellitus and/or because of obesity. Nine children were obese and 12 had high waist-hip ratio in this study.[5] Obesity trends of general population also affect the predisposition of babies to diabetes. Babies of obese mothers are more insulin resistant, as estimated by the homoeostatic model assessment of insulin resistance (HOMA-IR). This observation is also supported by recent data from the Hyperglycemia and Adverse Pregnancy Outcome (HAPO) study[6] which shows an association between increased maternal BMI and fetal hyperinsulinemia, an effect independent of maternal glycemia. Studies also show that maternal obesity (prepregnancy BMI >27–30 kg/m^2) and excessive weight gain during pregnancy predisposes to T2DM by 11 years of age.

A study from Srinagar[7] in 2001 by Zargar et al. with 724 young diabetics with age less than 40 years, showed a prevalence rate of 24% for T2DM. Another risk factor prevalent in India is small for gestational age status. This is mostly attributed to poor maternal nutrition but may be due to various medical causes. Many studies have shown a link between being born small for gestational age and likelihood of diabetes, also there are evidences from molecular studies showing a genetic variation of islet cell proteins, such as KCNJ11, among others. Babies born small for gestational age, common in India, are more prone to insulin resistance, especially if they are given energy dense feeds and experience rapid catch-up growth.

PRESENTATION

Diabetes in children is usually heralded by characteristic symptoms of polyuria, polydipsia, nocturia, enuresis, and weight loss. It may also present with recurrent infections. Diabetic ketoacidosis (DKA), although less common in children with T2DM, may be a presenting feature. Diabetic ketoacidosis and less commonly nonketotic hyperosmolar syndrome may develop and lead to coma or death if not promptly treated. If the blood glucose level is elevated in a child with symptoms of hyperglycemia, a prompt referral to a center with experience in managing children with diabetes is essential. Median age of diagnosis of youth-onset T2DM is 13.5 years and most cases present in the second decade of life, and are rare before puberty. The median of age of onset is 1 year higher in boys than girls. Both these facts suggest a role of physiologic pubertal insulin resistance in unmasking the diabetic state. There is usually a strong family history of diabetes in these children. Youth-onset T2DM occurs in all races, but at a much greater prevalence in those of non-White European descent, e.g., those of Black African descent, native North American, Hispanic (especially Mexican)-American, Asian, South Asian (Indian Peninsula), and Native Pacific islanders. In Hong Kong, 90% of youth-onset diabetes is T2DM, in Taiwan, 50%, and nearly 60% in Japan.[8] In the United States and Europe, nearly all youth with T2DM have BMI above 85th percentile for age and sex. However, this is not true in Asia. In Japan, 15% of children with T2DM are not obese.[8] In Asian Indian urban children, half of those with T2DM had normal weight and ketoacidosis or hyperosmolar state are seen in up to 25% of patients.[8] These latter two presentations can entail significant risk for morbidity and mortality if not recognized and treated.

PATHOGENESIS OF TYPE 2 DIABETES MELLITUS

Pathogenesis of T2DM is an interplay of increased insulin resistance, islet cell insulin secretory defect, and defect in incretin production or action. The relative importance of impaired insulin release and insulin resistance in the pathogenesis can be variable. A seven-year prospective study on 714 Mexican-Americans who were nondiabetics showed that decreased insulin resistance[9] and insulin secretion were independent risk factors for T2DM. A prospective study of over 6,500 British civil servants without diabetes at baseline evaluated the change in insulin sensitivity in those patients who developed diabetes on follow-up. Five hundred and five subjects became diabetic during a median follow-up of 9.7 years.[10] Compared to those who did not develop diabetes, those who developed it had a marked decrease in insulin sensitivity since 5 years before the onset of diabetes. Insulin secretion increased 3–4 years prior to diagnosis but later decreased till the diagnosis of diabetes. Landmark studies on Pima Indians have shown that the transition from normal glucose tolerance to IGT to diabetes is associated with decrease in insulin-stimulated glucose disposal as well as glucose-stimulated insulin secretion. Recently, focused research has been done on the role of incretin hormones in the pathogenesis of diabetes. Impaired incretin effect, most likely due to impaired islet responses to the incretin hormones, has been shown to be an early sign of impaired glucose metabolism. A further impairment of incretin effect is seen as glucose intolerance worsens.

AUTOIMMUNE TYPE 2 DIABETES MELLITUS

Some authors have reported the phenomenon of autoimmune T2DM. This has sometimes been referred to as type 1.5, type 3, or double diabetes. However, it is now becoming clearer that these individuals are best understood as having autoimmune T1DM presenting in overweight or obese individuals with underlying insulin resistance. Youth and adults in United States and Europe, who are clinically diagnosed with T2DM, are found to have T1DM-associated autoantibodies in 15–40% of cases, including many who are not receiving insulin 1 year after diagnosis.[8] The β-cell function is significantly less in antibody positive youth with T2DM phenotype, resulting in more rapid development of insulin dependence. The clinician is obliged to weigh the evidence in each individual patient to distinguish between T1DM and T2DM. There are various challenges for differentiating these two types of diabetes in clinical practice. The few reasons for this are: with increasing obesity in childhood, as many as 30% of newly diagnosed T1DM (or monogenic diabetes) patients may be obese, depending on the rate of obesity in the background population. A significant number of pediatric patients with T2DM demonstrate ketonuria or ketoacidosis at diagnosis. However, persistence of C-peptide above the normal level for age would be unusual in T1DM after 12–14 months.

DIFFERENCES OF PEDIATRIC FROM ADULT TYPE 2 DIABETES MELLITUS

As the complications of diabetes correlate with the duration of the disease, children with diabetes are at a higher risk of complications by the time they become adults. Also, there is a higher chance of progression of diabetic retinopathy at the time of puberty in children who have a prepubertal onset of diabetes. Girls with diabetes may be at a higher risk of polycystic ovary syndrome (PCOS), infertility, hypertension, and obstetric complications in the future. The differentiation between T1DM, T2DM, monogenic, and other forms of diabetes has important implications for both therapeutic decisions and educational approaches. Diabetes-associated autoantibodies: the presence of glutamic acid decarboxylase (GAD), tyrosine phosphatase, insulin autoantibodies, and/or zinc transporter-8 (ZnT8) confirms the diagnosis of T1DM, as one and usually more of these autoantibodies are present in 85–90% of individuals when fasting hyperglycemia is detected. An elevated fasting C-peptide level can distinguish young people with insulin resistant T2DM from T1DM. However, there is considerable overlap in insulin or C-peptide measurements between T1DM and T2DM in the first year after diagnosis; C-peptide measurements are not recommended in the acute phase. In insulin treated patients, C-peptide will be detected if endogenous insulin secretion is still present, when the glucose is sufficiently high (>150 mg/dL) to stimulate C-peptide. Regardless of the type of diabetes, the child who presents with severe hyperglycemia, ketonemia, and metabolic derangements will require insulin therapy initially to reverse the metabolic abnormalities.

Types of diabetes other than T1DM or T2DM should be considered in the child with diabetes, who have:
- No autoantibodies
- An autosomal dominant/family history of diabetes
- Diabetes diagnosed in the first 6 months of life
- Mild fasting hyperglycemia (100–150 mg/dL), which does not progress, especially if young, nonobese, and asymptomatic
- Associated conditions such as deafness, optic atrophy, or syndromic features
- A history of exposure to drugs known to be toxic to β-cells or cause insulin resistance.

CLINICAL FEATURES TO DIFFERENTIATE FROM TYPE 1 DIABETES MELLITUS (TABLE 1)

Type 1 diabetes mellitus usually has a rapid onset of osmotic symptoms within days to weeks from presentation. It is associated with weight loss, prostration, and usually progresses to ketoacidosis. However, weight loss is not specific to T1DM and children with T2DM also can present with weight loss or low BMI, especially if hyperglycemia is undetected for a long time. Even ketosis and ketoacidosis may be seen in patients with T2DM, which is usually precipitated by severe infections/stress. Other autoimmune diseases, like vitiligo, autoimmune thyroid disease, celiac disease, hypoadrenalism, etc., may be present in patients with T1DM, whereas T2DM may be accompanied by markers of insulin resistance like skin

TABLE 1: Features to differentiate between type1 and type 2 diabetes mellitus

Type 1 diabetes mellitus	Type 2 diabetes mellitus
Lean	Normal weight or obese
Young	Older
Weight loss	Insignificant
Severe hyperglycemic symptoms	Usually absent
Low C-peptide	Normal or high
No evidence of insulin resistance	May be present
Antibodies present	Not seen

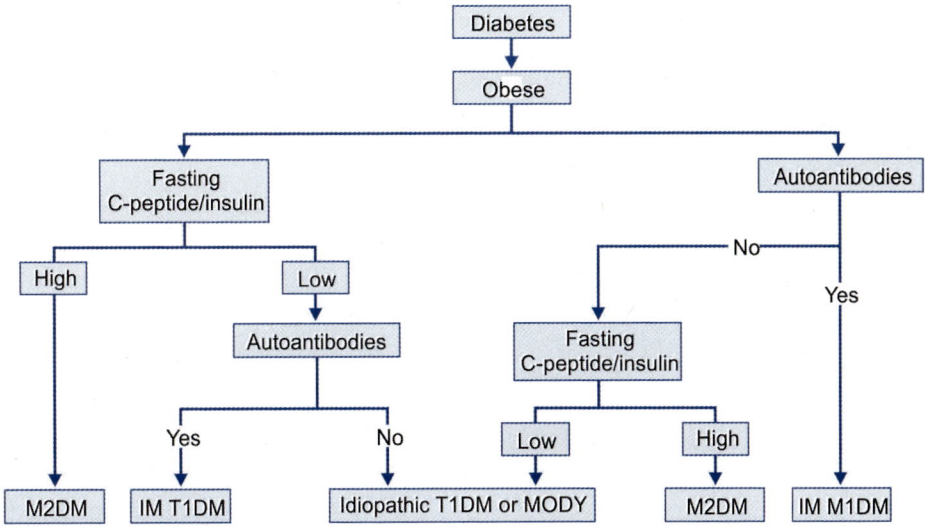

MODY, maturity onset diabetes of the young; T1DM, type 1 diabetes mellitus; T2DM, type 2 diabetes mellitus.

Fig. 1: Approach to young diabetes

tags and acanthosis nigricans, and patients may have comorbidities like dyslipidemia, hypertension, and PCOS. Finally, patients with T1DM may have a low insulin requirement (0.25–0.5 IU/kg/day) compared to those with T2DM with insulin resistance (>1 IU/kg/day). The approach for classifying young diabetes is shown in figure 1.

LABORATORY STUDIES TO DIFFERENTIATE FROM TYPE 1 DIABETES MELLITUS

Anti-glutamic acid decarboxylase-65 and other autoantibodies, like islet cell antibody, anti-insulin antibody, ZnT8, etc., may be positive in patients with T1DM. Serum C-peptide levels, if measured, are low in patients with T1DM, whereas in those with T2DM, it may be normal or increased.

MANAGEMENT OF TYPE 2 DIABETES MELLITUS IN CHILDREN

Unlike T1DM, where diabetes-related complications develop after many years of diabetes, the majority of patients with T2DM will have comorbidities, such as fatty liver, sleep apnea, hypertension at the time of diagnosis, and appear to develop microvascular and macrovascular complications at an accelerated rate. Therefore, the treatment of these associated disorders is often required at the time of initiation of therapy for dysglycemia. Reduction in the rate of complications may require a special attention to comorbidities in these patients.

While education on diet and physical activity is important in all youth with diabetes, the need for intensive lifestyle intervention is a dominant feature of therapy in youth with T2DM.

Goals of Treatment

The goals of treatment of T2DM in children include following:
- Normalization of glycemia
- Education for diabetes self-management
- Weight loss
- Reduction in carbohydrate and calorie intake
- Increase in exercise capacity
- Control of comorbidities, including hypertension, dyslipidemia, nephropathy, sleep disorders, and hepatic steatosis.

Education[8]

The education and treatment team for T2DM ideally should include a nutritionist, psychologist and/or social worker, and exercise physiologist. Education in T2DM places greater emphasis on behavioral, dietary, and physical activity changes than is generally required for the management of T1DM. Education should be given by team members with expertise and knowledge of the unique dietary, exercise, and psychological needs of youth with T2DM. The education should be provided in a culturally sensitive and age-appropriate manner. The entire family needs education to understand the principles of treatment of T2DM and to understand the critical importance of the lifestyle changes required for the entire family to successfully manage youth with T2DM.

The anxiety of the patient and family where diagnosis is uncertain can be minimized by emphasizing the importance of normalizing blood glucose metabolism using whatever therapy is appropriate to the metabolic circumstances of the specific individual, regardless of the "type" of diabetes.

Behavioral Change[8]

Lifestyle change is the cornerstone of treatment of T2DM and clinicians should initiate a lifestyle modification program, including nutrition and physical activity, for children and adolescents at the time of diagnosis of T2DM. The aim should be to promote a healthy lifestyle through behavior change which should include diet and exercise, weight management, and cessation of smoking.

Lifestyle intervention can decrease the incidence of diabetes in high-risk patients and those with impaired glucose tolerance.

Changes should be made slowly, in small achievable increments. The patient and his/her family should receive training on monitoring the quantity and quality of food, eating patterns, and physical activity.

Dietary Management[8]

Dietary recommendations should be culturally appropriate and acceptable to the family. The family should make dietary changes consistent with standard recommendations. Emphasis should be placed on reducing carbohydrate and total and saturated fat intake, increasing fiber intake and physical activity, with individualized counseling for weight reduction. Dietary modification should include:

- Eliminating sugar-containing drinks, including soft drinks and juices. This should be the initial focus with emphasis on substituting these with water, diet soft drinks, and other calorie-free beverages, which will help in weight loss
- Increasing the intake of vegetables and fruits
- Reducing use of processed, prepackaged, and convenience food
- Reducing intake of refined simple sugars, e.g., processed candy and high fructose corn syrup
- Serving food in a plate or bowl, as opposed to directly eating from a box or can
- Reducing take-out and dine-out meals and increasing meals eaten at home
- Modifying the diets with increased portions of fresh vegetables and reducing portions of carbohydrate-rich food, namely, white rice, noodles, and starches
- Changing staple foods to brown rice and whole grain items from white rice and white flour
- Limiting food and drink that are rich in fat and have high calories
- Teaching family members to understand and interpret the nutrition fact labels
- Encouraging setting of goals (e.g., reducing intake of high-calorie drinks, etc.) and achieving them; avoid blaming in case of failure
- Emphasizing on the importance of eating meals on schedule, in one place, as a family
- Considering cultural food preferences and taking into account the use of food during festivals and family events
- Maintaining food and activity logs.

Exercise Management[8]

Regular exercise improves blood glucose control, reduces cardiovascular risk factors, helps to lose weight, and improves well-being. Children and adolescents with T2DM should be encouraged to exercise daily, for an hour at least (moderate-to-vigorous intensity). Exercise regimens should be enjoyable and should be individualized for each patient, taking into account the family resources and environment.

A family member or friend should participate in physical activity with the patient. Reduction in sedentary time, including viewing television, computer-related activities, texting, and video games is an important step in exercise management. Screen time should be limited to less than 2 hours a day.

Pharmacotherapy[8]

The aim of therapy in youth-onset T2DM is to decrease insulin resistance, increase endogenous insulin secretion, or provide exogenous insulin. Among oral agents, only metformin is approved for use in most countries, and sulfonylureas are approved in a few countries, in adolescents. The evidence for use of other agents in adolescents and children is limited at this time. Insulin is also an approved agent.

Initial treatment[8] should include metformin and/or insulin, either alone or in combination. Choice of agent will be determined by symptoms, level of hyperglycemia, and whether ketosis/ketoacidosis is present or not.

If the patient is metabolically stable, i.e., HbA1c less than 9% with no symptoms, the treatment of choice is metformin monotherapy, starting with 500 mg once daily for a week. Uptitrate by 500 mg once a week, over 3–4 weeks, until the maximal dose of 1,000 mg twice daily is reached.

Insulin will be required if the patient is not metabolically stable. Basal insulin, once daily, with a starting dose of 0.3–0.6 units/kg, is effective in attaining glycemic control. Metformin can be started along with insulin, unless acidosis is present.

In order to eliminate insulin therapy, transition to metformin can usually be achieved over 2–6 weeks. Decrease the dose of insulin 30–50% each time that metformin dose is increased.

About 90% of youth with T2DM can be successfully treated initially with metformin alone. If the glucose values remain in the diabetic range during titration of metformin and insulin, the diagnosis of T2DM should be reconsidered and lifestyle changes reinforced.

The goal of initial treatment is to attain HbA1c less than 6.5%. Another oral or injected agent may be beneficial in addition to or instead of metformin and insulin if target is not achieved, but there are very limited studies of the use of these agents and they are generally not approved in the pediatric population.

Metformin[8]

Metformin acts on insulin receptors in muscle, and fat tissue, but has a predominant action on the liver. Hepatic glucose production is reduced by decreasing gluconeogenesis. Insulin stimulated glucose uptake is increased in muscle and fat. An initial anorexic effect may promote weight loss. Long-term use is associated with a 1–2% reduction in HbA1c. Intestinal side effects (transient abdominal pain, diarrhea, nausea) may occur with metformin use which may be eliminated in most patients with slow dosage titration over 3–4 weeks, and instructions to take the medication with food. Intestinal side effects (transient abdominal pain, diarrhea, nausea) may occur with metformin use. With slow dose titration, over 3–4 weeks and instructions to consume the medicine with food, these side effects can generally be negated. Use of extended release formulations may attenuate these side effects further.

Metformin should not be administered to those with significant renal impairment, hepatic disease, cardiac or respiratory insufficiency, or those who are receiving radiographic contrast materials. Consider discontinuing metformin temporarily during a gastrointestinal illness.

Insulin[8]

Relatively small doses of supplemental insulin are usually effective, despite prevailing hyperinsulinemia and insulin resistance. If glycemic control is not attained with oral agents, a long-acting basal insulin analog may help in achieving control. Continue metformin, along with insulin, in order to improve insulin sensitivity.

Thiazolidinediones, if used along with insulin, may pose an increased risk for fluid retention. Premeal meglitinide and rapid-acting insulin are good choices if postprandial hyperglycemia occurs. Side effects of insulin are hypoglycemia (less common in T2DM), and weight gain (more significant in T2DM). Sulfonylureas, pioglitazone, and α-glucosidase inhibitors are not approved for use in children in many countries but sulfonylureas may be specifically be useful in some forms of maturity-onset diabetes of the young and congenital diabetes mellitus (associated with defects in potassium-sensitive adenosine triphosphate channel).

Bariatric Surgery[11,12]

Adolescents having obesity-related comorbidities (including T2DM), can be considered for bariatric surgery. However, gastric bypass (the most commonly performed surgical procedure) can be associated with many complications, including malabsorption and even death.

Various studies have shown the effectiveness of bariatric surgery procedures, namely, persistent weight loss after 10 years, reduced mortality, and even a high remission rate for recent onset T2DM.

However, this mode of treatment is still uncommon in children and should be undertaken in specialized centers with an established system to collect outcome data.

COMPLICATION TESTING SPECIFIC TO TYPE 2 DIABETES MELLITUS IN YOUNG PEOPLE[8]

The International Society for Pediatric and Adolescent Diabetes (recommends the following for complication screening at diagnosis and during follow-up in children with T2DM:
- Nephropathy should be assessed by testing for micro- or macroalbuminuria, at the time of diagnosis and then every year
- Blood pressure should be measured at every visit. An elevated reading of blood pressure should be confirmed on two separate days, in addition
- Dyslipidemia should be evaluated soon after diagnosis, when blood glucose targets are achieved and then every year thereafter
- Nonalcoholic fatty liver disease should be evaluated for at the time of diagnosis, and then every year thereafter
- It is prudent to enquire regularly about puberty, menstrual irregularities, and obstructive sleep apnea starting at the time of diagnosis
- Retinopathy should be evaluated at the time of diagnosis, and then every year thereafter.

Although not recommended in guidelines, regular screening for neuropathy, musculoskeletal, and infectious complications, like tuberculosis, are suggested by some workers in young patients with diabetes.

CONCLUSION

Type 2 diabetes mellitus in children is an emerging public health problem and a huge challenge for physicians, parents, and research fellows. The prevalence of T2DM in children ranges from 4.1 per 1,000 12–19 year olds in the United States to 50.9 per 1,000 15–19-year-old Pima Indians of Arizona. Approximately, 8% and 45% of recently diagnosed cases of diabetes among children and adolescents in the United States, respectively, are T2DM. The clinical profile is highly variable from asymptomatic to various nonspecific or severe hyperglycemic symptoms. At diagnosis, the affected child may present with weight loss, ketosis, and acidosis. Insulin and C-peptide levels are often raised and antibodies absent, which may help differentiate T1DM from T2DM, but insulin secretion may be well-blunted at diagnosis. These individuals will have severe hyperglycemia and most of patients will have hypertension, hypertriglyceridemia, albuminuria, sleep apnea, and depression, and these comorbidities worsen over time. We need to have a well-coordinated, multidisciplinary approach for the treatment and prevention of this rapidly increasing incidence of T2DM in children.

REFERENCES

1. American Diabetes Association. Standards of Medical Care in Diabetes. Diabetes Care. 2017;40(Suppl 1).
2. D'Adamo E, Caprio S. Type 2 diabetes in youth: Epidemiology and pathophysiology. Diabetes Care. 2011;34(Suppl 2):S161-5.
3. Jagadesan S, Harish R, Miranda P, et al. Prevalence of overweight and obesity among school children and adolescents in Chennai. Indian Pediatr. 2014;51:544-9.
4. Marwaha RK, Tandon N, Singh Y, et al. A study of growth parameters and prevalence of overweight and obesity in school children from Delhi. Indian Pediatr. 2006;43(11):943-52.
5. Bhatia V. IAP National Task Force for Childhood Prevention of Adult Diseases: Insulin Resistance and Type 2 Diabetes Mellitus in Childhood. Indian Pediatr. 2004;41:443-45.
6. The HAPO Study Cooperative Research Group, Metzger BE, Lowe LP, Dyer AR, et al. Hyperglycemia and adverse pregnancy outcomes. N Engl J Med. 2008;358(19):1991-2002.
7. Zargar AH, Bhat MH, Laway BA, et al. Clinical and aetiological profile of early onset diabetes mellitus: data from a tertiary care centre in the Indian subcontinent. J Postgrad Med. 2001;47(1):27-9.
8. Zeitler P, Fu J, Tandon N, et al. ISPAD Clinical Practice Consensus Guidelines 2014 Compendium. Type 2 diabetes in the child and adolescent. Pediatr Diabetes. 2014;15(Suppl 20):26-46.
9. Haffner SM, Miettinen H, Gaskill SP, et al. Decreased insulin secretion and increased insulin resistance are independently related to the 7-year risk of NIDDM in Mexican-Americans. Diabetes. 1995;44:1386.
10. Tabák AG, Jokela M, Akbaraly TN, et al. Trajectories of glycaemia, insulin sensitivity, and insulin secretion before diagnosis of type 2 diabetes: an analysis from the Whitehall II study. Lancet. 2009;373:2215.
11. Sjöström L, Narbro K, Sjöström CD, et al. Effects of bariatric surgery on mortality in Swedish obese subjects. N Engl J Med. 2007;357:741-52.
12. Dixon JB, O'Brien PE, Playfair J, et al. Adjustable gastric banding and conventional therapy for type 2 diabetes. JAMA. 2008;299:316-23.

31 CHAPTER

Type 1 Diabetes Mellitus: A Perspective from Guidelines

Sanjay Kalra, Yashdeep Gupta

INTRODUCTION

The management of diabetes in children is challenging, to say the least. The diabetes care provider has to balance biomedical aspects with psycho-socio-environmental reality; patient's needs with family's wishes; firmness with empathy; scientific facts with (well-meaning) misinformation; and accuracy with appropriateness. This, as the reader is well aware, is easier written than done.

Guidelines available from leading professional organizations help pediatric diabetes care providers meet these challenges in daily practice. In this chapter, we describe three major recommendations for management of pediatric diabetes. This review emphasizes the philosophy and principles of diabetes care in children, focusing on the subtle differences between pediatric diabetes recommendations. It highlights the multiple factors which make diabetes in children a unique condition, and showcases the specific interventions which contribute to making childhood diabetology a satisfying and rewarding specialty.

AMERICAN DIABETES ASSOCIATION: STANDARDS OF CARE 2017

The American Diabetes Association (ADA) describes management of diabetes in children and adolescents in a separate chapter.[1] It emphasizes the need to consider aspects such as growth and sexual maturation related changes in insulin sensitivity, neurological vulnerability to hypoglycemia, hyperglycemia, and ketoacidosis. Ability to provide self-care, availability of supervision, and the role of the family is also highlighted.

Focus is laid on the need for a multidisciplinary approach, which is able to provide essential services such as diabetes self-management education (DSME) and support (DSMS), medical nutrition therapy, and psychosocial support. The team should be able to address not only biomedical, but also psychosocial needs, while assisting the growing child in achieving an age- and development-appropriate balance between independent self-care and adult supervision.

Glycemic Targets

Children of all age groups who live with diabetes should aim for glycosylated hemoglobin (HbA1c) goal of less than 7.5%. Safety is paramount, and goals may be revised in stepwise manner, as tolerated. Hypoglycemia unawareness, and inability to recognize, communicate, and manage symptoms of hypoglycemia in younger children (<6 years) must be considered. A lower goal (<7.0%) is considered reasonable, provided it can be achieved without excessive hypoglycemia. The ADA recommends a preprandial glucose target of 90–130 mg/dL. Postprandial glucose measurement is advised to resolve discrepancy between preprandial blood glucose values and HbA1c levels, and to titrate preprandial insulin doses of a basal-bolus regime.

Autoimmune Conditions

The ADA recommends screening at diagnosis, and periodically for autoimmune conditions such as thyroid disease and celiac disease. Estimation of serum thyroid-stimulating hormone (TSH) is recommended soon after diagnosis of type 1 diabetes mellitus (T1DM), and after glycemic control is achieved. If normal, it should be monitored every 1–2 years, or earlier, if symptoms or signs of a thyroid disorder develop. Thyroid antibodies (antithyroid peroxidase, antithyroglobulin) should be estimated soon after diagnosis. A high titer is predictive of development of thyroid dysfunction, and calls for regular monitoring.

Celiac disease should be screened in children with a first-degree relative with celiac disease, growth failure, and weight loss, failure to gain weight, diarrhea, flatulence, abdominal pain, or signs of malabsorption. It is also indicated in case of hypoglycemia or deterioration in glycemic control. Screening can be done by testing tissue transglutaminase or deamidated gliadin antibodies (with normal total serum immunoglobulin A), and confirmed by biopsy or endomysial antibody positivity. Screening should be done at diagnosis, and repeated within 2 and 5 years thereafter.

Cardiovascular Risk Factors

The ADA recommends measurement of blood pressure at each routine visit, with measurements repeated on three separate days if found to be high. Systolic or diastolic blood pressure greater than equal to 90th percentile for age, sex, and height is the threshold for lifestyle modification therapy, while values greater than equal to 95th percentile are the therapeutic threshold for pharmacological intervention. Renin angiotensin system blockers are the drug of choice, with the goal of treatment being a blood pressure less than 90th percentile. Angiotensin converting enzyme inhibitors are preferred as initial therapy, with angiotensin receptor blockers being prescribed if the former are not tolerated.

A fasting lipid profile is indicated in children greater than equal to 10 years of age, after diagnosis, as soon as glucose control has been established. The test is repeated every 3–5 years if initial results are normal [low-density lipoprotein (LDL) cholesterol <100 mg/dL], and annually if lipids are abnormal.

Initial therapy includes achievement of optimal glucose control and a diet with restricted cholesterol (200 mg/day) and saturated fat (7% of total calories). Statins are suggested in children more than 10 years who fail to achieve an LDL cholesterol less than 160 mg/dL, or in children more than 10 years with one or more additional cardiovascular disease risk factors who have an LDL cholesterol >130 mg/dL. The goal of therapy is to lower LDL cholesterol to less than 100 mg/dL.

Smoking is an important contributor to macrovascular (cardiovascular disease), microvascular (albuminuria), and oncological complications. Cigarette smoking should be enquired about and activity discouraged in routine diabetes care. Secondhand smoke exposure should also be assessed, and avoided.

Microvascular Complications

Glomerular filtration rate should be estimated at initial evaluation, and periodically thereafter. The frequency will be based on clinical factors such as age, duration of diabetes, and treatment. Annual screening for albuminuria, using a random spot urine sample for albumin-to-creatinine ratio, should be performed in children with a history of diabetes more than 5 years.

Albuminuria (>30 mg/g albumin/creatinine ratio) should be confirmed in at least two of three urine samples, obtained over a 6 month period, after improving glycemic control and normalizing blood pressure. This should be treated with angiotensin converting enzyme (ACE) inhibitors.

The recommendations for retinopathy screening are to conduct a dilated, comprehensive eye examination at age more than or equal to 10 years or after puberty has started, whichever is earlier, once the youth has had diabetes for 3–5 years. Annual follow-up is suggested, but less frequent examinations may sometimes suffice.

The recommendations for foot examination are similar. All children with a history of diabetes for 5 years should undergo annual comprehensive foot examination from puberty or 10 years age onwards, whichever is earlier.

This should include inspection, palpation of pulses, elicitation of patellar and Achilles reflexes, and determination of sensory acuity.

Type 2 Diabetes Mellitus

While ADA mentions T2DM separately, it iterates that the provision of multidisciplinary care, and treatment goals, are similar. The difficulty in differential diagnosis of T1DM from T2DM is addressed by advising insulin in such patients. Metformin is suggested only when ketosis/ketoacidosis have resolved, but the need for combination therapy in most youth is highlighted. No other oral hypoglycemia agent is approved for use in children. Medical nutrition therapy and lifestyle modification is reinforced.

Type 2 diabetes mellitus children should undergo blood pressure, fasting lipid, albumin excretion, and retinopathy screening at diagnosis. Later on, monitoring should be done as per guidelines for children with T1DM.

Psychosocial Issues

Diabetes self-management education and DSMS should be offered not only to children, but their parents and care givers as well. Such intervention should be culturally sensitive, developmentally appropriate, individualized as per need, and be in concordance with national standards. Periodic assessment and audits are necessary in order to ensure effectiveness, and mild-course corrections will often be needed as the child grows. School or day care personnel should also be involved in diabetes management.

Psychosocial issues, including personal and family stresses, should be assessed at diagnosis and during follow-up of diabetes. Such issues, if left unaddressed, may impact adherence to therapy, and hinder achievement of optimal outcomes. Children with diabetes should be screened for diabetes distress, fear of hypoglycemia (and hyperglycemia), anxiety, depression, and eating disorders. Referral to a qualified mental health professional should be advised if necessary. Diabetes-specific family conflict leads to poor adherence and glycemic control, and needs to be resolved as well.

Transition

The ADA makes special mention of the challenges involved in transition of care from pediatric to adult healthcare providers. This transition occurs at a time when the adolescent faces multiple personal, psychological, financial, and social changes. As glycemic control may deteriorate, healthcare providers and families should begin to prepare in early to mid-adolescence, for a transition to adult healthcare. All healthcare providers should assist this move.

GLOBAL INTERNATIONAL DIABETES FEDERATION (IDF)/ INTERNATIONAL SOCIETY FOR PEDIATRIC AND ADOLESCENT DIABETES GUIDELINES

The IDF/ISPAD suggest three levels of care in their detailed guidelines for management of T1DM in childhood and adolescence.[2] Recommended care is that which is evidence-based, and is cost-effective in most nations. Limited care seeks to achieve the major objectives of diabetes management, and is relevant for health care settings with very limited resources. Only low cost, or highly cost-effective interventions are offered. Comprehensive care has some evidence to back it, and is provided in resource-rich healthcare settings, with the aim of achieving best possible outcomes.

The IDF/ISPAD guidelines define and describe various types of childhood diabetes at length. Separate chapters are devoted to the framework of diabetes care, and various nonpharmacological as well as pharmacological aspects of management. Specific situations such as diabetic ketoacidosis, sick day management, surgery, and adolescence are covered separately, as are complications.

The document lists the nonemergency and emergency presentations of diabetes, and enumerates the diagnostic tests and criteria that should be followed. It discourages intervention in the "preclinical" stage of T2DM.

CHAPTER 31: Type 1 Diabetes Mellitus: A Perspective from Guidelines

Education

The right to accessible planned DSME is documented by IDF/ISPAD. Diabetes self-management education should be available to all growing persons with diabetes, and their parents/care givers. An interdisciplinary team should provide learner-centered, adaptable, individualized education, which facilitates behavioral change to ensure optimal diabetes management. This should be a continuous process, repeated at regular intervals.

This team should ideally include a pediatrician, a diabetes specialist, a nurse educator, a dietician, a pediatric social worker, and/or a psychologist/psychiatrist. The importance of the family and the child as an integral part of the care team is emphasized. It must be noted that an endocrinologist, "diabetologist", or "pediatric endocrinologist" is not mentioned as a team member for ambulatory care by IDF/ISPAD.

The specific needs of minority children, children of recent immigrants, children in school settings and organized camps, and those in transition to adult care are mentioned.

Nonpharmacological Therapy

The importance of nutrition and exercise is highlighted by devoting separate chapters to these aspects of treatment. Foods rich in sucrose and saturated fat should be limited or avoided. The dynamic relationship between carbohydrate intake, physical activity, and insulin requirement should be explained. The total calorie intake should be achieved from carbohydrate (>50%), fat (<35%; saturated fat <10%), and protein (10–15%). Sucrose should not provide more than 10% of total energy intake. Tailored advice about exercise, including insulin dose adjustment and snack intake is mentioned.

Insulin

Children with T1DM should be treated with insulin. Various regimes and preparations are mentioned, but use of a basal bolus regime is recommended. The IDF/ISPAD guidelines acknowledge the use of various regimes and preparations, in differing requirements and distributions, as per individual needs.

Detailed algorithms and clinical pathways are presented for the management of diabetic ketoacidosis and its complications. The need for a pediatric endocrinologist or pediatric critical care specialist is mentioned in comprehensive care of diabetic ketoacidosis. Guidance is also published for management of children undergoing surgery.

Hypoglycemia

Hypoglycemia prevention is strongly supported by IDF/ISPAD, as its occurrence is fairly predictable, it is associated with psychosocial dysfunction, it can lead to permanent long-term sequelae, and it is potentially life threatening. Education, self-management, and physician-directed management is covered. It is noteworthy that access to glucagon is recommended for all parents and care givers in recommended care. The use of insulin analogs is supported as a hypoglycemia-reducing strategy in comprehensive care.

Sick day management is covered in detail. Apart from frequent glucose monitoring, diagnosis, and resolution of underlying disease, continuation of insulin and fluid replacement, mini-glucagon regimes are suggested for management of hypoglycemia.

Monitoring

Self-monitoring of blood glucose (SMBG) is described as an essential tool for diabetes management. Ideally, SMBG should be done 4–6 times a day. Ketone testing, preferably blood ketone testing, is indicated in children who are unwell, symptomatic, or persistently hyperglycemic. Glycosylated hemoglobin should be monitored 4–6 times a year in younger children. Adolescents with stable T2DM should have 2–4 HbA1c tests per annum, as they may experience sudden change in ß-cell function, which may necessitate institution of insulin therapy. A target HbA1c less than 7.5% is recommended for all age groups. However, targets include the requirement for minimal levels of severe hypoglycemia, and absence of hypoglycemia unawareness. In case these are present, glycemic targets must be relaxed till hypoglycemia episodes and their unawareness, abate.

Chronic Complications

Prevention and management of macro- and microvascular complications is covered in detail by IDP/ISPAD. Measurement of blood pressure is recommended annually, with a target of less than 95th percentile for age.

Screening for retinopathy, neuropathy, and microalbuminuria should start from 11 years of age, after 2 years duration of diabetes. Fasting lipids should be tested at age 12 years, and repeated every 5 years if normal. Children with family history of hypercholesterolemia, early cardiovascular disease, or unknown family history should be screened at age 2 years and above.

Type 2 Diabetes Mellitus

In metabolically stable children with T2DM, metformin is indicated, beginning with 250 mg once daily, and titrating twice a week, to a maximum of 1,000 mg twice a daily. Insulin should be used in metabolically unstable children, but can usually be tapered off over 2–6 weeks.

Testing for albuminuria, dyslipidemia, nonalcoholic fatty liver disease, and retinopathy should be performed at diagnosis, and annually thereafter. Blood pressure should be monitored at every visit. History should be elicited with regards to symptoms of polycystic ovary syndrome and obstructive sleep apnea at diagnosis, and regularly thereafter.

Monogenic Diabetes

Monogenic diabetes should be confirmed by molecular genetic testing. Some forms, such as hepatocyte nuclear factor (HNF)-1α maturity onset diabetes of the young (MODY), HNF-4α MODY, and KIR 6.2 mutations, are sensitive to sulfonylureas. Glucose kinase deficiency may present as mild fasting hyperglycemia and may require insulin only during pregnancy. Transient neonatal diabetes should be identified and managed appropriately.

Transition

The distinct needs of adolescents with diabetes are highlighted. Emphasis is laid on understanding their needs, and on developing communication skills necessary to connect with this age group.

CANADIAN DIABETES ASSOCIATION

The Canadian Diabetes Association (CDA) publishes well-written guidelines, in which T1DM in children and adolescents merits a separate chapter.

The Canadian recommendations focus on the need for an interdisciplinary healthcare team to deliver intensive diabetes education to children and their families. It lists the topics on which education must be shared, and uses the term "anticipatory guidance" to help decide issues to be discussed.

Glycemic Targets

Canadian guidelines suggest age specific glycemic targets for children and adolescents, making them more stringent as age advances. Children below 6 years should aim for an HbA1c less than 8.0% (fasting/preprandial glucose 6.0–10.0 mmol/L), which may be relaxed to less than 8.5% if excessive hypoglycemia occurs. Children aged 6–12 years should target an HbA1c of less than 7.5 % (relaxed to <8.0% if excessive hypoglycemia occurs) and fasting/preprandial glucose values of 4.0–10.0 mmol/L. In adolescents (aged 13–18), a tighter goal is targeted, HbA1c should be kept less than 7.0%, and fasting/preprandial glucose at 4.0-7.0 mmol/L. This target is appropriate for most adolescents, and can be lowered to HbA1c less than 6.0%, fasting/preprandial glucose 4.0–6.0 mmol/L, and 2 hour postprandial glucose 5.0–8.0 mmol/L, if safely achieved.

Management

The CDA describes basal bolus regimes, using insulin analogs, and continuous subcutaneous insulin infusion (CSII) as options for children, and reports that CSII provides better metabolic control.

It promotes self-monitoring of blood glucose, and the use of subcutaneous continuous glucose sensors. Nutrition therapy is reinforced, with insulin suggested to be matched to carbohydrate content.

Management of hypoglycemia, chronic poor metabolic control, and diabetic keto-acidosis are discussed. Prevention measures such as smoking prevention/cessation, contraception/sexual health counseling, and psychological issues are discussed in detail.

Autoimmune Conditions

Children should be screened at diagnosis of T1DM and every 2 years, for thyroid disease, using TSH and thyroid peroxidase antibodies. Screening should be done when symptoms such as goiter, or positive antibodies are present. Children should also be screened for celiac disease using tissue transglutaminase + immunoglobulin A if symptoms of classic or atypical celiac disease are present (screening for asymptomatic celiac disease is controversial). Symptoms include recurrent gastrointestinal symptoms, poor linear growth, poor weight gain, fatigue, anemia, unexplained frequent hypoglycemia, or poor metabolic control.

Chronic Complications

Screening for nephropathy, with first morning (preferred) or random albumin to creatinine ratio is recommended annually, beginning at 12 years of age in children with T1DM > years duration. Yearly screening of retinopathy, with standard field stereoscopic color fundus photography, or direct ophthalmoscopy or indirect slit-lamp fundoscopy through dilated pupils, or digital fundus photography, is commenced at 15 years. Screening may be done at 2 yearly intervals in children with diabetes less than 10 years, good glycemic control, and a healthy retina at initial assessment. Postpubertal adolescents with poor metabolic control should be screened every year, after 5 years of living with T1DM, by history and physical examination.

A fasting lipid profile is indicated at 12 and 17 years of age, after metabolic control has stabilized. Children below 12 years with a body mass index more than 95th percentile and family history of premature cardiovascular disease, should be screened as well. All children with T1DM should have their blood pressure checked at least twice a year a, with appropriate are similar to those in other guidelines.

CONCLUSION

This chapter summarizes the important recommendations related to T1DM management, as laid down by leading professional bodies. It does not suggest the use of one guideline over another. On the contrary, the authors support an in-depth understanding of these well written guidelines, and their translation into clinical practice, in a manner that is relevant, pragmatic, and cost-effective for the local healthcare system environment

REFERENCES

1. American Diabetes Association. Children and adolescents. Sec. 12. In Standards of Medical Care in Diabetes 2017. Diabetes Care. 2017;40(Suppl. 1):S105-S113.
2. Hanas R, Donaghue K, Klingensmith G, Swift P, Colagiuri S. Global IDF/ISPAD guideline for diabetes in childhood and adolescence. Brussels: International Diabetes Federation. 2011.
3. Canadian Diabetes Association Clinical Practice Guidelines Expert Committee. Canadian Diabetes Association 2013 Clinical Practice Guidelines for the Prevention and Management of Diabetes in Canada. Can J Diabetes. 2013;37(Suppl 1):S1-S212.

APPENDIX

APPENDIX

TABLE A1: Monogenic subtypes of neonatal and infancy-onset diabetes[2,3]

Gene	Locus	Inheritance	Other clinical features
Abnormal pancreatic development			
PLAGL1/HYMAI	6q24	Variable (imprinting)	TNDM ± macroglossia ± umbilical hernia
ZFP57	6p22.1	Recessive	TNDM (multiple hypomethylation syndrome) ± macroglossia ± developmental delay ± umbilical defects ± congenital heart disease
PDX1	13q12.1	Recessive	PNDM + pancreatic agenesis (steatorrhea)
PTF1A	10p12.2	Recessive	PNDM + pancreatic agenesis (steatorrhea) + cerebellar hypoplasia/aplasia + central respiratory dysfunction
PTF1A enhancer	10p12.2	Recessive	PNDM + pancreatic agenesis without CNS features
HNF1B	17q21.3	Dominant	TNDM + pancreatic hypoplasia and renal cysts
RFX6	6q22.1	Recessive	PNDM + intestinal atresia + gall bladder agenesis
GATA6	18q11.1-q11.2	Dominant	PNDM + pancreatic agenesis + congenital heart defects + biliary abnormalities
GATA4	8p23.1	Dominant	PNDM + pancreatic agenesis + congenital heart defects
GLIS3	9p24.3-p23	Recessive	PNDM + congenital hypothyroidism + glaucoma + hepatic fibrosis + renal cysts
NEUROG3	10q21.3	Recessive	PNDM + enteric anendocrinosis (malabsorptive diarrhea)
NEUROD1	2q32	Recessive	PNDM + cerebellar hypoplasia + visual impairment + deafness
PAX6	11p13	Recessive	PNDM + microphthalmia + brain malformations
MNX1	7q36.3	Recessive	PNDM + developmental delay + sacral agenesis + imperforate anus
NKX2-2	20p11.22	Recessive	PNDM + developmental delay + hypotonia + short stature + deafness + constipation
Abnormal β-cell function			
KCNJ11	11p15.1	Spontaneous or dominant	PNDM/TNDM ± DEND
ABCC8	11p15.1	Spontaneous, dominant, or recessive	TNDM/PNDM ± DEND
INS	11p15.5	Recessive	Isolated PNDM or TNDM
GCK	7p15-p13	Recessive	Isolated PNDM
SLC2A2 (GLUT2)	3q26.1-q26.3	Recessive	Fanconi-Bickel syndrome: PNDM + hypergalactosemia, liver dysfunction

Continued

Continued

Gene	Locus	Inheritance	Other clinical features
SLC19A2	1q23.3	Recessive	Roger's syndrome: PNDM + thiamine-responsive megaloblastic anemia, sensorineural deafness
Destruction of β-cells			
INS	11p15.5	Spontaneous or dominant	Isolated PNDM
EIF2AK3	2p11.2	Recessive	Wolcott-Rallison syndrome: PNDM + skeletal dysplasia + recurrent liver dysfunction
IER3IP1	18q21.2	Recessive	PNDM + microcephaly + lissencephaly + epileptic encephalopathy
FOXP3	Xp11.23-p13.3	X-linked, recessive	IPEX syndrome (autoimmune enteropathy, eczema, autoimmune hypothyroidism, and elevated IgE)
WFS1	4p16.1	Recessive	PNDM*+ optic atrophy ± diabetes insipidus ± deafness

CNS, central nervous system; DEND, developmental delay, epilepsy, and neonatal diabetes syndrome; IgE, immunoglobulin E; IPEX, immune dysregulation, polyendocrinopathy, enteropathy, X-linked syndrome; TNDM; transient neonatal diabetes mellitus.

*The mean age of diagnosis among patients with WFS1 mutations is approximately 5 years.

TABLE A2: Clinical and molecular characteristics of maturity-onset diabetes of the young subtypes[23]

MODY gene	Chromosomal location	Frequency (% from MODYs)	Pathophysiology	Other features	Treatment
HNF4A	20q13	5	β-cell dysfunction	Neonatal hyperinsulinemia, low triglycerides	Sensitive to sulfonylurea
GCK	7p13	15–20	β-cell dysfunction (glucose sensing defect)	Fasting hyperglycemia from newborn	Diet
HNF1A	12q24	30–50	β-cell dysfunction	Glycosuria	Sensitive to sulfonylurea
PDX1/IPF1	13q12	<1	β-cell dysfunction	Homozygote: Pancreatic agenesis	Diet or OAD or insulin
HNF1B	17q12	5	β-cell dysfunction	Renal anomalies, genital anomalies, pancreatic hypoplasia	Insulin
NEUROD1	2q31	<1	β-cell dysfunction	Adult onset diabetes	OAD or insulin
KLF11	2p25	<1	β-cell dysfunction	Similar to type 2 diabetes mellitus	OAD or insulin

Continued

Continued

MODY gene	Chromosomal location	Frequency (% from MODYs)	Pathophysiology	Other features	Treatment
CEL	9q34	<1	Pancreas endocrine and exocrine dysfunction	Exocrine insufficiency, lipomatosis	OAD or insulin
PAX4	7q32	<1	β-cell dysfunction	Possible ketoacidosis	Diet or OAD or insulin
INS	11p15	<1	Insulin gene mutation	Can also present PNDM	OAD or insulin
BLK	8p23	<1	Insulin secretion defect	Overweight, relative insulin secretion defect	Diet or OAD or insulin
ABCC8	11p15	<1	ATP-sensitive potassium channel dysfunction	Homozygote: permanent neonatal diabetes; heterozygote: transient neonatal diabetes	OAD (sulfonylurea)
KCNJ11	11p15	<1	ATP-sensitive potassium channel dysfunction	Homozygote: neonatal diabetes	Diet or OAD or insulin

MODY, maturity-onset diabetes of the young; *HNF4A*, hepatocyte nuclear factor 4 α; *GCK*, glucokinase; *PDX1*, pancreatic and duodenal homeobox 1; *IPF1*, insulin promoter factor 1; *OAD*, oral antidiabetic agents; *NEUROD1*, neurogenic differentiation 1; KLF11, Kruppel-like factor 11; *CEL*, carboxyl ester lipase; *PAX4*, paired-box-containing gene 4; *INS*, insulin; *PNDM*, permanent neonatal diabetes; *BLK*, B-lymphocyte kinase; *ABCC8*, ATP-binding cassette, subfamily C (CFTR/MRP), member 8; ATP, adenosine triphosphate; *KCNJ11*, potassium channel, inwardly rectifying subfamily J, member 11.

TABLE A3: Monogenic diabetes—insulin resistance syndromes[2,3]

Insulin resistance syndrome subtype	Gene (inheritance)	Leptin	Adiponectin	Other clinical features
Primary insulin signaling defects				
Receptor defect Post receptor defects	*INSR* (AR or AD) *AKT2*, *TBC1D4* (AD)	Decreased	Normal or elevated	No dyslipidemia No fatty liver
Adipose tissue abnormalities				
Monogenic obesity	*MC4R* (AD) *LEP*, *LEPR*, *POMC* (AR) Others	Increased (low in *LEP*)	–	Tall stature (*MC4R*) Hypogonadism (*LEP*) Hypoadrenalism (*POMC*)

Continued

Continued

Insulin resistance syndrome subtype	Gene (inheritance)	Leptin	Adiponectin	Other clinical features
Congenital generalized lipodystrophy	*AGPAT2*, *BSCL2* (AR) Others	Decreased	Decreased	Severe dyslipidemia (high triglycerides, low HDL cholesterol) Fatty liver
Partial lipodystrophy	*LMNA*, *PPARG*, *PIK3R1* (AD) Others	Variable	–	Myopathy and cardiomyopathy (*LMNA*) Pseudoacromegaly (*PPARG*) SHORT syndrome with partial lipodystrophy, insulin resistance and diabetes (*PIK3R1*)
Complex syndromes				
Alstrom	*ALMS1* (AR)	–	–	–
Bardet-Biedl	*BBS1* to *BBS18* (mostly AR)	–	–	–
DNA damage repair disorders	*WRN* (AR) *BLM* (AR)	–	–	–
Primordial dwarfism	*PCNT* (AR)	–	–	–

Insulin resistance syndromes can be divided into three groups depending on the pathogenesis: (i) Insulin signaling defects, (ii) Adipose tissue abnormalities, and (iii) Insulin resistance as part of the disease. Targeted genetic testing will be facilitated by prior clinical and biochemical characterization. Monogenic insulin resistance is not common, when compared to monogenic B cell failure.

INDEX

Page numbers followed by *f* refer to figure, *b* refer to box, and *t* refer to table.

A

Abscess, intra-abdominal 173
Acanthosis nigricans 6*t*, 28, 52, 60, 128*b*, 293
Acarbose 124
Acidosis 159, 169, 173
  correction of 169
  degree of 169
  lactic 27
  metabolic 161, 162, 173
Addison's disease 11, 50
Adenosine triphosphate 24, 238
Aldosteronoma 4
Alpha glucosidase inhibitors 127
Ambulatory glucose profile 142, 143*f*
Anesthetic technique 179
Angiotensin
  converting enzyme 301
    inhibitor 212
  receptor blocker 212
Anomalies
  genital 27, 310, 312
  renal 242*t*
  uterine 27, 312
Antibodies 61
Antihypertensive drugs 212*t*
Anti-insulin receptor antibodies 5
Anxiety 97, 173
Apneusis 169
Appendicitis 173
Arrhythmias, cardiac 192
Arterial blood gas level 162
Artificial pancreas 218
Asthma 173
Atresia, intestinal 242
Atrophy 27
Autoimmune
  diseases 11
  disorder 105
Autoimmunity 6
Autosomal dominant 23

B

Bardet-Biedl syndrome 61
Bariatric surgery 297
Basal insulin analogs 109*f*
Beta-cell dysfunction monogenic diabetes 22, 23
Bicarbonate
  serum 44, 50, 151, 162, 165
  therapy 173
Biphasic human insulin 106, 109*f*
Bipolar disorders 251
Blood glucose 173, 184
  charting 54
  level measurement 136*f*
  monitoring, home 58
  self-monitoring of 51, 54, 83, 117, 118, 132, 196, 244, 304
Blood pressure 42, 208*t*, 212
  controls 76
  diastolic 42, 169
  evaluation 208
  high 42, 207, 210*t*
  monitoring 209
  normal 42
  systolic 42, 207, 211*t*
Body mass index 68, 222, 289
  chart 276, 278
Bowel obstruction 162
Brain malformations 242
Bromocriptine 124

C

Calcium channel blocker 212
Carbohydrate 68, 69, 71, 78, 274, 275*f*, 294
  gram increments of 72
  replacement, pre-exercise 79*t*
Carbon dioxide 164
Carboxyl ester lipase 5
Cardiovascular disease 201, 215, 223, 301
Celiac disease 11, 46, 73, 300

Cerebral edema
  development of 169
  signs of 168
  symptoms of 168
Chennai Urban Rural Epidemiology Study 14
Cheyne-Stokes respiration 169
Cholesteryl ester transfer protein 202
Chronic distal symmetric polyneuropathy 217
Cognitive behavioral therapy 99
Complete blood count 162
Complex metabolic disorder 3
Continuous glucose monitoring system 57, 131, 132, 134, 134*f*, 135, 136, 136*f*, 139, 139*f*, 140, 140*f*, 141, 142*f*, 143, 143*f*, 146*f*, 191
Coronary artery calcification 223
Cranial nerve palsy 168, 169
Cushing's syndrome 4
Cysts, renal 22, 27
Cytomegalovirus 5
Cytotoxic T-lymphocyte-associated antigen 4 281

D

Deafness 27
  syndrome 22
Dehydration 162, 232
Deoxyribonucleic acid 281, 284, 285
Depression 97, 257
Detemir 108, 144, 187*t*, 195, 254*t*
Diabetes 3, 8, 9, 17, 22, 23, 26, 67, 82, 94-96, 101, 222, 231, 238, 249, 251
  childhood 3, 8, 9, 59, 62
  classification of 4
  congenital 242

Control and Complication
  Trial 53, 67, 105, 191, 223
diagnosis of 8
drug or chemical-induced 21
education 82, 263
Epidemiology Study Group 14
familial 22
family history of 17
fibrocalculous pancreatic 61
immune-mediated 21
insipidus 22, 27, 242
latent autoimmune 10
lipoatrophic 4
management of 172, 299
mellitus 3, 8, 22, 27, 53, 160,
  172
  gestational 5, 15, 21, 29
  insulin dependent 13, 288
  neonatal 4, 17, 18, 22-24, 61,
    238, 242t, 246
  transient 4, 22-24, 24t,
    238
  type 1 9, 10, 12-14, 13t, 21,
    31, 41, 48, 59, 60, 62, 67,
    68, 71, 73, 76, 82, 94, 105,
    117, 123, 124t, 128, 144,
    145, 159, 173, 173t, 177,
    191, 194, 197, 201, 207,
    215, 218, 219, 222, 224,
    226, 226f, 238, 250, 263,
    280, 281, 281f, 288, 292,
    293, 299, 300
  type 2 9, 14, 15, 21, 49, 53,
    59, 60, 62, 177, 189, 222,
    239, 255, 288, 290, 291,
    292t, 293, 297, 301
mitochondrial 21, 22, 61
monitor 57
monogenic 6t, 17, 21-23, 28,
  28t, 29, 304
neonatal 22-26, 242
pancreatic 61
self-management 294
syndrome of 22, 242t
types of 3, 61
Diarrhea 242
Diazoxide 5
Digital monitoring 57
Dilantin 5
Dipeptidyl peptidase 4
  inhibitor 124, 125
Down's syndrome 5, 61

Dyslipidemia 128, 203, 294
Dysplasia, renal 27
Dysrhythmia, cardiac 170
Dystrophy, myotonic 5

E

Eating disorders 251, 257
Edema
  cerebral 168, 169
  pulmonary 170
Electrolyte
  disturbances 173
  serum 173
Encephalopathy 27
Enterovirus 5, 12
Epilepsy 24, 242
Epiphyseal dysplasia 25, 242
Episodic liver 242
Erythrocytosis, post-
  transplant 151
Euglycemia, maintenance of 179
European Diabetes Study
  Group 222
European Nicotinamide Diabetes
  Intervention Trial 284
Exercise 85
  capacity 294
  intensive, effect of 77
  management 195, 295
Exocrine
  dysfunction 25, 242
  pancreas
    diseases of 4, 21
    monogenic diseases of 22

F

Fasting glucose
  control 110
  impaired 289
Fatigue 161
Fatty acids
  monounsaturated 70
  polyunsaturated 70
Fatty liver disease,
  nonalcoholic 128
Fever 70, 161, 162
Fibrosis, cystic 4, 28
Fluid and electrolyte balance 181
Free fatty acid 161
Friedreich ataxia 5, 61
Fructosamine 56

G

Gallbladder hypoplasia 242
Gastritis, autoimmune 11
Gastroenteritis 162, 173
Gastroparesis 145
Genetic syndromes 21-23, 26,
  27t
Genital anomalies 27
Gerhardt's tests 50
Glargine 108, 144, 187t, 195,
  254t
Glomerular filtration rate 154
Glucagon like peptide 1 receptor
  agonist 124, 125
Glucagonoma 4
Glucocorticoids 5
Glucokinase
  gene mutations 22
  monogenic diabetes 29
Gluconeogenesis 178
Glucose 85, 138, 184
  capillary 137f
  counter-regulation of 192
  dependent insulinotropic
    polypeptide, lower 125
  homeostasis 76, 179
  measurement 139f
  metabolism 178
  meter 136f
  monitoring 85, 196, 268
  sensor 133f
  serum 162, 173
  tolerance, impaired 289
Glutamic acid decarboxylase 49,
  243, 291
Gluten-free diet 73
Glycation, advanced 180
Glycemia
  monitoring 56
  normalization of 294
Glycemic 180
  control, inadequate 145
  monitoring 53, 54, 57, 58
  parameter 51
  targets 181, 300, 305
Glycogenolysis 178
Glycosuria 41, 173
Gout 27
Growth 32
  disorders 31
  hormone 34

H

Head trauma 161
Headache 80, 169
Hemochromatosis 4
Hemoglobin, glycosylated 33, 44, 51, 55, 85, 110, 131, 162, 186, 276, 277f, 288
Hepatocyte nuclear factor 5, 59, 304
Hernia, umbilical 242
Human leukocyte antigen 46, 159, 280, 281
Huntington's chorea 5
Hyperactivity disorder, attention deficit 251
Hyperglycemia 8, 41, 85, 151, 159, 160, 162, 173, 178f, 180, 232, 268, 290
   chronic 3
   exercise 79
   familial mild 22, 23, 26
   mild fasting 17, 22
   perioperative 179
   postprandial 128
   recurrent 145
   severe 105
Hyperinsulinemia 28
Hyperkalemia 170
Hyperpnea 173
Hypertension 51, 128, 207, 209, 210, 213, 294
Hyperthyroidism 4
Hypertrichosis 28
Hypertriglyceridemia 28
Hyperuricemia 27
Hyperventilation 161
Hypocalcemia 170
Hypocapnia 169
Hypoglycemia 56, 78, 84, 85, 121, 131, 137, 170, 180, 191-194, 232, 268, 303
   asymptomatic 191
   causes of 170
   documented symptomatic 191
   epidemiology of 191
   exercise induced 78
   iatrogenic 191, 193, 194
   minimizing risk of 194
   perioperative 180
   preprandial 128
   severe 191
   treatment of 197
Hypokalemia 170
Hypoplasia
   cerebellar 242
   pancreatic 242
Hypothyroidism 242
   congenital 242

I

Immunodysregulation polyendocrinopathy enteropathy X-linked syndrome 5, 22, 25, 26, 242
Immunosuppressants 149, 150
   regimen, glucocorticoid free 152
   therapy 150
Insulin 44, 116, 233, 268, 296, 303
   absorption 116
   action 21
   adjustments 78
   autoantibody 243, 283
   carbohydrate ratio 72
   cloudy 111f
   infusion, continuous subcutaneous 105, 116, 131, 185, 305
   injection 113f, 144
      technique 112
   mixing of 112
   promoter factor 5
   pump 131, 144, 185
      technology 131
      therapy 117
   receptor 28
   regimes 110
   resistance 4, 17
      monogenic diabetes 22, 28
      severe 28
      syndromes 28, 28t
   secretion 85
   sensitizers 123
   storing of 112
   therapy 83, 105, 106, 244
   types of 85, 106
Interstitial fluid glucose
   concept of 137f
   level 136f
Islet autoantibodies, pancreatic 26
Islet cell
   antibody 243
   transplantation 148, 151, 153
      types of 152
      preparation of 152
      procedure for 153
      outcomes 153
         complications 153
         efficacy 154

J

Joint mobility
   limited 217
   lower 217

K

Ketoacidosis 168, 178f
   alcoholic 162
   diabetic 18, 24, 42, 43, 44t, 50, 59, 159, 160, 161f, 162t, 163, 164f, 165f, 166, 167f, 168, 169, 172, 173, 173t, 181, 202, 232, 290
Ketone 85
Ketonemia 41, 162, 173
Ketones, serum 44
Ketosis 6, 61, 85, 159, 173
Klinefelter syndrome 5, 61
Kussmaul's respiration 42, 161, 173

L

Laurence-Moon-Biedl syndrome 5
Leprechaunism 4
Lethargy 161, 169
Lipodystrophy 28
Lipoproteins
   high density 201, 203, 225
   low-density 201, 203, 300
   very low-density 201, 203
Liver function test 27, 205
Lypoglycemia 110

M

Macroglossia 242
Malaise 161
Maturity onset diabetes of young 5, 16, 16t, 26, 27, 27t, 49, 177, 293, 304
   prevalence of 17
Mauriac syndrome 31

Meal-time flexibility 110
Medical nutrition therapy 67, 68, 88
Megaloblastic anemia, thiamine responsive 27
MELAS (mitochondrial myopathy, encephalopathy, lactic acidosis, and stroke) syndrome 27t
Mental status 44
Metabolic syndrome 224, 226
complications of 224
Metformin 28, 123, 124, 296
Micro-insulin autoantibody 49
Microphthalmia 242
Monogenic insulin resistance syndromes 62
Myopathy 205, 312
mitochondrial 27

N

National Glycohemoglobin Standardization Program 288
National Kidney Disease Education Program 45
National Urban Diabetes Survey 14
Nausea 161
Neoplasia 4
Nephropathy 51, 212, 294
diabetic 215
Neuropathy, diabetic 217
Nicotinic acid 5
Nocturnal enuresis 251
Non-human leukocyte antigen genes 282
Noninsulin
glucose lowering drugs, classification of 124t
therapy 123, 128
Nonpharmacological therapy 303

O

Obesity 6, 15, 60, 28
central 128
management 256f
signs of 17
Obsessive compulsive disorders 251
Optic atrophy 22, 27, 61, 242
Oral glucose tolerance test 288
Orthostatic hypotension 42

P

Pain, abdominal 61, 161, 173
Pancreas 27, 148
atrophy of 25
transplantation 148
Pancreatectomy 4
Pancreatic function tests 61
Pancreatitis 4, 61, 162
Pancreatopathy, fibrocalculous 4
Papilledema 168
Pediatric diabetes 67
Pentamidine 5
Peptide based vaccine strategy 284, 285
Pheochromocytoma 4
Phobic disorders 251
Phosphate 164
Pioglitazone 124
Planter pressure 217
Plasma
acetone level 44
capillary 136
glucose 44
concentration 44
self-monitoring of 141
oncotic pressure 170
Pneumonia 162, 173
Polycystic ovarian syndrome 28, 128, 226, 291
Polydipsia 50, 161
Polyendocrine syndrome, autoimmune 5
Polyphagia 161
Polyuria 50, 161
Porphyria 4
Postprandial glucose control 110
Potassium 24, 164, 184, 238
channel genes 17
replacement 162t
serum 162
Prader-Willi syndrome 4
Pramlintide 124, 127
Prehypertension 209, 210
Proinflammatory cytokine 226
Proteins 70
Psychiatric
comorbidity, management of 249
disorders 251
problems, management of 251
Psychotic disorders 251
Pyloric stenosis 162

Q

Qualitative lipid abnormalities 203

R

Rabson-Mendenhall syndrome 4
Rapid acting insulin analogs 108, 108f, 117
Renal development disorders 27
Reticulum, endoplasmic 282
Retinitis pigmentosa 61
Retinopathy 51
diabetic 216
Ribonucleic acids 281
Roger syndrome 27t
Rothera's tests 50
Rubella
congenital 5
virus 12

S

Salicylate toxicity 162
Seizures, infantile 242
Selective serotonin reuptake inhibitors 257
Sensory neural deafness 27
Sick-day
guidelines 55
management 84, 231
Skin tags 128
Sleep disorders 251, 294
Sodium 184
glucose cotransporter 124, 126
Somatostatinoma 4
Steatorrhea 61
Steatosis, hepatic 294
Stiff man syndrome 5
Stress 173
disorder, post-traumatic 251
pathophysiology of 178f
Stroke 27
Sulfonylurea 24, 124
receptor mutations 24, 24t

T

Tachycardia 161
Tachypnea 161, 169
Thiamine-responsive megaloblastic anemia syndrome, part of 242
Thiazides 5

Thiazolidinediones 28, 124
Thyroid
　disease 46
　　autoimmune 11
　disorder 50
　hormone 5
　stimulating hormone 300
Toxic ingestion 173
Toxins 12
Trauma 4
Truncal ataxia 27
Trypanophobia 251
Tumor necrosis factor 226
Turner syndrome 5, 61
Tyrosine phosphatases islet
　antigen 172

U

United Kingdom Prospective
　Diabetes Study 67
Uremia 217
Urine
　albumin creatinine ratio 45
　C-peptide creatinine
　　ratio 45
　ketones 44

V

Venous plasma 136*f*
Viral infections 12
Vital signs 42
Vomiting 161, 169, 173

W

Wolcott Rallison syndrome 18,
　22, 25, 240, 242
Wolfram syndrome 5, 22, 61

Y

Young diabetes registry 18